AF251782

Intracranial Pressure and its Effect on

VISION

in Space and on Earth

Vision Impairment in Space

Intracranial Pressure and its Effect on VISION in Space and on Earth

Vision Impairment in Space

Editors

Brandon R Macias
UC San Diego, USA

John HK Liu
UC San Diego, USA

Christian Otto
NASA Johnson Space Center, USA

Alan R Hargens
UC San Diego, USA

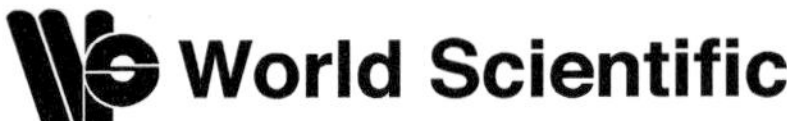

World Scientific

NEW JERSEY · LONDON · SINGAPORE · BEIJING · SHANGHAI · HONG KONG · TAIPEI · CHENNAI · TOKYO

Published by

World Scientific Publishing Co. Pte. Ltd.

5 Toh Tuck Link, Singapore 596224

USA office: 27 Warren Street, Suite 401-402, Hackensack, NJ 07601

UK office: 57 Shelton Street, Covent Garden, London WC2H 9HE

Library of Congress Cataloging-in-Publication Data

Names: Macias, Brandon R., editor. | Liu, John H. K., editor. | Otto, Christian, 1968–   editor. |
    Hargens, Alan R., editor.
Title: Intracranial pressure and its effect on vision in space and on earth :
    vision impairment in space / [edited by] Brandon R. Macias, John H.K. Liu,
    Christian Otto, Alan R. Hargens.
Description: New Jersey : World Scientific, 2017. | Includes bibliographical references and index.
Identifiers: LCCN 2016040511 | ISBN 9789814667104 (hardback : alk. paper)
Subjects: | MESH: Intraocular Pressure--physiology | Intracranial Pressure--physiology |
    Space Flight | Weightlessness--adverse effects | Vision Disorders--physiopathology
Classification: LCC RE725 | NLM WW 103 | DDC 617.7--dc23
LC record available at https://lccn.loc.gov/2016040511

British Library Cataloguing-in-Publication Data
A catalogue record for this book is available from the British Library.

Typeset by Stallion Press
Email: enquiries@stallionpress.com

Printed in Singapore

Contents

Introduction to Visual Impairment and Intracranial Pressure

1

Brandon R. Macias, PhD and Alan R. Hargens, PhD

Department of Orthopaedic Surgery, University of California, San Diego, 9452 Medical Center Drive, La Jolla, California 92037-0863, USA

As the spaceflight community prepares for long-duration exploration class missions of distant objects beyond low Earth orbit, a new and perplexing spaceflight-induced ocular syndrome has emerged. Vestibular dysfunction, loss of mechanical weight bearing, subjective sensation of a headward fluid shift, reduction in muscle volume, and bone loss were intensely studied in the past five decades. These spaceflight adaptations are obvious to most of us now, reduced muscle activity results in muscle atrophy, and reduced mechanical loading of bone results in bone loss. Body fluid redistribution and cardiovascular adaptations during spaceflight result in postflight orthostatic intolerance, but are now mostly met with effective countermeasure strategies.

Our International Space Station, home to more than 200 crew members to date, provides novel data that challenge the scientific community to elucidate the mechanisms responsible and to provide effective countermeasures for spaceflight-induced ocular adaptations. Recent ophthalmic evaluations of astronauts after their six-month missions to the International Space Station reveal unexpected vision problems (Mader *et al.*, 2011). While there are many possible explanations for these vision problems in astronauts, altered posterior ocular fluid volume and pressure (above levels in the upright posture) due to a headward fluid shift during microgravity (Watenpaugh and Hargens, 1996) is proposed as the leading mechanism for the observed disc edema, globe flattening, choroidal folds, and hyperopic shifts (Mader *et al.*, 2011). On Earth adults spend about two-thirds of their existence in upright sitting or standing postures. During microgravity exposure, without countermeasures or artificial gravity, posture-associated hydrostatic gradients are lost. The documented spaceflight-induced vision deficits may be produced by a redistribution of fluid altering ocular and cerebral tissue transmural pressures. The Starling–Landis fluid pressure factors that regulate fluid shifts between blood and interstitial fluid are affected by the absence of gravity (Fig. 1). In microgravity, the loss of tissue weight

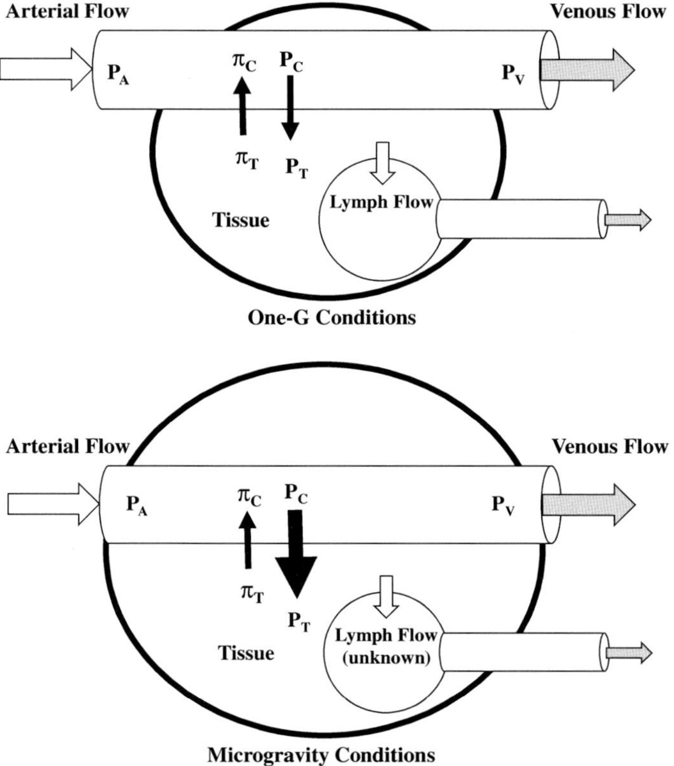

Figure 1. Hypothesized increase in head-ward capillary transmural pressure (blood to tissue) during microgravity produces cranial edema. One-G conditions reflect relative values on Earth. Pre-capillary sphincters and myogenic activities regulate microvascular blood flow within physiological limits. Therefore, the Starling–Landis pressures do not directly correlate with hydrostatic pressure gradients. Arterial pressure (P_A) is the primary contributor to the capillary blood hydrostatic pressure, resulting in fluid filtration out of the capillary and into the interstitial space. Tissue fluid accumulation in the interstitial space increases tissue fluid pressure (P_T) when transvenular flow is impaired by elevated venous pressure (Pv). Reduced tissue mechanical loads and hydrostatic gradients during microgravity likely disrupt cephalic lymphatic flow, exacerbating (P_T).

also reduces tissue fluid pressure and thus increases transcapillary filtration, tissue edema, and potentially cerebrospinal fluid pressure at the optic nerve head. During simulated microgravity, transcapillary filtration increases in upper regions of the body because capillary blood pressure increases, causing facial edema (Parazynski *et al.*, 1991). We have assembled a series of chapters to provide a scientific overview of key elements of spaceflight-induced vision impairment.

Our understanding of ocular structure and function in space has grown significantly with the deployment of new technologies on the International Space Station. These new spaceflight results build on a foundation of classical data since the early 1960s that characterize tissue fluid pressure and transport mechanisms between blood-tissue-lymph. Ludwig, Starling, Guyton, and Scholander and others lay the ground work of methods and data that describe our unique adaptation to life in a one gravity environment. The following chapters are a summary of early attempts by the space medicine community to understand adaptations to microgravity and solve spaceflight-induced vision impairment.

References

Mader, TH, CR Gibson, AF Pass, LA Kramer, AG Lee, J Fogarty, WJ Tarver, JP Dervay, DR Hamilton, A Sargsyan, JL Phillips, D Tran, W Lipsky, J Choi, C Stern, R Kuyumjian and JD Polk (2011). Optic disc edema, globe flattening, choroidal folds, and hyperopic shifts observed in astronauts after long-duration space flight. *Ophthalmology*, 118, 2058–2069. doi:10.1016/j.ophtha.2011.06.021.

Parazynski, SE, AR Hargens, B Tucker, M Aratow, J Styf and A Crenshaw (1991). Transcapillary fluid shifts in tissues of the head and neck during and after simulated microgravity. *Journal of Applied Physiology*, 71, 2469–2475.

Watenpaugh, DE and AR Hargens (1996). The cardiovascular system in microgravity. In *Handbook of Physiology, Environmental Physiology*, MJ Fregly and CM Blatters (eds.), pp. 631–674. Bethesda, MD: American Physiological Society.

Early Evidence of Vision Impairment after Long-Duration Spaceflight

2

Thomas H. Mader, MD and C. Robert Gibson, OD†*

**COL (R) US Army, Cooper Landing, Alaska*
†Coastal Eye Associates, Webster, Texas 77598, USA

1. Introduction

Since the early days of the space program, there have been sporadic reports of vision anomalies during spaceflight. In the late 1980s NASA incorporated a questionnaire into the postflight eye examination, regarding anecdotal evidence of inflight visual changes during short- and long-duration spaceflight. This postflight survey of approximately 300 astronauts documented that reduced near visual acuity was observed in nearly 25% of short-duration shuttle fliers and 53% of astronauts on long-duration International Space Station (ISS) missions. These visual changes were noted to be hyperopic in nature and more clinically apparent in those older astronauts with decreased accommodation. Once these changes were discovered, NASA offered astronauts over the age of 40 plus lens "Space Anticipation Glasses" in order to be prepared for a possible hyperopic shift during the mission. This visual shift appears to occur gradually, is variable in magnitude, and may persist for years following return to Earth.

In response to persistent reports of vision changes NASA began a stepwise process to determine the etiology of these visual anomalies. This began with pre- and postmission visual acuities, dilated fundus examinations with binocular ophthalmoscopy, cycloplegic refraction, and fundus photos of astronauts before and after each space mission. Following the postflight photographic documentation of one astronaut with choroidal folds and a cotton wool spot (CWS), as well as two astronauts with disc edema, NASA flight medicine personnel determined that more extensive pre- and postflight evaluations were appropriate in order to help sort out the possible etiology of these more recent findings. Therefore, preflight and postflight brain and optic nerve (ON) magnetic resonance imaging (MRI), optical coherence tomography (OCT), and ultrasound were initiated as well as inflight fundus photography, OCT and ocular ultrasound. These baseline studies set the stage for the more precise documentation of ocular, ON, and brain anomalies that might occur in association with these visual changes. Using this methodology over the next few years, seven astronauts were documented to have ophthalmic findings consisting of disc edema in five, globe flattening in five, choroidal folds in five, CWSs in three, nerve fiber layer thickening by OCT in six, and decreased vision in six (Mader *et al.*, 2011). The crucial element that drives these changes appears to be the cephalad fluid shift that occurs during microgravity exposure (Mader *et al.*, 2011). Disc edema, globe flattening, and choroidal expansion directly impact the optical system of the eye and lead to visual changes during long-term microgravity exposure. Therefore, we will begin our discussion with an analysis of the physiologic mechanisms thought to cause these anatomic changes and how these alterations may impact the vision of astronauts.

2. Anatomic Changes during Long-Duration Spaceflight

2.1. *Disc edema*

Disc edema has been documented by photos and OCT in eight astronauts. Disc edema by itself has not been known to cause visual anomalies in astronauts, but it may alter the anatomy such that vision changes are more likely to occur. Three basic theories have been proposed to explain the etiology of the disc edema documented during and following long-duration spaceflight. These theories are not mutually exclusive and the true etiology may be multifactorial. The first possible explanation is that prolonged microgravity exposure causes a rise in intracranial pressure (ICP), leading to an idiopathic intracranial hypertension (IIH)–like syndrome (Mader *et al.*, 2011). IIH is well documented to cause globe flattening, choroidal folds, and enlargement of the subarachnoid space (SAS) of the ON as documented by OCT, MRI, and ultrasound (Kalina and Mills, 1980; Nettleship, 1884; Jacobson, 1995; Dailey *et al.*, 1986; Cassidy and Sanders, 1999; Sharma *et al.*, 1999; Lavinsky *et al.*, 2007; Friedman, 2007; Griebel and Kosmorsky, 2000). These findings are similar to those observed in astronauts. The specific mechanism of a rise in ICP during extended microgravity is open to question but may involve a rise in cephalad venous pressure brought about by microgravity fluid shifts. There is a cephalad fluid shift of 1 to 2 liters during microgravity exposure (Nicogossian and Parker, 1982). Although this shift does not appear to have an effect on the cerebral arterial vasculature (Frey *et al.*, 1993; Iwasaki *et al.*, 2007), it does cause jugular venous distension (Harris *et al.*, 1997; Thornton *et al.*, 1977; Herault *et al.*, 2000; Arbeille *et al.*, 2001), which suggests an elevation of cervical and cerebral venous pressure. The cerebral venous system does not contain valves, so the effect of a rise in venous pressure may impact this entire venous system (Kim and Parsa, 2012; Mader *et al.*, 2012). Cerebrospinal fluid (CSF) is largely produced in the choroid plexus of the brain and drained through the cerebral venous system. This CSF drainage is dependent upon a pressure gradient from the relatively high-pressure cerebral CSF to the lower pressure cerebral venous system (Davson and Dome, 1973; Alperin *et al.*, 2005; Andersson *et al.*, 2008; Kapoor *et al.*, 2008). If a rise in venous pressure did occur during microgravity exposure it would presumably lessen the magnitude of the gradient and possibly lead to impairment of CSF drainage (Mader *et al.*, 2011). This CSF drainage impairment, coupled with cerebral venous congestion, may cause a rise in CSF pressure (Kapoor *et al.*, 2008; Mader *et al.*, 2011).

In this scenario, the elevated subarachnoid pressure is thought to be directly transmitted, bilaterally, from the intracranial compartment into the intraorbital compartment through the subarachnoid sheath of the ON (Liu and Kahn, 1993). This could result in optic nerve sheath (ONS) distention, pressure on the ON, stasis of axoplasmic flow, axonal swelling, and visible disc edema (Tso and Hayreh, 1977; Jacobson, 1995). Lumbar puncture performed on four astronauts with disc edema documented opening pressures of 22, 21, 28, and 28.5 cm H_2O performed 60, 19, 12, and 57 days postmission, respectively (Mader *et al.*, 2011). The two higher measurements are clearly above 25 cm H_2O and thus meet the Modified Dandy Criteria for IIH. Since these moderately elevated measurements were documented weeks after return to Earth it is possible that even higher ICPs may have existed during the space mission. Pituitary indentation, presumably caused by chronic pituitary gland compression from increased ICP, documented by MRI in an astronaut exposed to long–duration microgravity, also supports this theory (Kramer *et al.*, 2012). Arguments against elevated ICP as the sole etiology include the fact that transient visual obscurations and sixth nerve palsies have thus far never been documented in an astronaut. These are typically seen in 68% and 30% of IIH patients, respectively (Giuseffi *et al.*, 1991; Friedman, 2007). Asymmetrical disc edema, ONS distension, and globe flattening documented in some astronauts also suggest that elevated ICP may not be the etiology (Mader *et al.*, 2011; Mader *et al.*, 2013; Mader *et al.*, 2016). Increased ICP should be propagated down both ONSs in an equal fashion and cause a similar degree of change bilaterally.

Several factors should be examined when we consider elevated ICP as the sole etiology of our findings. More than 90% of terrestrial IIH patients experience headaches (Giuseffi *et al.*, 1991). Terrestrial IIH headaches are characteristically pressure-like, throbbing, usually unremitting, occur with retro-ocular pain and may be accompanied by nausea (Degnan and Levy, 2011). They are frequently described as the worst headache ever experienced (Wall, 2010). This degree of headache intensity is usually associated with moderate to severe papilledema. None of the eight astronauts thus far documented with disc edema reported inflight headaches when asked this question during their postflight eye exam. However, one study of 17 astronauts (16 male, 1 female) documented that 71% reported having experienced at least one headache episode, of moderate to severe intensity, while in space whereas they had not suffered from headache on Earth (Vein *et al.*, 2009). It should be noted that the incidence of headache is low in males with IIH (Bruce *et al.*, 2009) but these data suggest they are more common in male astronauts. Although these flight-related headaches do not appear to approach the intensity of most terrestrial IIH headaches, it is possible that they could represent symptoms caused by a chronic low-grade microgravity-induced increase in ICP. Thus far the majority of disc edema in astronauts has been mild to moderate. Also, terrestrial IIH is far more common in overweight females with a female/male ratio of 8:1 (Durcan *et al.*, 1988) whereas spaceflight-related cases of disc edema, globe flattening, and NFL thickening have thus far only been described in males of normal weight. All this information suggests the possibility that a microgravity-induced elevation of ICP may produce low-grade IIH-like symptoms in the astronaut population with no sexual or body build predilection.

The second possible etiology of this disc edema is that it occurs as a result of localized events at the level of the intraorbital ON with or without a rise in ICP (Mader *et al.*, 2011; Mader *et al.*, 2013). There is generally thought to be homogeneity of pressure between the intracranial CSF and the CSF within the SAS of the ON (Killer *et al.*, 2006). However, the unique cul-de-sac-like anatomic connection between the intracranial SAS and the SAS of the ON is thought to create a rather fragile flow equilibrium (Killer *et al.*, 2007). Lymphatics in the dura of the ON have also been proposed as a CSF outflow pathway that may be impacted by microgravity exposure (Killer *et al.*, 2007). It is possible that microgravity exposure may lead to lymphstasis that could also be a contributing factor in ONS pressures (Mader *et al.*, 2011). Poor exchange of fluid between the intracranial and intraorbital CSF has been proposed as a possible mechanism to explain persistent papilledema in patients with IIH despite a functioning lumbar peritoneal shunt (Kelman *et al.*, 1991; Killer *et al.*, 2007; Killer *et al.*, 2009). Also recent

CT cisternography studies of patients with increased ICP suggest that CSF turnover in the SAS of the ON is reduced in patients with papilledema and the chemical composition of the CSF differs between the spinal CSF and that surrounding the ON (Killer *et al.*, 2011). It has been hypothesized that such biomechanically altered CSF may cause metabolic toxicity to the ON and set the stage for focal arteriolar closure that may appear clinically as CWSs (Killer *et al.*, 2009). CWSs are not commonly associated with increased ICP but have been reported in four astronauts. Regardless of specific etiology, perhaps during prolonged microgravity conditions impaired fluid exchange may occur and CSF in the SAS of the ON may gradually become partially or completely sequestered, producing a type of ON compartment syndrome that could result in ONS distention, ON compression, and resultant disc edema with or without a rise in ICP (Mader *et al.*, 2011). The documentation of one astronaut with a lumbar puncture opening pressure of 18 cm H_2O eight days after landing in conjunction with moderate bilateral enlargement of the ONSs, unilateral disc edema, and choroidal folds lends support to this theory (Mader *et al.*, 2013). The main argument against the compartment syndrome theory is that we have no confirmation of normal lumbar puncture opening pressures during spaceflight. In another case, persistent, asymmetric disc swelling and globe flattening for six months following long duration spaceflight were documented with lumbar puncture opening pressures of 22 and 16 cm H20 performed seven days and 12 months post-mission respectively, again suggesting asymmetrical increases in local SAS pressures (Mader, *et al.*, 2016).

The third possible cause of disc edema is the combination of elevated CSF pressure in conjunction with a relatively low intraocular pressure (IOP) across the lamina cribrosa (Mader *et al.*, 2011; Berdahl *et al.*, 2012). Some head–down studies document that the initial IOP spike observed in assuming the head–down position is followed by a leveling or lowering of IOP over a period of days (Mader *et al.*, 1990; Chiquet *et al.*, 2003). Parabolic flight studies have documented a quick increase in IOP after only 20 seconds of microgravity exposure (Mader *et al.*, 1993). IOP data from Space Shuttle missions have noted a similar IOP spike upon entering microgravity followed by a lowering of pressures to near normal (Draeger *et al.*, 1987). This initial quick increase in IOP is thought to occur as a result of choroidal expansion brought about by cephalad fluid shifts (Mader *et al.*, 1990). It is further hypothesized that the decrease in IOP after the initial spike may occur as a result of a compensatory decrease in aqueous volume (Mader *et al.*, 1990). Although one case report documented disc edema in the presence of normal IOPs during a six–month mission (Mader *et al.*, 2013) it is possible that some degree of IOP lowering may occur in other astronauts. Ocular hypotony, defined as a profound drop in IOP to below 6 mmHg, is well known to cause disc edema similar to that observed in astronauts (Costa and Arcieri, 2007; Westfall *et al.*, 2004).

2.2. *Globe flattening*

As described previously, increased ICP may occur following prolonged microgravity exposure. In this scenario, the CSF pressure is transmitted down the SAS to the intraorbital ONS. Alternatively a rise in ONS pressure may arise from a local compartmentalization with or without a rise in ICP. Regardless of the specific etiology, this elevated intrasheath pressure may lead to changes in eye and ON anatomy that may directly impact vision.

Increased nerve sheath volume from any cause may exert an anterior force on the globe that indents the posterior sclera, resulting in posterior globe flattening, decreased axial length, and choroidal folds. This form of choroidal folding is caused by the physical indentation of the posterior globe that causes redundancy and folding of the choroid. A postmission decrease in axial length has been independently documented by MRI (Fig. 1), ocular ultrasound, and optical biometry (IOL Master) techniques (Mader *et al.*, 2011; Kramer *et al.*, 2012). Decreased axial length shortens the distance between the cornea and the retina and will cause an astronaut to become more hyperopic.

Given the importance of this anatomic concept, a brief explanation of the optical system of the eye is appropriate. The hyperopic eye does not possess enough optical power for its axial length. In hyperopia, with accommodation relaxed, an object at infinity focuses behind the retina. Highly farsighted eyes tend to be shorter than non–farsighted eyes.

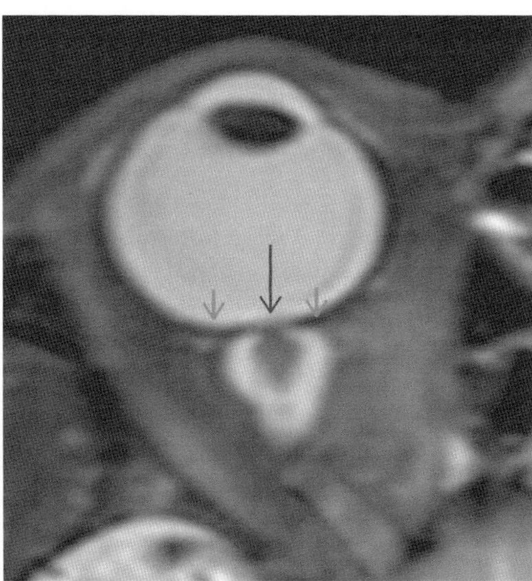

Figure 1. Post-mission 3T ocular MRI documenting a decrease in axial length (small arrows), optic disc edema (large arrow) and marked distention of the optic nerve sheath.

A flattening of the back of the eyeball, as occurs in some astronauts (i.e., globe flattening), will also cause hyperopia. A 0.33 mm anterior displacement of the retina would lead to a 1.00 D shift toward hyperopia. Thus, if globe flattening occurs in a previously normal (emmetropic) astronaut, he will become farsighted. His major complaint will be worsening of near vision.

In Fig. 2 below light enters the eye from optical infinity and focuses on the retina, yielding clear vision (normal vision — "emmetropia"). Figure 3 shows light from optical infinity focusing behind the retina due to the eye's weak optical system; this is hyperopia. To correct this, a plus power "space anticipation lens" that CONverges light can be used by astronauts thereby strengthening the (weak) eye to focus light directly onto the retina.

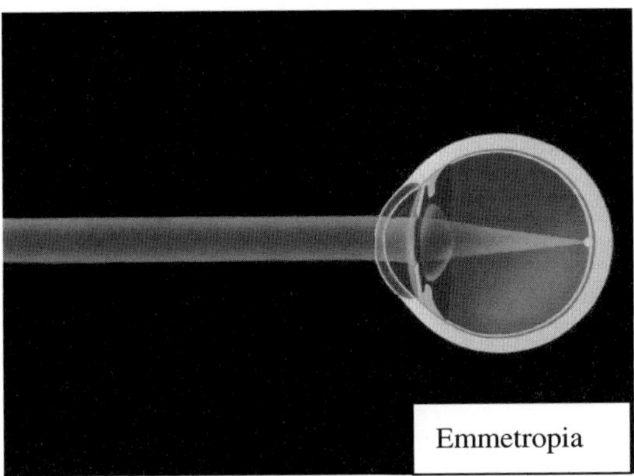

Figure 2.   Schematic of emmetropia.

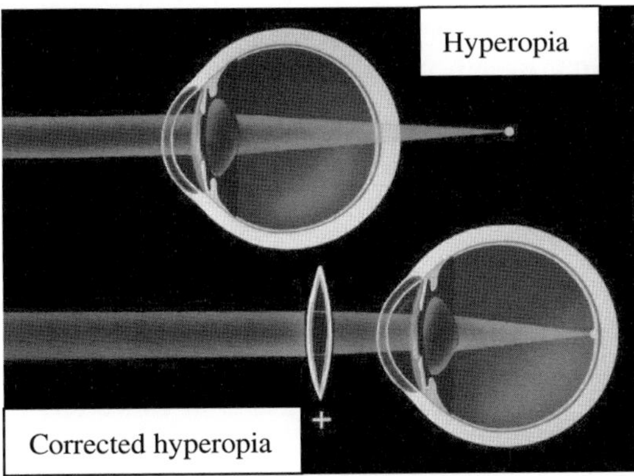

Figure 3.   Schematic of hyperopia and corrected hyperopia.

When the eye views an object at near, an *accommodative demand* is placed on the crystalline lens. *Accommodation* is the mechanism by which the eye changes refractive power by altering the shape of its crystalline lens. *Accommodative effort* occurs when the ciliary muscle contracts and the zonule fibers relax in response to parasympathetic innervation. The outward-directed tension on the lens capsule is decreased and the lens becomes more "round," increasing its power. The movement of the equatorial edge of the lens is away from the outer covering of the eye (sclera) during accommodation, and toward the sclera again when accommodation is relaxed. However, as we age, we lose the ability to use the crystalline lens to change focus (accommodative amplitude), a process called *presbyopia*. Depending on a person's prescription and ability to focus (based on their age), a farsighted person may see clearly at distance without correction, but have to work harder to see up close. In other words, a hyperopic person will see well if they have the ability to focus "through" their refractive error. This is dependent upon the degree of the hyperopia and the age of the person. A 20-year-old will typically have 10.00 D of accommodative amplitude, a 40-year-old ~4.00 D, and a 50 year old ~2.00 D. From age 40–55, the crystalline lens loses about 0.25 D of accommodative amplitude each year. A person with normal near vision as a young man or woman will require stronger and stronger reading glasses (plus lenses) as they age. Presbyopia is not the same phenomenon as farsightedness (hyperopia), but it does affect a person's ability to compensate for hyperopia. Thus, older presbyopic astronauts with little ability to accommodate may be particularly bothered by hyperopic changes and will seek plus lens correction during space missions.

The myopic eye possesses too much optical power for its axial length. In myopia, with accommodation relaxed, light rays from an object at infinity converge too soon and thus focus in front of the retina. A subtle steepening in the curvature of the cornea can cause this. Another way to become myopic is for the eyeball to grow too long. Highly nearsighted eyes tend to be longer than non-nearsighted eyes. The uncorrected myope usually can see at near better than at a distance, hence the term "nearsighted".

In the figures below we see two images. In Fig. 4, light enters the eye from optical infinity (>20 ft) and focuses on the retina, yielding clear vision (normal vision — "emmetropia") without using accommodation of the crystalline lens. Fig. 5 shows light from optical infinity focusing in front of the retina due to the eye having too much optical power for its axial length. This is myopia. To correct this we put a minus power lens in front of the eye that DIverges light to exactly compensate for what the eye overCONverges. This lens placement results in convergence of the light rays directly onto the retina and normal visual acuity. Interestingly, if globe flattening occurs in a myopic astronaut, his uncorrected distance visual acuity will improve because the retina will be moved nearer to where the light is focused.

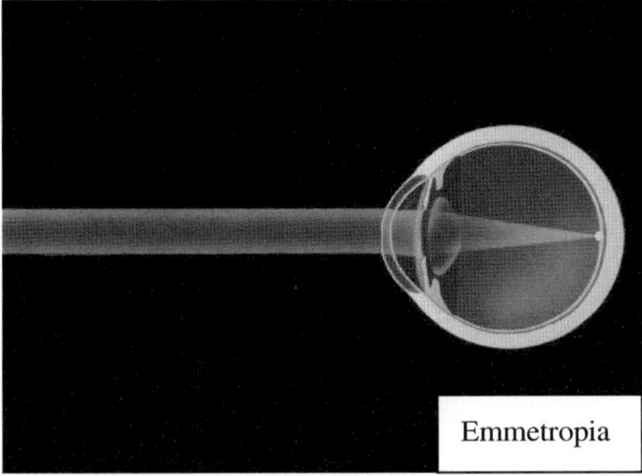

Figure 4. Schematic of emmetropia.

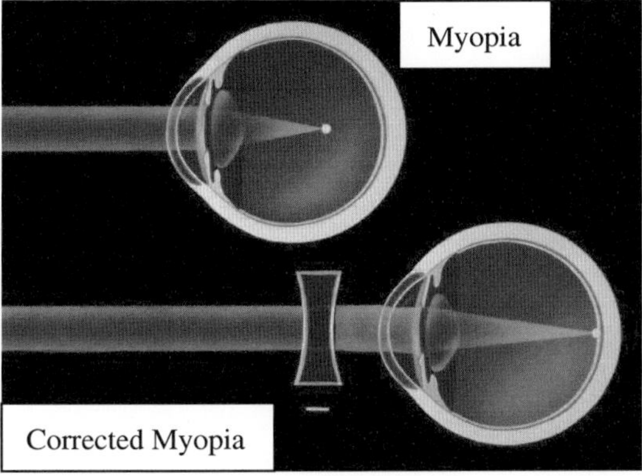

Figure 5. Schematic of myopia and corrected myopia.

Globe flattening is well documented to occur in some astronauts and would likely explain their visual changes. However, not all astronauts with visual symptoms during and after long-duration spaceflight have evidence of globe flattening. Thus, it appears that other factors may be involved in these visual anomalies.

2.3. *Choroidal expansion*

The choroid is the highly vascular layer of the eye that lies just posterior to the retina. Its function is to provide oxygen-rich blood and nutrients to the outer retina and to carry away waste products. The area supplied by the choroid includes the very metabolically active photoreceptor/retinal pigment epithelium (RPE) complex. Since the outer retinal layers are avascular, this exchange takes place through the process of diffusion. The retina oxygenation process is dependent upon a very steep concentration gradient that is maintained by a very high rate of choroidal blood flow that approaches ten times that of the brain. It seems likely that this spongy choroidal vascular system may be very sensitive to the fluid shifts produced by microgravity exposure. The choroid is supplied by the anterior and posterior ciliary arteries and drained by the vortex vein system. As noted above, during even transient microgravity exposure, there is a cephalad fluid shift that may increase venous pressure in the head and neck (Mader *et al.*, 1993). This rise in venous pressure presumably raises the vortex vein pressure, thus partially inhibiting the normal venous drainage from the choroidal vasculature. This lack of normal drainage leads to an expansion of the choroid. The clinical presentation of choroidal expansion appears to be dependent upon the anatomic microstructure of the choroidal attachment to the underlying RPE (Newell, 1973). During choroidal expansion, if the choroid is not attached to the underlying Bruch's membrane, the RPE slides over the choriocapillarus, folds are not produced, and the fundus has a homogeneous smooth appearance. However, choroid–Bruch's adhesions that are normal in some people prevent this easy sliding and lead to the choroidal fold striations that have been documented in astronauts. The dark lines correspond with the troughs of the folds where there is compaction of the RPE and the light lines correspond to the crest of the folds, where the RPE is somewhat stretched and attenuated. Thus the clinical appearance of the swollen choroid may vary according to individual microanatomy. Regardless of clinical appearance, choroidal expansion may have an impact on visual acuity during microgravity exposure.

Choroidal engorgement may gradually push the macula slightly forward, thus shortening the distance between the lens and the macula (Mader *et al.*, 2011). This change in the eye's optical system is similar to the change that may take place during globe flattening. Additionally, this choroidal pooling may gradually expand the delicate collagen lamella of the choroid beyond its normal structural boundaries, resulting in a choroid that may become permanently distended, even on return to the 1G environment with normalization of venous pressure (Mader *et al.*, 2011). Choroidal folds have been documented to be present in astronauts several years after long-duration missions (Mader *et al.*, 2011). Therefore, in a space traveler, there might not be a fixed distance between the lens and the retina as there is on Earth. Perhaps choroidal expansion and a commensurate hyperopic shift are common during spaceflight and may exist for months to years following return to Earth.

3. Other Possible Causes of Visual Changes

3.1. *Corneal refractive changes*

It has been well documented that an alteration in the anterior curvature of the cornea may result in visual changes. This subject has been studied in great detail in patients who have had refractive surgery as well as in normal controls (Mader *et al.*, 1996; Ng *et al.*, 1996; Mader and White, 1995; Winkle *et al.*, 1998; White and Mader, 2000; Nelson *et al.*, 2001; Bosch *et al.*, 2010; Mader and White, 2010). To briefly summarize, patients who had undergone radial keratotomy (RK) experienced corneal flattening during exposure to more than approximately 12 hours of hypoxia. In one study, RK, photorefractive keratectomy (PRK), and normal patients were exposed to 14,000 feet for three days and a hyperopic shift was observed in RK patients with no refractive change in PRK patients or normal controls (Mader *et al.*, 1996). Hypoxic corneal expansion is thought to occur in the mechanically unstable areas of the RK incisions, causing a circumferential elevation of the peripheral cornea, a flattening of the corneal surface, and a resultant hyperopic shift. RK subjects as well as normal controls were also studied in an altitude chamber at a simulated altitude of 12,000 feet (Ng *et al.*, 1996). This study confirmed that only a few hours of hypobaric hypoxic exposure had little to no effect on either RK or normal control corneas. This suggested that the refractive changes in RK corneas during exposure to hypoxia were of a slow metabolic origin and not related to the direct effect of lower atmospheric mechanical pressure (Ng *et al.*, 1996). The effect of hypoxia on the corneas of patients who had undergone LASIK and PRK was also examined using goggles that subjected corneas to very low oxygen concentrations (Nelson *et al.*, 2001). LASIK patients who had their central corneas incised by LASIK incisions suffered mild edema in the central cornea, a slight central elevation, and a resultant very mild myopic shift (Nelson *et al.*, 2001). In this case, the central cornea had more optical power and effectively shifted the focal point of the eye anteriorly. A later study of LASIK patients during 30-minute exposure at a simulated altitude of 35,000 feet in a hypobaric chamber showed no significant change in refraction (Wright *et al.*, 2012). LASIK corneas have not yet been studied under prolonged microgravity conditions. PRK patients who had undergone a uniform ablation of their anterior corneas and normal cornea controls had no visual or keratometric changes during any hypoxic studies (Mader *et al.*, 1996). Normal and PRK corneas do increase in thickness during exposure to hypoxia, but since there is no preferential corneal swelling around incisions, there is no change in the anterior corneal curvature and thus no change in vision (Mader *et al.*, 1996). We also studied an astronaut with bilateral PRK and found no visual changes following 12 days in microgravity (Gibson *et al.*, 2012). Finally, a 60-year-old astronaut who had undergone bilateral intraocular lens implants was also examined before, during, and after 18 days in orbit (Mader *et al.*, 1999). His vision was completely stable during this time. All of this information suggests that the corneal surface in normal or PRK corneas is stable during exposure to hypoxia or microgravity. The subjects with potential visual concerns would be those with a history of incisional procedures that may mechanically weaken the cornea in a nonuniform fashion, such as RK, old cornea lacerations, or a corneal transplant (Koe *et al.*, 2001). In summary, evidence suggests that those astronauts with normal corneas or those who have had PRK would not be subject to corneal or refractive changes during microgravity exposure.

3.2. *Crystalline lens changes*

Another hypothesis to explain visual acuity changes in microgravity would be the axial movement of the crystalline lens during microgravity exposure. It is thought that perhaps increased blood volume in the anterior choroid/ciliary body area may displace the lens/iris diaphragm, thus causing a refractive change. It is also possible, although unlikely, that the fluid shifts within the eye could lead to lenticular changes which could cause alterations in refractive power.

3.3. *Other ramifications of a dynamic choroid*

Increased choroidal volume does not occur as an isolated event and may impact other intraocular structures. In the normal living adult human eye, under one-G conditions, the choroid is a low pressure vascular space about 300–400 microns in thickness that produces no anatomic displacement of intraocular structures. The choroid is one of the most highly vascularized tissues of the body, is drained by the vortex venous system, and supplies oxygen and nutrients to the retina. Since the choroid lacks autoregulation, it may be subject to shifts in vascular volume during position changes or microgravity exposure (Mader *et al.*, 1990; Kergoat and Lovasik, 2005; Shinojima *et al.*, 2012). One 48-hour, 10-degree, head-down bed rest study documented an immediate increase in IOP when going from the sitting to the head-down position (Mader *et al.*, 1990). This spike in IOP was thought to result from a sudden increase in choroidal volume brought about by the head-down position. This increase in IOP underwent some diurnal changes but stayed evenly elevated during the entire duration of head-down tilt. Immediately upon sitting up, after 48 hours of head-down tilt, the choroidal vascular engorgement was abolished and the IOP underwent a statistically significant decrease to below that of pre-head-down IOP values. This finding strongly suggests that over 48 hours, some component of ocular volume decreased in the face of increasing choroidal volume (Mader *et al.*, 1990). It seems likely that as the choroid expanded during the 48 hours of head-down tilt a compensatory decrease in anterior chamber (AC) volume may have occurred. It is unclear if this AC volume loss results from decreased aqueous production or increased outflow. Thus, following the initial choroidal expansion, there appears to be a gradual redistribution of fluid within the compartments of the eye. As previously mentioned, chronic engorgement of the choroid, as manifested by choroidal folds, has also been well documented in astronauts after return to Earth following long-duration spaceflight (Mader *et al.*, 2011). Furthermore, it has been recently reported that an astronaut with documented choroidal folds on his first six-month space mission developed more widespread choroidal folds during a second six-month mission (Mader *et al.*, 2013). This suggests that if the choroid was previously expanded during one mission, it may be subject to more extensive expansion on a repeat mission (Mader *et al.*, 2013).

These shifts in the volume of intraocular compartments may adversely impact the eyes of some astronauts during extended microgravity. As noted above, under microgravity conditions an increase in choroidal volume and a compensatory decrease in AC volume may occur (Mader *et al.*, 1990). The anterior force on the vitreous from the expanded choroid may displace the lens slightly forward. Normally aqueous is produced by the ciliary body, flows through the pupil into the AC, and drains into the trabecular meshwork. As discussed by Tiederman (1991), even a slight anterior movement of the front surface of the lens leads to an anterior bowing of the iris toward the trabecular meshwork. A pathologic rise in IOP may occur when the trabecular meshwork is obstructed by an anterior circumferential elevation of the peripheral iris. Shallowing of the AC in response to a rise in choroidal volume has been proposed as a possible mechanism for some cases of terrestrial narrow angle glaucoma (Quigley *et al.*, 2003). For example, pathologic conditions such as uveal effusion (Maumenee and Schwartz, 1985), suprachoroidal hemorrhage (Alexandrakis *et al.*, 1998), orbital pseudotumor (Bernardino *et al.*, 2001), and arterial venous fistulas (Fourman, 1989) can cause an increase in choroidal volume and a resultant anterior force that can produce shallowing of the AC with resultant angle closure glaucoma. Other studies have also documented the dynamic behavior of the choroid and its possible role in angle closure (Lowe, 1970; Alsbirk, 1976; Silver and Geyer, 2000; Arora *et al.*, 2012a,b). Mild anatomic shallowing of the AC from plateau iris or other iris-crowding configurations is a common and usually clinically insignificant finding in the 1G environment. However, in zero G, these same anatomic configurations may become salient features and predispose some astronauts to trabecular meshwork obstruction and a pathologic rise in IOP. People of East Asian descent and eyes with shorter axial length have flatter corneas, shallower anterior chambers, thicker lenses, and may also be predisposed to such changes (Alsbirk, 1976; Quigley *et al.*, 2003). Pharmacologic mydriasis as performed for inflight fundus photos could also increase the likelihood of angle closure in some astronauts (Patel *et al.*, 1995). Trabecular meshwork obstruction could be clinically manifest by symptoms of subacute, chronic, or acute narrow angle glaucoma. These symptoms may include severe eye pain and decreased vision, as well as nausea and vomiting. Pressure spikes as high as 22.6 mmHg have been recorded on initial entry into microgravity (Draeger *et al.*, 1987). Since no overt narrow angle glaucoma has ever been reported during microgravity exposure, this is presumably a rare event in healthy astronauts with normal AC depth. However, given the potentially harmful nature of such an occurrence, documentation of microgravity-induced anatomic changes of the iris, lens, and anterior chamber depth by OCT would be a worthwhile consideration for future ISS research. This may help us to determine the mechanism of microgravity fluid shifts within the eye and help identify astronauts at risk for angle closure during microgravity exposure.

References

Alexandrakis, G, NA Chaudhry, PE Liggett, *et al.* (1998). Spontaneous suprachoroidal hermorrhage in age-related macula degeneration presenting as angle-closure glaucoma. *Retina*, 15, 485–486.

Alperin, N, SH Lee, M Mazda, *et al.* (2005). Evidence for the importance of extracranial venous flow in patients with idiopathic intracranial hypertension (IIH). *Acta Neurochirurgica Supplement*, 95, 129–132.

Alsbirk, PH (1976). Primary angle-closure glaucoma: Oculometry, epidemiology, and genetics in a high risk population. *Acta Ophthalmologica*, 54, 5-31.

Andersson, N, J Nalm and A Eklund (2008). Dependency of cerebrospinal fluid outflow resistance on intracranial pressure. *Journal of Neurosurgery*, 109, 918–922.

Arbeille, P, G Fomina, J Roumy, *et al.* (2001). Adaptation of the left heart, cerebral and femoral arteries, and jugular and femoral veins during short- and long-term headdown tilt and space flights. *European Journal of Applied Physiology*, 86, 157–168.

Arora, KS, JL Jefferys, EA Maul and HA Quigley (2012a). Choroidal thickness change after water drinking is greater in angle closure than in open angle eyes. *Investigative Ophthalmology & Visual Science*, 53, 6393–6402.

Arora, KS, JL Jefferys, EA Maul and HA Quigley (2012b). The choroid is thicker in angle closure than in open angle and control eyes. *Investigative Ophthalmology & Visual Science*, 53, 7813–7818.

Berdahl, J, D Fleischman, RR Allingham and M Fautsch (2012). Disc swelling in space flight. *Ophthalmology*, 119, 1290.

Bernardino, CR, RS Davisdon, M Maus, *et al.* (2001). Angle-closure glaucoma in association with orbital pseudotumor. *Ophthalmology*, 108, 1603–1606.

Bosch, MM, D Barthelmes, TM Merz, PB Knecht, F Truffer, KE Bloch, MA Thiel, BL Petrig, AF Turk, OD Schoch, U Hefti and K Landau (2010). New insights into changes in corneal thickness in healthy mountaineers during a very-high-altitude climb to Mount Muztagh Ata. *Archives of Ophthalmology*, 128(2), 184–189.

Bruce, BB, S Kedar, GP Van Stavern, D Monaghan, MD Acierno, RA Braswell, P Preechawat, JJ Corbett, NJ Newman and V Blousse (2009). Idiopathic intracranial hypertension in men. *Neurology*, Jan, 72(4), 304–309.

Cassidy, LM and MD Sanders (1999). Choroidal folds and papilloedema. *British Journal of Ophthalmology*, 83, 1139–1143.

Chiquet, C, MA Custeaud, AP Le Traon, *et al.* (2003). Changes in intraocular pressure during prolonged (7-day) head-down tilt bed rest. *Journal of Glaucoma*, 12, 204–8.

Costa, VP and ES Arcieri (2007). Hypotonymaculopathy. *ACTA Ophthalmologica Scandinavica*, 85, 586–597.

Dailey, RA, RP Mills, GK Stimac, *et al.* (1986). The natural history and CT appearance of acquired hyperopia with choroidal folds. *Ophthalmology*, 93, 1336–1342.

Davson, H and FR Domer, JR (1973). Hollingsworth. The mechanism of drainage of the cerebrospinal fluid. *Brain*, 96, 329–336.

Degnan, AJ and LM Levy (2011). Pseudotumorcerebri: brief review of clinical syndrome and imaging findings. *American Journal Neuroradiology*, Dec, 32(11), 1986–1993.

Draeger, J, H Wirt and R Schwartz (1987). Tonometry under microgravity conditions. In: *Proceeding of the Norderney Symposium on Scientific Results of the German Spacelab Mission: D1*, PR Sahm, R Jansen, MH Keller (eds.), pp. 503–509. Norderney, Germany, August 27–29, 1986. Koln, Germany: WissenschaftlicheProjektfuhrung DI c/o DFVLR.

Durcan, FJ, JJ Corbett and M Wall (1988). The incidence of pseudotumorcerebri. Population studies in Iowa and Louisiana. *Archives of Neurology*, Aug, 45(8), 875–877.

Fourman S (1989). Acute closed-angle glaucoma after arteriovenous fistulas. *American Journal of Ophthalmology*, 107, 156–159.

Frey, MA, TH Mader, JP Bagian, *et al.* (1993). Cerebral blood velocity and other cardiovascular responses to 2 days of head-down tilt. *Journal of Applied Physiology*, 74, 319–25.

Friedman, D (2007). Idiopathic intracranial hypertension. *Current Pain and Headache Reports*, 11, 62–68.

Gibson, CR, TH Mader, S Schallhorn, K Pseudovs, W Lipsky, E Raid, RT Jennings, JA Fogarty, RA Garriott, OK Garritott and SL Johnston (2012). The visual stability of laser vision correction in an astronaut on a Soyuz Mission to the International Space Station (ISS). *Journal of Cataract Refractive Surgery*, Aug, 38(8), 1486–1491.

Giuseffi, V, M Wall, PZ Siegel and PB Rojas (1991). Symptoms and disease associations in idiopathic intracranial hypertension (pseudotumorcerebri): A case-control study. *Neurology*, 41, 239–244.

Griebel, SR and GS Kosmorsky (2000). Choroidal folds associated with increased intracranial pressure. *American Journal of Ophthalmology*, 129, 513–516.

Harris, BA, RD Jr. Billica, SL Bishop, *et al.* (1997). Physical examination during space flight. *Mayo Clinic Proceedings*, 72, 301–308.

Herault, S, G Fomina, I Alferova, *et al.* (2000). Cardiac, arterial and venous adaptation to weightlessness during 6-month MIR spaceflights with and without thigh cuffs (bracelets). *European Journal Applied Physiology*, 81, 384–390.

Iwasaki, K, BD Levine, R Zhang, *et al.* (2007). Human cerebral autoregulation before, during and after spaceflight. *Journal of Physiology*, 579, 799–810.

Jacobson, DM (1995). Intracranial hypertension and the syndrome of acquired hyperopia with choroidal folds. *Journal of Neuro-Ophthalmology*, 15, 178–185.

Kalina, RE and RP Mills (1980). Acquired hyperopia with choroidal folds. *Ophthalmology*, 87, 44–50.

Kapoor, KG, SE Katz, DM Grzybowski and M Lubow (2008). Cerebrospinal fluid outflow: An evolving perspective. *Brain Research Bulletin*, 77, 327–334.

Kelman, SE, RC Sergott, GA Cioffi, *et al.* (1991). Modified optic nerve decompression in patients with functioning lumboperitoneal shunts and progressive visual loss. *Ophthalmology*, 98, 1449–1453.

Kergoat, H and JV Lovasik (2005). Seven-degree head-down tilt reduces choroidal pulsatile ocular blood flow. *Aviation, Space, and Environmental Medicine*, 76, 930–934.

Killer, HE, GP Jaggi, J Flammer, *et al.* (2006). The optic nerve: A new window into cerebrospinal fluid composition? *Brain*, 129, 1027–1030.

Killer, HE, GP Jaggi, J Flammer, *et al.* (2007). Cerebrospinal fluid dynamics between the intracranial and the subarachnoid space of the optic nerve. Is it always bidirectional? *Brain*, 130, 514–520.

Killer, HE, GP Jaggi and NR Miller (2009). Papilledema revisited: Is its pathophysiology really understood? *Clinical & Experimental Ophthalmology*, 37, 444–447.

Killer, HE, GP Jaggi, NR Miller, AR Huber, H Landolt, A Mironov, P Meyer and L Remonda (2011). Cerebrospinal fluid dynamics between the basal cisterns and the subarachnoid space of the optic nerve in patients with papilloedema. *British Journal of Ophthalmology*, 95, 822–827.

Kim, DH and CF Parsa (2012). Space flight and disc edema. *Ophthalmology*, 119, 2420–2421.

Koe, MT, RL Goodman, SG Waller and DA Johnson (2001). Case report: myopic shift in a stable corneal graft following high altitude exposure. *Aviation, Space, and Environmental Medicine*, 72, 1145–1147.

Kramer, LA, AE Sargsyan, KM Hasan, JD Polk and DR Hamilton (2012). Orbital and intracranial effects of microgravity: Findings at 3-T MR Imaging. *Radiology*, 263, 1–9.

Lavinsky, J, D Lavinsky, F Lavinsky and A Frutuoso (2007). Acquired choroidal folds: a sign of idiopathic intracranial hypertension. *Graefes Archive for Clinical and Experimental Ophthalmology*, 245, 883–888.

Liu, D and M Kahn (1993). Measurement and relationship of subarachnoid pressure of the optic nerve to intracranial pressures in fresh cadavers. *American Journal of Ophthalmology*, 116, 548–556.

Lowe, RF (1970). Aetiology of the anatomical basis for primary angle–closure glaucoma. Biometrical comparisons between normal eyes and eyes with primary angle–closure glaucoma. *British Journal of Ophthalmology*, 54, 161–169.

Mader, TH and LJ White (2010). Corneal thickness changes in very-high-altitude mountaineers. *Archives of Ophthalmology*, 128(9), 1224–1225.

Mader, TH, AG Lee, CR Gibson, LA Kramer and AF Pass (2012). A Sargsyan. Author reply. Space flight and disc edema. *Ophthalmology*, 119, 2421–2422.

Mader, TH, CR Gibson, AF Pass, AG Lee, HE Killer, H-C Hansen, JP Dervay, MR Barratt, WJ Tarver, AE Sargsyan, LA Kramer, R Riascos, DG Bedi and DR Pettit (2013). Optic disc edema in an astronaut after repeat long-duration space flight. *Journal of Neuro-Ophthalmology*, 33(3), 249–255.

Mader, TH, CR Gibson, AF Pass, *et al.* (2011). Optic disc edema, globe flattening, choroidal folds, and hyperopic shifts observed in astronauts after long-duration space flight. *Ophthalmology*, 118, 2058–2069.

Mader, TH, CR Gibson, CA Otto, *et al.* (2016). Persistent asymmetric optic disc swelling after long-duration space flight: implications for pathogenesis. *Journal of Neuro-Ophthalmology*, doi: 10.1097/WNO.0000000000000467.

Mader, TH, CR Gibson, M Caputo, *et al.* (1993). Intraocular pressure and retinal vascular changes during transient exposure to microgravity. *American Journal of Ophthalmology*, 115, 347–350.

Mader, TH, D Koch, K Manual, CR Gibson, RK Effenhauser and S Musgrave (1999). Stability of vision during space flight in an astronaut with bilateral intraocular lenses. *American Journal of Ophthalmology*, 127, 342–343.

Mader, TH, GR Taylor, N Hunter, M Caputo and RT Meehan (1990). Intraocular pressure, retinal vascular, and visual acuity changes during 48 hours of 10 degree head-down tilt. *Aviation. Space and Environmental. Medicine*, 61, 810–813.

Mader, TH and LJ White (1995). Refractive changes at extreme altitude following radial keratotomy. *American Journal of Ophthalmology*, 119(6), 733–737.

Mader, TH, S Blanton, S Schallhorn, B Glibert, LJ White, V Parmley and JD Ng (1996). Refractive changes during 72 hour exposure to altitude following refractive surgery. *Ophthalmology*, 103(8), 1188–1195.

Maumenee, AE and MF Schwartz (1985). Acute intraoperative choroidal effusion. *American Journal of Ophthalmology*, 100, 147–154.

Nelson, M, S Brady, TH Mader, LJ White, V Parmley, RK and Winkle (2001). Refractive changes caused by hypoxia after laser In situ keratomileusis surgery. *Ophthalmology*, 108, 542–544.

Nettleship, E (1884). Peculiar lines in the choroid in a case of postpapilliticatrophy. *Transactions Ophthalmological Society UK*, 4, 167–168.

Newell, FW (1973). Choroidal folds. The seventh Harry Searls Gradle Memorial Lecture. *American Journal of Ophthalmology*, 75, 930–942.

Ng, JD, LJ White, V Parmley, J Hubickey, Carter J and TH Mader (1996). Effects of simulated altitude on post radial keratotomy corneas. *Ophthalmology*, 103(3), 452–457.

Nicogossian, AE and JF Jr Parker (1982). *Space physiology and medicine*. Washington, DC: NASA, Technical Information Branch, 158. NASA SP–447.

Patel, KH, JC Javitt, JM Tielsch *et al.* (1995). Incidence of acute angle-closure glaucoma after pharmacologic mydriasis. *American Journal of Ophthalmology*, 120(6), 709–717.

Quigley, HA, DS Friedman and NG Congdon (2003). Possible mechanisms of primary angle-closure and malignant glaucoma. *Journal of Glaucoma*, 12, 167–180.

Sharma, M, NJ Volpe, T Patel and A Kimmel (1999). Intracranial hypertension associated with acquired hyperopia and choroidal folds. *Retina*, 19, 260–262.

Shinojima, A, K Iwasaki and K Aoki, *et al.* (2012). Subfoveal choroidal thickness and foveal retinal thickness during head-down tilt. *Aviation, Space, and Environmental Medicine*, 83, 388–393.

Silver DM and O Geyer (2000). Pressure-volume relation for the living human eye. *Current Eye Research*, 20, 115–120.

Thornton, WE, GW Hoffler and JA Rummel (1977). Anthropometric changes and fluid shifts. In *Biomedical Results from Skylab*. Washington, DC: Scientific and Technical Information Office, R Johnston, L Dietlein (eds.), NASA. Available at: http://lsda.jsc.nasa.gov/books/skylab//Ch32.htm. Accessed [29 May 2011].

Tiedeman, JS (1991). A physical analysis of the factors that determine the contour of the iris. *American Journal of Ophthalmology*, 111, 338–343.

Tso, MO and SS Hayreh (1977). Optic disc edema in raised intracranial pressure. IV. Axoplasmic transport in experimental papilledema. *Archives of Ophthalmology*, 95, 1458–1462.

Vein, AA, H Koppen, J Haan, GM Terwindt and MD Ferrari (2009). Space headache: a new secondary headache. *Cephalagia*, Jun, 29(6), 683–686.

Wall, M (2010). Idiopathic intracranial hypertension. *Neurologic Clinics*, Aug, 28(3), 593–617.

Westfall, AC, JD Ng, JR Samples and JL Weissman (2004). In reply to: Brodsky MC. Flattening of the posterior sclera: Hypotony or elevated intracranial pressure [letter]? *American Journal of Ophthalmology*, 138, 511–512.

White, LJ and TH Mader (2000). Refractive changes at high altitude after LASIK. *Ophthalmology*, 107, 2118.

Winkle, RK, TH Mader, V Parmley, K Polse and LJ White (1998). The etiology of refractive changes at high altitude following radial keratotomy: hypoxia versus hypobaria. *Ophthalmology*, 105, 282–286.

Wright, AM, J Gooch, R Harvey, R Davis and C Reilly (2012). Stability of laser-assisted in situ keratomileusis (LASIK) at altitude. *Aviation, Space, and Environmental Medicine*, 83, 958–961.

Eye, Orbit, and Pituitary MRI: Relevance to Space Medicine — 3

Larry A. Kramer, MD

Department of Diagnostic Imaging and Intervention,
University of Texas Health Science Center-Houston, 6431 Fannin St,
Houston, TX 77030, USA

1. Introduction

Magnetic resonance imaging (MRI) has been utilized in the practice of medicine since the early 1980s within a short time after the availability of commercial scanners. MRI was rapidly adopted in neuroimaging in large part due to the excellent soft tissue contrast resolution of the brain and orbits not possible with the computed tomography (CT) developed just a decade earlier. The ability of MRI to directly acquire images in multiple planes such as axial, coronal, sagittal, or essentially in unlimited obliquities is uniquely beneficial to evaluation of the orbits and pituitary gland, which can be difficult to analyze solely on the basis of axial imaging, a technological limitation of CT. The lack of ionizing radiation is an additional advantage of MRI compared to CT. MRI evaluation of the highly radiosensitive structure such as the eye is typically performed with multiple thin specialized sequences required for detailed evaluation of the orbit without concern for radiation-induced injury of the lens or cornea. The lack of ionizing radiation also permits frequent repetition of imaging studies necessary for longitudinal studies for research applications and health surveillance without radiation exposure limitations.

Although MRI has been applied in the study of the effects of microgravity on astronauts since the early 1990s, such as quantification of loss of muscle mass (Jaweed *et al.*, 1992), it was nearly two decades later that a clinical MRI evaluation

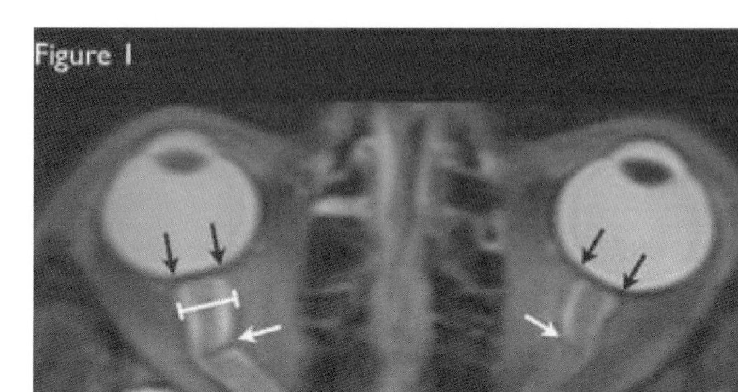

Figure 1. Example of a postflight MRI of the orbits. Axial 3D T2-weighted image of the orbits in an astronaut presenting with choroidal folds. MRI reveals a range of unexpected orbital abnormalities including posterior globe flattening bilaterally (black arrows), dilated right optic nerve sheath to 10 mm (line with bars), bilateral kink the optic nerve sheath (white arrows).

of an astronaut was requested to better understand the etiology of an unusual phenomenon of choroidal folds (Jacobson, 1995). Choroidal folds are undulations in the retinal and choroidal layers of the posterior globe that can be related to compression of the posterior globe by a mass or intracranial hypertension (Griebel and Kosmorsky, 2000; Lavinsky *et al.*, 2007) and can result in metamorphopsia, a distortion of vision that cannot be corrected by refraction techniques. The discovery of choroidal folds in a postflight astronaut temporally related to a recent exposure to microgravity could be considered a sentinel event. The identification of multiple abnormal MRI findings in this singular case (Fig. 1) engendered a new role of MRI in space medicine in the backdrop of increasing clinical and quantitative evidence of visual impairment in astronauts (Mader *et al.*, 2011).

2. MRI Technique

High-resolution MRI images of the orbits can be obtained with high field strength magnets preferably at 3 Tesla and having eight-channel or greater sensitivity encoding head coils. The combination of high field strength and multichannel coils results in improved signal-to-noise ratios allowing high-quality high-resolution thin images of the orbits. The brain and pituitary gland can be imaged with less demanding sequences more commonly utilized in routine clinical applications.

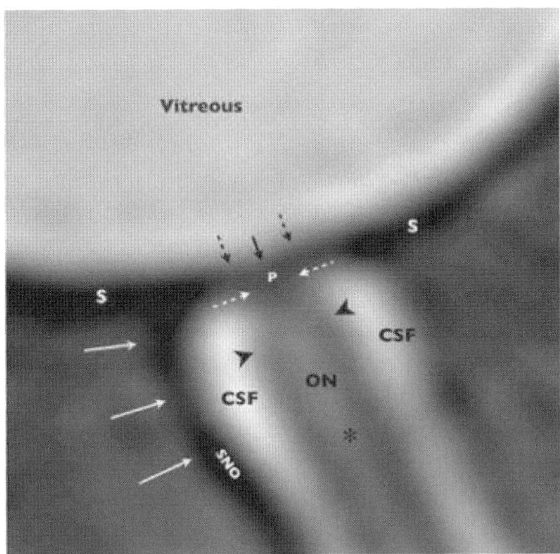

Figure 2.   Example of high-resolution MRI anatomy of the optic nerve and posterior globe. T2-weighted axial image of the optic papilla (P) with associated normal depression (physiologic cup) (small black arrow) and raised annular ridge (small dashed arrows). The cerebral spinal fluid (CSF) in the perineural subarachnoid space is hyperintense relative to the ONS and optic nerve (ON). Note the intermediate signal intensity of the optic nerve with associated central hyperintensity (*). The bulbar section of the ONS is indicated by the white arrows. The estimated location of the non–myelinated laminar optic nerve at the lamina cribosa is indicated by the white dashed arrows. The estimated location of the retrolaminar myelinated optic nerve is indicated by the black arrow heads. The sclera (S) and optic nerve sheath (ONS) are contiguous structures. Image courtesy of the journal *Radiology*.

Ideally, 3D sequences should be acquired with isotropic pixel dimensions of 1 mm or less and using a technique that suppresses surrounding intraconal fat signal. The isotropic pixel dimension permits reformatting of the data set along the longitudinal axis of the optic nerve sheath without loss of resolution to optimize diameter measurements of the optic nerve sheath and improve visualization of the optic papilla. Identification of the physiologic cup of the optic nerve (Fig. 2) helps to best localize the center point of the optic nerve and optic nerve sheath for consistent and accurate diameter measurements.

Fluid-sensitive 3D T2-weighted fast spin–echo sequences give excellent contrast between the optic nerve sheath, cerebral spinal fluid (CSF), sclera, optic papilla, and intraorbital optic nerve (Figs 2–3). Similar contrast is maintained between the pituitary gland and suprasellar cistern useful to evaluate the morphology of the dome of the pituitary gland and the position of the pituitary stalk (Fig. 4).

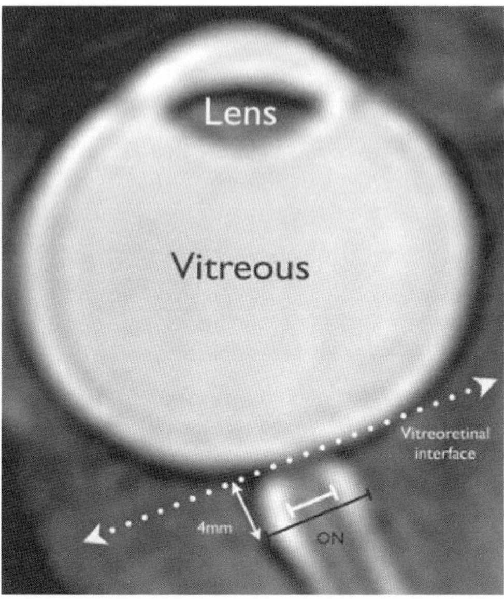

Figure 3. Example of the vitreoretinal interface and the measurement location of the optic nerve and optic nerve sheath diameter measurements. The vitreoretinal interface (VRI) (dashed line with arrows) shown in the illustration above represents a plane perpendicular to the optic nerve (ON) at the border between the optic nerve papilla and the vitreous. The optic nerve sheath diameter is measured from inner margin to inner margin of the sheath (solid black line with bars) 4 mm posterior to the vitreoretinal interface (solid white line with arrows). Note optic nerve (ON) diameter is measured 3 mm posterior to the VRI (solid white line with bars). Image courtesy of the journal *Radiology*.

A full description of the all sequence types and pulse sequence parameters is beyond the scope of this chapter; however, a detailed MRI protocol of the brain and pituitary gland with high-resolution imaging of the orbits is available in a publication entitled; "Orbital and intracranial effects of microgravity: Findings at 3-T MR imaging" (Kramer *et al.*, 2012).

3. Normal Anatomy of the Orbit and Pituitary Gland

Using the high-resolution 3D T2-weighted fast spin-echo sequences the myelinated optic nerve is visualized as an intermediate signal structure surrounded by hyperintense CSF and encapsulated by the low signal intensity of the optic nerve sheath (Fig. 2). Myelination of the nerve fibers is known to decrease the T2 signal intensity of neural tissue (Barkovich, 2000). The normal myelinated retrolaminar

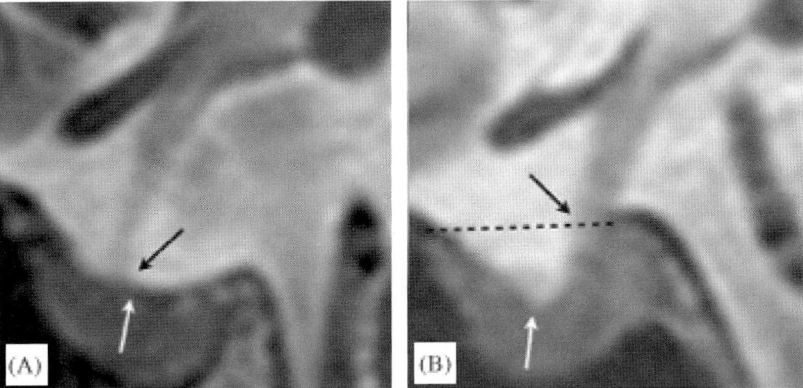

Figure 4. Sagittal T2-weighted image through pituitary gland and stalk in two different astronauts. (A) Note upward convexity of the dome of the pituitary gland (white arrow) and midline position of the pituitary stalk (black arrow) defined as a normal pituitary gland. (B) Note posterior displacement of the pituitary stalk (black arrow) and prominent concavity of the dome of the pituitary gland (arrow) with significant loss in height relative to the height of the sella (white arrow) consistent with elevated intracranial pressure and arachnoid herniation into the pituitary fossa (dashed line). Image courtesy of the journal *Radiology*.

portion of the optic nerve (Fig. 2) measures 3 mm in diameter (Sternberg, 1992) (Fig. 3). The optic nerve gradually thins as it approaches the optic canal due to reduction in the percentage of connective tissue relative to myelinated axons (Karim, 2004). The nonmyelinated retrolaminar optic nerve (Fig. 2) just posterior to the lamina cribosa measures 1.5 mm (Krstic, 1991). The optic nerve shows mild redundancy without evidence of abrupt angulation or excessive tortuosity.

The optic nerve sheath contrasts with the T2 hyperintensity of the perineural CSF and to lesser degree from the surrounding intraconal fat, which is T2 hypointense due to purposeful suppression of fat signal. The terminal expansion of the optic nerve sheath is referred to as the bulbar region and is the preferred site of diameter measurement most commonly utilized to evaluate for indirect imaging evidence of intracranial hypertension with either ultrasound, CT, or MRI as it has been shown to be a region of greatest distention in response to volume expansion (Hansen and Helmke, 1997). Although the retinal layer of the posterior globe cannot be clearly resolved from the choroidal layer or sclera, the inner margin of the posterior globe relative to the T2 hyperintense vitreous is defined as the vitreoretinal interface (Fig. 3). The vitreoretinal interface can be used a reference point in which to reproducibly measure the optic nerve sheath diameter at a consistent point along the bulbar portion of the optic nerve sheath (Fig. 2). The optic nerve sheath diameter measured 4 mm posterior to the vitreoretinal interface should not exceed 5.8 mm in the absence of intracranial hypertension (Geeraerts *et al.*, 2008) (Fig. 3). A central region of the relative T2 hyperintensity can be resolved in the optic nerve and is believed to represent unmyelinated perivascular optic nerve fibers found in this region (Fig. 2). The optic nerve sheath shows mild redundancy without evidence of abrupt angulation or a kink allowing sufficient laxity for ocular motion.

The contour of the posterior globe consisting of the sclera has low T2 signal intensity and is readily delineated from the adjacent intraorbital fat and T2 hyper-intense vitreous. The sclera measures approximately 1 mm in thickness (Norman *et al.*, 2010). The posterior margin of the sclera should demonstrate a smooth rounded convexity (Figs. 2 and 3).

The lens is well visualized between the T2 hyperintense fluid-filled anterior aqueous and posterior vitreous compartments of the globe having low T2 signal intensity on all pulse sequences (Fig. 3). The lens can be utilized as the center point of the globe anteriorly and to measure anterior displacement of the retina.

The CSF surrounding the optic nerve communicates with the intracranial CSF via the optic canal and adjacent suprasellar cistern and is thus capable of transmitting intracranial CSF pressure to the intraorbital space (Liu and Kahn, 1993; Hansen and Helmke, 1997). Within the optic nerve sheath there is an extensive system of thin arachnoid trabeculae, pillars, and septae that likely alters the flow of CSF in the perineural space (Killer, 2003). These ultrafine structures cannot be resolved with current MRI technique.

The pituitary gland is well characterized morphologically using sagittal T2-weighted images delineating the dome of the pituitary gland, the pituitary stalk, and the suprasellar cistern. The CSF in the suprasellar cistern is T2 hyperintense and readily differentiated from the pituitary stalk and gland, which are intermediate in signal intensity. The T2 hypointense structure surrounding the pituitary gland represents the cortical margin of the pituitary fossa. The pituitary dome is normally convex or flat and the pituitary stalk is vertical and midline (Fig. 4A). The pituitary gland height is generally less than 8 mm in males and 9 mm in females (Suzuki *et al.*, 1990).

4. Anatomic Alteration of the Globe, Optic Nerve Sheath, Optic Nerve in Astronauts Exposed to Microgravity

Microgravity is ubiquitous in the space environment and can be measured in units of time. A total lifetime cumulative exposure to microgravity can be determined for each astronaut from one or multiple missions. Total exposure in astronauts can be characterized as short duration equating to less than 30 days such as found in shuttle missions or long duration such as can be found in six-month missions on the international space station. Although anatomic alterations described in astronauts may be related in part to exposure to microgravity due to fluid shifts, venous outflow resistance, or decreased CSF reabsorption (Otto, 2013), other aberrations of the space environment such as elevated levels of ionizing radiation and carbon dioxide may also be contributory.

With well-established normal qualitative and quantitative assessment of the globe, optic nerve sheath, and optic nerve, abnormalities have been identified in greater prevalence in astronauts compared to the normal population. Since baseline high-resolution MRI evaluation of the orbits is not available in the majority of astronauts prior to microgravity exposure, the true prevalence of abnormalities and its relationship to microgravity exposure is still unknown. In addition, postflight MRI has not been consistently obtained in the immediate postflight period and thus a natural decay of imaging abnormalities could potentially result in a lower prevalence of abnormalities due to this mechanism. Longitudinal studies following immediate postflight imaging will help determine the true prevalence and the half-life of imaging findings. In a limited number of cases pre- and postflight MRI studies are available and have documented modification of orbital structures following exposure to microgravity and were optimally obtained within a relatively short time interval between reentry and MRI evaluation. Although postflight questionnaires have suggested that up to 29% of short-duration and 60% of long-duration astronauts have experienced a change in visual acuity (Mader *et al.*, 2011), the actual prevalence of imaging abnormalities with subjective and clinical correlation is unknown due to incomplete imaging data sets.

The posterior globe contour composed of the fibrous sclera has a smooth rounded convexity and is directly attached to the optic nerve sheath at the level of the optic papilla. Flattening of the posterior globe was present in 8% of short-duration astronauts and 40% of long-duration astronauts (Kramer *et al.*, 2012) and was centered at the optic nerve sheath attachment. There is also documentation of the development of posterior globe flattening in an individual astronaut when preflight and postflight data are compared (Fig. 5). The significance of posterior globe flattening is that in the absence of a mass lesion compressing the posterior globe or ocular hypotony (Westfall *et al.*, 2004) it is an imaging finding that is 100% specific for intracranial hypertension (Agid *et al.*, 2006). It is also clinically associated with hyperoptic shift as the retina and therefore the optical focal point is displaced towards the lens. It is therefore not unexpected that hyperoptic shift is a phenomenon documented to occur during space flight (Mader *et al.*, 2011). It should be noted that microgravity is actually associated with elevated

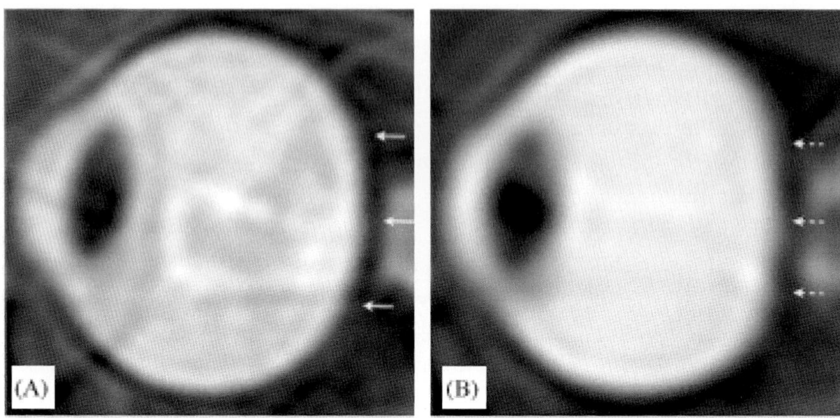

Figure 5. Sagittal oblique T2-weighted images through left eye of same astronaut. (A) Image before long-term exposure to microgravity. Note normal convexity of posterior globe (white arrows). (B) Image after long-term exposure to microgravity. Note flattening of the posterior scleral margin (white dashed arrows). Image courtesy of the journal *Radiology*.

intraocular pressures (Schwartz *et al.*, 1993; Draeger *et al.*, 1995), which in contrast to ocular hypotony could theoretically resist posterior globe flattening. The difference in pressure across the lamina cribosa between the CSF in the optic nerve sheath and the vitreous is referred to as the translaminar pressure difference (Berdahl *et al.*, 2012). In the presence of elevated intracranial CSF pressures, the intraorbital CSF pressures via continuity with the intracranial space are in turn elevated. Intracranial hypertension hypothetically elevates translaminar pressure and directs hydrostatic forces at the insertion of the optic nerve sheath at the posterior scleral attachment. Hypothetically this is the cause of the posterior globe flattening associated with intracranial hypertension although this hypothesis has not been verified experimentally.

Optic nerve sheath diameter is an indirect parameter of intracranial hypertension (Hansen and Helmke, 1997). The perineural space of the intraorbital optic nerve is in direct continuation of the intracranial CSF space as verified by a cadaver study (Liu and Kahn, 1993). Optic nerve sheath diameter measured at the bulbar expansion of the optic nerve sheath can be evaluated with ultrasound, MRI, or CT. With the best available data to date, the 90% probability level of intracranial hypertension using optic nerve sheath diameter measured at 4 mm posterior to the vitreoretinal interface (Fig. 3) using T2-weighted MRI images is 5.82 mm or greater (Geeraerts *et al.*, 2008). Using high-resolution MRI technique 42% of short-duration and 60% of long-duration astronauts had abnormally dilated optic nerve sheath diameters indicating exposure to elevated intracranial pressures (Kramer *et al.*, 2012). It should be noted that the threshold of optic nerve sheath diameter was based on a publication utilizing a lower resolution data set then utilized with astronauts (Geeraerts *et al.*, 2008). Thus the prevalence of abnormal dilatation of the optic nerve sheath indicative of intracranial hypertension could be modified based on revision of normative data using high-resolution technique as the threshold for intracranial hypertension would likely increase as edge detection optic nerve sheath improves and partial volume averaging effect is diminished.

It should also be noted that optic nerve sheath dilatation was identified in some instances greater than 100 days postflight indicating either persistent intracranial hypertension or remodeling of the optic nerve sheath. Dilatation of the optic nerve sheath may at some point exceed the tensile strength of the optic nerve sheath proper. In addition, the thin arachnoid trabeculae, pillar, and septae found in the perineural space (Killer, 2003) may undergo breakdown as the optic nerve sheath dilates beyond the tensile strength of these microstructures. These microstructures may restrain of the optic nerve sheath to the optic nerve and resist deformation. A final possibility of the persistent optic nerve sheath dilatation is reduced CSF exchange between the intracranial subarachnoid space and the perineural space of the intraorbital of nerve sheath due to sequestering of the CSF of the optic nerve sheath referred to compartmentalization (Killer *et al.*, 2007).

Although nonspecific, optic disc protrusion is another potential marker of intracranial hypertension (Agid *et al.*, 2006). When optic nerve protrusion is associated with intracranial hypertension it is referred to as papilledema (Dhungana *et al.*, 2010). Papilledema is believed to occur due to mechanical effects of elevated perineural CSF pressures altering axoplasmic transport in the optic nerve resulting in axonal swelling and interstitial edema (Hayreh, 1977; Tso and Hayreh, 1977; Dhungana *et al.*, 2010). The net result is the reversal of the normal concavity of the optic disc with protrusion of the optic disc into the vitreous (Fig. 6). Although vision may remain normal with papilledema it can eventually lead in rare severe cases to optic nerve ischemia with associated blindness (Green *et al.*, 1980). MRI evidence of optic disc protrusion has only been found in up to 27% of long-duration and not in short-duration astronauts. Thus long chronic exposure to the microgravity appears to be an important component to developing papilledema.

In addition to optic disc protrusion the retrolaminar portion of the optic nerve is subject to abnormal expansion. There is a linear relationship between optic nerve sheath dilatation measured at 4 mm posterior to the vitreoretinal interface and optic nerve diameter thickening measured at 3 mm posterior to the vitreoretinal interface (Kramer *et al.*, 2012). The greater the dilatation of the optic nerve sheath indicating increasing level of perineural CSF pressures, the greater the

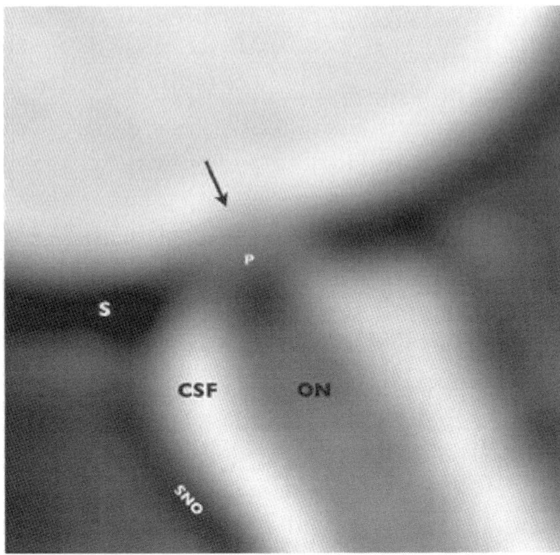

Figure 6.   Example of Optic Disc Protrusion. T2-weighted axial image of the optic papilla (P) showing protrusion (small black arrow) with loss of the physiologic cup. The sclera (S) is seen as hypointense signal and is in continuity with the optic nerve sheath (ONS). Perineural cerebral spinal fluid (CSF). Optic nerve (ON). Image courtesy of the journal *Radiology*.

diameter of the optic nerve is found, measuring up to 50% larger in diameter in a retrospective study compared to normal (Kramer *et al.*, 2012). Optic nerve expansion may also be indicative of the impaired axoplasmic transport and interstitial edema associated with papilledema. In one case the optic nerve was also severely thickened in the posterior portion of the orbit just proximal to a severe kink the optic nerve sheath with expansion of central T2 hyperintensity of the optic nerve (Fig. 7). A possible explanation is that the kink, in conjunction with the perineural microstructures, obstructs the distal CSF flow and alters the pressure gradient along the optic nerve sheath. In this case it is proposed that higher pressures occurring in the proximal optic nerve sheath cause greater localized interstitial edema within proximal optic nerve.

The least sensitive sign of the intracranial hypertension is morphologic distortion of the optic nerve or the optic nerve sheath represented as tortuosity of the optic nerve or similarly tortuosity of the optic nerve sheath with a kink (Suzuki *et al.*, 2001; Agid *et al.*, 2006; Lim *et al.*, 2010; Kramer *et al.*, 2012). In the normal situation there is mild redundancy in the optic nerve and optic nerve sheath with a mild undulation. With chronic elevated perineural pressure it is conceivable that

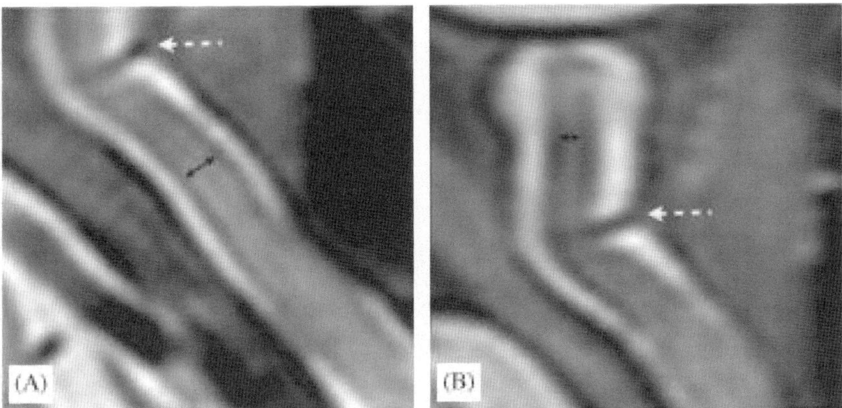

Figure 7.   Example of expanded optic nerve in an astronaut with visual abnormality. (A) T2-weighted axial images through an abnormal mid optic nerve. Note width of central T2 hyperintensity (small double arrow) and kink (dashed white arrow). (B) Note optic nerve central T2 hyperintensity (small double arrow) distal to the kink (dashed white arrow) assumes a more normal diameter. Image courtesy of the journal *Radiology*.

the optic nerve sheath is gradually lengthened in addition to known cross-sectional dilatation. The expansion of the length of the optic nerve sheath results in greater redundancy within the intraconal space and therefore an increasing amount of folding or tortuosity of the optic nerve and optic nerve sheath is necessary to conform to this limited space. Increasing expansion of the optic nerve due to impaired axoplasmic flow could also result in redundancy of the optic nerve. In the study of astronauts a kink was defined as an abrupt angulation of the optic nerve sheath as an indication of tortuosity since it is less subjective than optic nerve redundancy (Fig. 8). An optic nerve sheath kink was present in 8% of short-duration and 20% of long-duration astronauts indicating that chronically elevated intracranial pressure contributes to this phenomenon.

5. Anatomic Alteration of the Pituitary Gland in Astronauts Exposed to Microgravity

Although the orbits and visual status of astronauts has been the area of greatest concern due to the clinical presentation of change in visual acuity, the pituitary gland can also be affected by intracranial hypertension although this effect is subclinical. A potential mechanism is prolapse of the arachnoid through a defect in

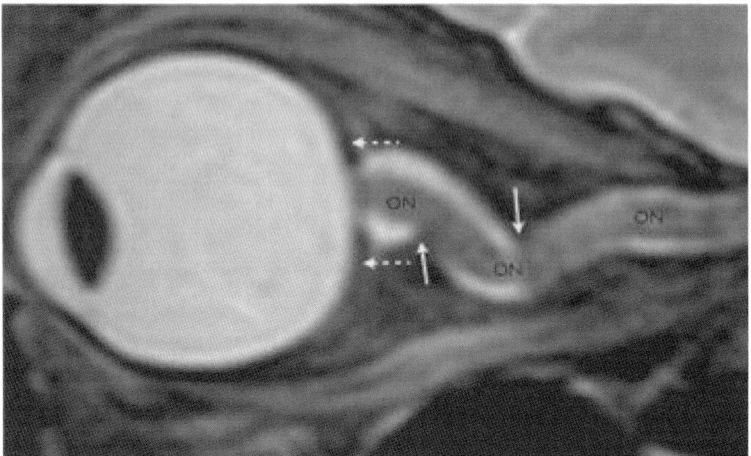

Figure 8.   Example of tortuosity of the optic nerve and optic nerve sheath. Sagittal oblique T2-weighted image through right eye showing two abruptly angulated margins of the optic nerve sheath compatible with kinks (white arrows). The optic nerve (ON) is also tortuous. Note posterior globe flattening (dashed arrows). Image courtesy of the journal *Radiology*.

diaphragmatic sella, which can gradually remodel the pituitary gland within the pituitary fossa through transmission of intracranial pressure to the intrasellar subarachnoid space (Yuh *et al.*, 2000; Maira *et al.*, 2005). The most common site of herniation is through the anterior diaphragm sella and thus the midline positioned pituitary stalk is subsequently displaced posteriorly (Jinkins *et al.*, 1996). This posterior displacement can occur up to the level of the posterior clinoid processes. The combination of moderate to greater concavity of the pituitary dome and posterior displacement of the pituitary stalk has a 92% specificity of acute intracranial hypertension relative to controls (Yuh *et al.*, 2000) (Fig. 5B). This is in contradistinction to empty sella syndrome in which there is complete flattening of the pituitary gland with midline positioning of the pituitary stalk. Empty sella syndrome not specific for intracranial hypertension (Maira *et al.*, 2005) (Fig. 9).

6. Dose Response Effect of Microgravity Exposure

When all the MRI findings are combined and the astronauts are divided into short- and long-duration subgroups there is an increasing prevalence of abnormal findings associated with increasing exposure to microgravity (Kramer *et al.*, 2012). All imaging findings associated with intracranial hypertension were found in astronauts with long-duration exposure. However, cases of optic disc protrusion

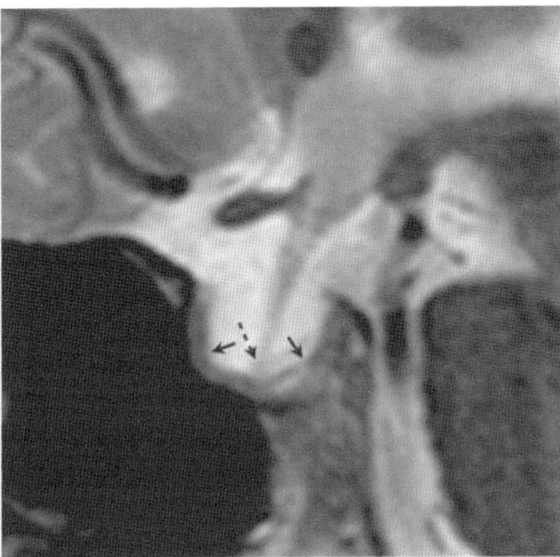

Figure 9. Example of Empty Sella Syndrome. Sagittal T2-weighted image through pituitary gland and stalk. Note severe downward concavity of the dome of the pituitary gland (arrow) and midline position of the pituitary stalk (dashed arrow) defined as an empty sella. Image courtesy of the journal *Radiology*.

or moderate pituitary concavity with posterior pituitary stalk displacement was only found in long-duration astronauts suggesting greater chronicity is required to reach a threshold of pathologic change detectable by imaging.

7. Conclusion

The constellation of the MRI findings identified in astronauts exposed to microgravity is very similar to patients with chronically elevated intracranial pressures as is documented with idiopathic intracranial hypertension (Agid *et al.*, 2006). The combination of the posterior globe flattening, optic disc protrusion, optic nerve sheath dilatation and tortuosity with a kink, optic nerve thickening, and moderate or greater pituitary concavity with posterior displacement of the pituitary stalk are all consistent with imaging findings of intracranial hypertension. The confounding factor is that these imaging findings have been only previously described with diseases associated with normal gravity. It therefore remains uncertain if the etiology of these imaging findings is potentially due to a novel pathological process found in microgravity or if intracranial hypertension is in fact the common denominator. If intracranial hypertension is confirmed to occur in microgravity by direct measurement or other noninvasive means the exact mechanism by which intracranial pressure increases will need to be further elucidated in order to determine risk stratification and to develop effective strategies to mitigate the disease process.

References

Agid, R, RI Farb, RA Willinsky, DJ Mikulis and G Tomlinson (2006). Idiopathic intracranial hypertension: The validity of cross-sectional neuroimaging signs. *Neuroradiology*, 48(8), 521–527.

Barkovich, AJ (2000). Concepts of myelin and myelination in neuroradiology. *AJNR American Journal of Neuroradiology*, 21(6), 1099–1109.

Berdahl, JP, DY Yu and WH Morgan (2012). The translaminar pressure gradient in sustained zero gravity, idiopathic intracranial hypertension, and glaucoma. *Medical Hypotheses*, 79(6), 719–724.

Dhungana, S, B Sharrack and N Woodroofe (2010). Idiopathic intracranial hypertension. *Acta Neurologica Scandinavica*, 121(2), 71–82.

Draeger, J, R Schwartz, S Groenhoff and C Stern (1995). Self-tonometry under microgravity conditions. *Aviation, Space, and Environmental Medicine*, 66(6), 568–570.

Geeraerts, T, VFJ Newcombe, JP Coles, *et al.* (2008). Use of T2-weighted magnetic resonance imaging of the optic nerve sheath to detect raised intracranial pressure. *Critical Care*, 12(5), R114.

Green, GJ, S Lessell and JI Loewenstein (1980). Ischemic optic neuropathy in chronic papilledema. *Archives of Ophthalmology*, 98(3), 502–504.

Griebel, SR and GS Kosmorsky(2000). Choroidal folds associated with increased intracranial pressure. *American Journal of Ophthalmology*, 129(4), 513–516.

Hansen, HC and K Helmke (1997). Validation of the optic nerve sheath response to changing cerebrospinal fluid pressure: Ultrasound findings during intrathecal infusion tests. *Journal of Neurosurgery*, 87(1), 34–40.

Hayreh, SS (1997). Optic disc edema in raised intracranial pressure. V. Pathogenesis. *Archives of Ophthalmology*, 95(9), 1553–1565.

Jacobson, DM (1995). Intracranial hypertension and the syndrome of acquired hyperopia with choroidal folds. *Journal of Neuro-Ophthalmology*, 15(3), 178–185.

Jaweed, M, P Narayana, J Slopis and I Butler (1992). Magnetic Resonance Imaging (MRI) of skeletal muscles in astronauts after 9 days of space flight. Aerospace Medical Association 63rd Annual Scientific Meeting. Miami Beach, Florida: Aerospance Medical Association.

Jinkins, JR, S Athale, L Xiong, WT Yuh, MI Rothman and PT Nguyen (1996). MR of optic papilla protrusion in patients with high intracranial pressure. *AJNR American Journal of Neuroradiology*, 17(4), 665–668.

Karim S (2004). Demonstration of systematic variation in human intraorbital optic nerve size by quantitative magnetic resonance imaging and histology. *Investigative Ophthalmology Visual Science*, 45(4), 1047–1051.

Killer, HE (2003). Architecture of arachnoid trabeculae, pillars, and septa in the subarachnoid space of the human optic nerve: anatomy and clinical considerations. *British Journal of Ophthalmology*, 87(6), 777–781.

Killer, HE, GP Jaggi, J Flammer, NR Miller, AR Huber and A Mironov (2007). Cerebrospinal fluid dynamics between the intracranial and the subarachnoid space of the optic nerve. Is it always bidirectional? *Brain*, 130(2), 514–520.

Kramer, LA, AE Sargsyan, KM Hasan, JD Polk and DR Hamilton (2012). Orbital and intracranial effects of microgravity: Findings at 3-T MR imaging. *Radiology*, 263(3), 819–827.

Krstic, RV (1991). *Human Microscopic Anatomy: An Atlas for Students of Medicine and Biology*, pp. 534–536. Berlin: Springer-Verlag.

Lavinsky, J, D Lavinsky, F Lavinsky and A Frutuoso (2007). Acquired choroidal folds: a sign of idiopathic intracranial hypertension. *Graefe's Archive for Clinical and Experimental Ophthalmology*, 245(6), 883–888.

Lim, MJ, K Pushparajah, W Jan, D Calver and JP Lin (2010). Magnetic resonance imaging changes in idiopathic intracranial hypertension in children. *Journal of Child Neurology*, 25(3), 294–299.

Liu, D and M Kahn (1993). Measurement and relationship of subarachnoid pressure of the optic nerve to intracranial pressures in fresh cadavers. *American Journal of Ophthalmology*, 116(5), 548–556.

Mader, TH, CR Gibson, AF Pass, *et al.* (2011). Optic disc edema, globe flattening, choroidal folds, and hyperopic shifts observed in astronauts after long-duration space flight. *Ophthalmology*, 118(10), 2058–2069.

Maira, G, C Anile and A Mangiola (2005). Primary empty sella syndrome in a series of 142 patients. *Journal of Neurosurgery*, 103(5), 831–836.

Norman, RE, JG Flanagan, SM Rausch, *et al.* (2010). Dimensions of the human sclera: Thickness measurement and regional changes with axial length. *Experimental Eye Research*, 90(2), 277–284.

Otto, C (2013). *Risk of Microgravity-induced Impairment and Elevated Intracranial Pressure (VIIP)*. Washington, DC: BiblioGov.

Schwartz, R, J Draeger, S Groenhoff and KD Flade (1993). [Results of self-tonometry during the 1st German-Russian MIR mission 1992]. *Ophthalmologe*, 90(6), 640–642.

Sternberg, SS (1992). *Histology for Pathologists*, p. 329. New York: Raven Press.

Suzuki, H, J Takanashi, K Kobayashi, K Nagasawa, K Tashima and Y Kohno (2001). MR imaging of idiopathic intracranial hypertension. *AJNR. American Journal of Neuroradiology*, 22(1), 196–199.

Suzuki, M, T Takashima, M Kadoya, *et al.* (1990). Height of normal pituitary gland on MR imaging: age and sex differentiation. *Journal of Computer Assisted Tomography*, 14(1), 36–39.

Tso, MO and SS Hayreh (1997). Optic disc edema in raised intracranial pressure. IV. Axoplasmic transport in experimental papilledema. *Archives of Ophthalmology*, 95(8), 1458–1462.

Westfall, AC, JD Ng, JR Samples and JL Weissman (2004). Hypotonus maculopathy: magnetic resonance appearance. *American Journal of Ophthalmology*, 137(3), 563–566.

Yuh, WT, M Zhu, T Taoka, *et al.* (2000). MR imaging of pituitary morphology in idiopathic intracranial hypertension. *Journal of Magnetic Resonance Imaging*, 12(6), 808–813.

Fluid Shifts and Cardiovascular-Related Factors That May Contribute to the VIIP Syndrome in Astronauts

4

Michael B. Stenger, PhD, Steven S. Laurie, PhD and Stuart M.C. Lee, PhD

Wyle Science, Technology and Engineering,
Johnson Space Center Cardiovascular Laboratory, 2101 E NASA Pkwy,
Houston, TX 77058, USA

1. Introduction

With the end of the Space Shuttle era, the National Aeronautics and Space Administration (NASA) is transitioning almost exclusively to long-duration International Space Station (ISS) missions while planning for future exploration-class missions to Mars, its moons, or nearby asteroids. However, a newly described medical condition affecting ocular structure and function that develops during and persists after long-duration spaceflight may have an impact on these activities. Vision disturbances were known to affect some astronauts during short-duration missions, but these changes were mostly transient and did not appear to have lasting impacts on the structure or function of the eye. In contrast, approximately 2/3 of American astronauts have developed changes in visual acuity after long-duration spaceflight since the persistence of these symptoms has been observed (Mader *et al.*, 2011; Barr *et al.*, 2014). This condition has been labeled by NASA as the visual impairment and intracranial pressure syndrome (VIIP). Recent findings include anatomical changes to the eye, including papilledema or choroidal folds, with some crewmembers also exhibiting increased lumbar puncture (LP) opening pressures postflight (Mader *et al.*, 2011), perhaps indicative of elevated intracranial pressure (ICP). Although VIIP shares some similarities with idiopathic intracranial hypertension in clinical populations, there is no clear understanding of the VIIP etiology in the astronaut population. Several hypotheses have been put forth, including the primary hypothesis that changes in vision originate from the spaceflight-induced cephalad fluid shift, which in turn might cause elevated intracranial and intraocular pressures. In addition, the vascular system of the head and neck is likely subjected to pressures and flows that are not normally present during daily activities on Earth and that might induce vascular dysfunction and remodeling. Such changes could impair cerebral drainage, increase fluid congestion, and contribute to tissue edema. While these hypotheses are attractive, bilateral asymmetries in ocular changes and the lack of VIIP symptoms in spaceflight analogs, such as head–down tilt bed rest, highlight the difficulties NASA faces in understanding and mitigating the VIIP risk during long-duration spaceflight. In this chapter we outline the current understanding of spaceflight-induced fluid shifts and how they may contribute to changes in intracranial or intraocular pressure, and highlight the potential contributions of the cardiovascular system to the development of VIIP.

2. Background

Spaceflight is known to cause a cephalad fluid shift secondary to the loss of the hydrostatic pressure gradient normally experienced on Earth. While the exact magnitude of this fluid shift has been difficult to characterize in spaceflight, Moore and Thornton suggested that a 2000-ml shift from the legs to the upper body occurs (Moore and Thornton, 1987). Ground-based analogs such as head–out water immersion and head–down tilt bed rest suggest that the fluid shift is between 700 and 3000 ml (Arborelius *et al.*, 1972; Nixon *et al.*, 1979; Montgomery, 1987). This fluid shift leads to transient increases in stroke volume (Lathers *et al.*, 1989; Liu *et al.*, 2012) and cardiac output (Norsk *et al.*, 2006), and may increase ICP (Keil *et al.*, 1992) or change intraocular pressure (Draeger *et al.*, 1995), although the magnitudes of these changes are unknown. As with many physiological adaptations, there is likely significant variability across astronauts in the type and volume of the fluid shift experienced during spaceflight (Montgomery, 1987), as well as in subsequent ocular structural and functional changes.

The manifestation of VIIP symptoms has not been documented using spaceflight analogs such as bed rest and dry water immersion, making it difficult to study these phenomena in a well-controlled model. This inability to replicate VIIP symptoms on Earth suggests that differences in physiological responses may exist between bed rest and spaceflight that underlie development of VIIP. For example, the fluid shift that occurs during bed rest results in a Henry–Gauer diuresis, while mechanisms counteracting the fluid shift during spaceflight are far less clear (Leach *et al.*, 1996). Extracellular fluid and plasma volume decrease in weightlessness, but the cephalad fluid shift likely leads to an increase in intracellular and interstitial fluid volume (Leach *et al.*, 1996). Coupled with this cephalad fluid shift, a decrease in vascular oncotic pressure may lead to an increase in transcapillary filtration in the upper body (Parazynski *et al.*, 1991). Further, the lack of gravity-driven hydrostatic gradients surrounding blood vessels may increase permeability of the blood–brain barrier (Lakin *et al.*, 2007). Some have suggested that these microgravity-induced adaptations lead to cerebral venous stasis and elevated intracranial and intraocular pressure, which are a possible cause of disc edema, globe flattening, choroidal folds, and hyperopic shifts seen in some long-duration astronauts (Mader *et al.*, 2011). Additional spaceflight factors that have been hypothesized to contribute to VIIP include elevated ambient levels of carbon dioxide on ISS, use of onboard exercise devices such as the Advanced Resistive Exercise Device (ARED), increased radiation exposure, or some combination of these or other factors.

The current state of knowledge about fluid shift/distribution in microgravity is largely based on results from short-duration spaceflight without corresponding measures of intraocular or ICP. Although it was well known that Shuttle astronauts experienced transient vision disturbances with spaceflight, some as large as 1.75 diopters in magnitude, NASA only recently began to routinely perform fundoscopy, optical coherence tomography, visual acuity tests, ocular ultrasound, and ocular tonometry as medical requirements on all long-duration crewmembers. It is not yet clear why some astronauts are more susceptible to vision disturbances, or why some of these changes become permanent in some but not all astronauts. Of the 33 US astronauts who have flown long-duration missions, at least seven have permanent vision changes after spaceflight (Mader *et al.*, 2011). The purpose of one current ISS research protocol is to measure the cephalad fluid shift during long-duration spaceflight, measure the compartmentalization of fluid in and out of the vascular and cellular spaces, and test the hypothesis that a relationship exists between the cephalad and vascular fluid shift and transient and permanent changes in eye morphology and visual acuity.

3. Cephalad Fluid Shift

The direction and magnitude of the gravitational vector and the resulting hydrostatic gradients influence the distribution of fluids throughout the body. On Earth, standing up from a supine position poses a substantial challenge to the human cardiovascular system to maintain arterial pressure and cerebral perfusion. Due to the increase in the hydrostatic pressure gradient acting along the length of the body, venous volume increases by approximately 500 ml (Rowell, 1993). This redistribution of fluid from the central circulation is immediately detected by baroreceptors (pressure) and, in time, by volume (osmolarity) receptors, activating reflex responses to increase heart rate, contractility, and vascular resistance to maintain blood pressure. When astronauts enter the weightless environment of spaceflight, the opposite effect occurs and a cephalad fluid shift ensues in the absence of the hydrostatic pressure gradient (Thornton *et al.*, 1977; Kas'ian *et al.*, 1980; Moore and Thornton, 1987; Thornton *et al.*, 1987; Kirsch *et al.*, 1993).

Early in the US space program, the spaceflight-induced cephalad fluid shift was documented using anthropometric measures. Although the technique lacked the specificity to distinguish between changes in fluid shifts and tissue loss, anthropometric measures were easily obtained by astronauts and flight surgeons. Decreased thigh circumference measurements obtained in Skylab 2 and 3 astronauts suggested that these crewmembers experienced a significant fluid shift and muscle atrophy during the course of their missions, but more extensive measures were obtained during Skylab 4 (Thornton *et al.*, 1977). Based upon measurements taken every 3 cm along the leg and the arm, and around the neck, chest, abdomen, and hip, Skylab 4 astronauts experienced a loss in leg volume during spaceflight that occurred too rapidly to be explained by loss of fat or lean tissue and was consistent with a cephalic fluid shift. However, there was little to no change in arm volume in these subjects from before flight to during flight or from during flight to after flight. Using infrared photography, it appeared that lower limb veins were not enlarged, as they would have been with standing. In contrast, veins in the upper body, including the jugular, temple, and forehead veins, were distended (Thornton *et al.*, 1977), leading researchers at the time to conclude that intravascular fluid shifted to above heart level and to hypothesize that increased transmural pressure led to extravascular fluid accumulation and cephalad edema.

Anthropometric measurements of the thigh and calf also were obtained in 11 astronauts during and after five early Space Shuttle flights using stocking plethysmography (Moore and Thornton, 1987; Thornton *et al.*, 1987). Upon entry into microgravity leg volume decreased by 11.6%, likely because of a rapid shift in fluid volume to the upper body, which was supported by photographs of puffy faces (Fig. 1) and reports of nasal congestion and "full headedness". The total fluid shift was measured to be 2 L, 1 L from each leg. The majority of the fluid shift came from the thighs, not the calves, and occurred in the first 6–10 hours after entering microgravity before a subsequent slow decline or plateau of the fluid shift occurred. Similar to observations after Skylab missions, when measurements were repeated within 1.5 h of landing with the astronauts standing, leg volume was

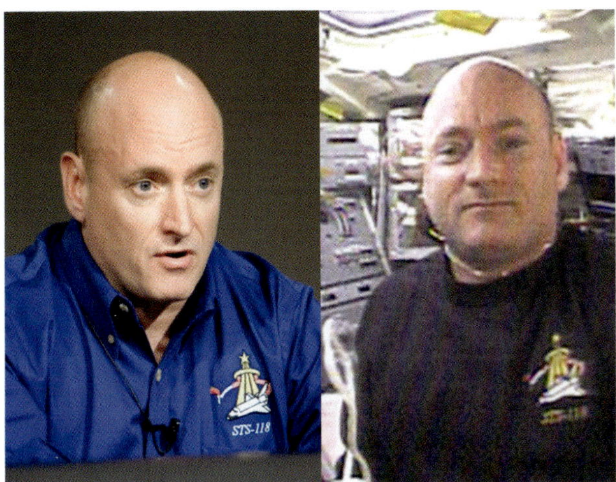

Figure 1. Commander Scott Kelly before and during Space Shuttle mission STS-118, demonstrating the characteristic facial "puffiness" that most astronauts experience as a result of the spaceflight-induced cephalad fluid shift.

decreased by only 4% on average, relative to before flight. The decreased volume upon landing was likely the combined result of lower plasma volume, decreased fat mass, and muscle atrophy. As in Skylab, one week after Shuttle landing, leg volume had recovered somewhat toward the preflight value; leg volume was 3% lower than before flight, at a time when plasma volume would have been recovered. Using a similar method, Kas'ian *et al.* measured leg volume changes on two cosmonauts during the 120-day Salyut-6 mission (Kas'ian *et al.*, 1980). They noted a decreased leg volume of 6%–7% within the first week of flight in both cosmonauts, which likely reflected the cephalad fluid shift and plasma volume loss. The continued decrease in leg volume continued through flight day 120, to an 18%–23% reduction in leg volume, presumably was due to muscle atrophy.

4. Intravascular Shift

One possible mechanism for changes in ICP is cerebral venous congestion secondary to the cephalad fluid shift and elevated cardiac filling pressure. During bed rest, the jugular vein becomes enlarged, while the femoral vein becomes smaller (Arbeille *et al.*, 2001), but after six months in space, veins from both the upper and lower body are distended by as much as 40% compared to supine rest measured before flight (Herault *et al.*, 2000; Arbeille *et al.*, 2001) (Fig. 2). These data highlight that despite the cephalad fluid shift induced by head–down tilt bed rest,

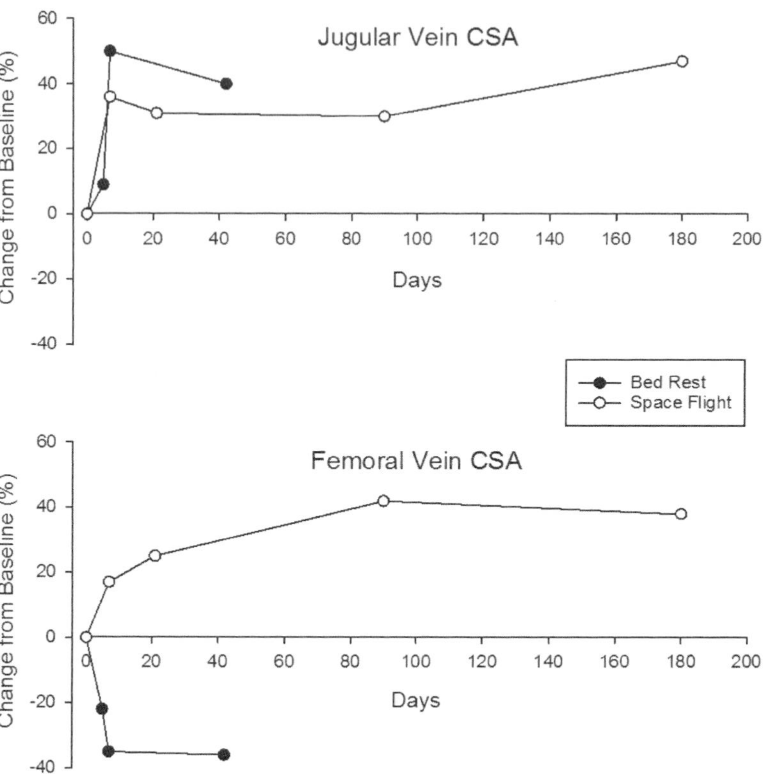

Figure 2.   Divergent responses in upper and lower body veins during spaceflight and bed rest. The jugular vein cross-section area (CSA) is distended in both real and simulated microgravity, while the femoral vein (CSA) is distended only in real microgravity (Redrawn from Arbeille *et al.*, 2001).

hydrostatic pressure tissue gradients still exist in bed rest, which may explain the divergence of femoral vein responses between spaceflight and bed rest studies (Arbeille *et al.*, 2001). Thus, it is important to appreciate that spaceflight causes a fluid shift unique to the microgravity environment that includes changes due to the removal of all hydrostatic gradients acting on all tissue.

5. Extravascular Shift

Parazynski and coworkers were the first to quantify all four Starling–Landis pressures during head-down tilt and the subsequent cephalad fluid shift. After 8 hours of 6° head-down tilt, facial capillary fluid pressure increased from 27.7 ± 1.5 mmHg to 33.9 ± 1.7 mmHg in seven men, whereas interstitial fluid pressure did not significantly change (Parazynski *et al.*, 1991). Although plasma oncotic pressure initially decreased, it returned to baseline by the end of 8 hours of bed rest, and subcutaneous and intramuscular colloid osmotic pressure in the face and neck did not change. These data suggested that an elevated net transcapillary pressure gradient in the head and neck is the reason for cephalic edema during bed rest and spaceflight and that capillaries above the heart may be more permeable to protein filtration than those below the heart, similar to the report by Leach *et al.* (1996). Interstitial pressure in the lower leg muscles and subcutaneous tissue decreased by 7.4 and 4.4 mmHg, respectively, after 8 hours of head down tilt (Hargens, 1983), leading to the hypothesis that lower leg vascular absorption decreases vascular oncotic pressure, and coupled with increased cephalic capillary pressure, results in filtration in the upper body. Several years later, this hypothesis was extended in a review article to suggest that the reduced tissue weight in microgravity results in lower interstitial fluid pressure, further shifting the Starling balance to net filtration during spaceflight (Hargens and Richardson, 2009).

Despite evidence for interstitial swelling in the forehead (Kirsch *et al.*, 1993) and many anecdotal reports of puffy faces, sinus congestion, and feeling of a full head during spaceflight, there currently are few data from spaceflight confirming filtration into the extravascular space in the head and neck. Using A-mode ultrasound, the spaceflight-induced fluid shift was quantified in one cosmonaut on the Mir '92 mission by measuring the interstitial thickness over the forehead and tibia before flight in the supine position, before flight in the head–down position, eight times during a seven–day flight, and after landing. Facial tissues swelled during the first three days of the mission, but may have been reduced by a lower body negative pressure session on day 4 of the mission. Tibial interstitial thickness was reduced by 20% and remained low for the duration of the flight and immediately upon landing. Similarly, we have observed decreases in lower body and increases in upper body interstitial thickness in subjects before and after 60 days of 6° head–down tilt bed rest (Platts *et al.*, 2009; Summers *et al.*, 2010). Changes in interstitial thickness during head-down tilt develop rapidly within the first 24 hours, especially when subjects experience a greater tilt angle (Diridollou *et al.*, 2000).

Spaceflight may further exacerbate cephalad edema by changing the permeability of the microvasculature to water. Lakin *et al.* suggested that cerebral fluid filtration increases if the space between endothelial cells of the cerebral blood vessels increases (Lakin *et al.*, 2007). This would be possible in spaceflight if the gravity-induced hydrostatic pressure gradients in the cerebral interstitium are removed. Long-duration bed rest increases the capacity for filtering fluid in the microvasculature (Christ *et al.*, 2001), and this may be enhanced in the presence of free oxygen radicals and activated leukocytes, such as during exposure to spaceflight radiation. Thus, radiation exposure during spaceflight may also alter endothelial protein structure, shrinking cells and increasing permeability between cell junctions. The synergistic effects of the spaceflight environment may lead to an increased extravascular fluid shift, which may also explain why VIIP is not reproducible in Earth analogs.

6. Compartmentalization

It is well known that plasma volume decreases with spaceflight (Johnson *et al.*, 1977; Buckey *et al.*, 1996b; Leach *et al.*, 1996; Waters *et al.*, 2002), although the exact mechanism of this plasma volume loss is not completely understood. Red blood cell mass also decreases during spaceflight (Johnson *et al.*, 1977; Udden *et al.*, 1995; Alfrey *et al.*, 1996), likely as a reflex response to hemoconcentration after plasma volume loss. Leach *et al.* initially reported that total body water was decreased after short-duration Shuttle flights (Leach *et al.*, 1991), but suggested that this may have been exaggerated by a reduction in water intake induced by space motion sickness. Several years later, plasma volume, total body water, and extra- and intracellular fluid volumes were reported in seven astronauts on NASA's dedicated Space and Life Sciences (SLS) missions, SLS-1 and SLS-2. Plasma and extracellular fluid volume decreased, while that of total body water was unchanged, suggesting that intracellular fluid volume increased (Leach *et al.*, 1996). The reduction in extracellular fluid volume occurred despite no report of natriuresis or diuresis, similar to previous results (Drummer *et al.*, 1993). It is generally accepted that the cause of reduced plasma volume during spaceflight is not diuresis, but rather a combination of decreased water balance (i.e., reduced intake) (Norsk, 2005) and extravasation into intracellular and interstitial compartments (Leach *et al.*, 1991). SLS crewmembers had a negative water balance and reduced total circulating protein (Leach *et al.*, 1996), indicating that a rapid filtration of protein out of the vascular space was responsible for the early plasma volume loss, and that a negative water balance perpetuates this relative hypovolemia. Intravenous infusion of isotonic saline attenuated diuresis during spaceflight compared to bed rest, suggesting the negative water balance in spaceflight may be more pronounced than what occurs during bed rest (Norsk, 2000). Similarly, oral water load during a Mir mission resulted in an attenuated diuresis compared to the results of an identical oral water load in bed rest (Christensen *et al.*, 2001). Studies currently underway on ISS will provide further insight into fluid compartmentalization in long-duration crewmembers.

7. Central Venous Pressure

Early in the Space Shuttle era, the spaceflight-induced cephalad fluid shift was assumed to cause an increase in central venous pressure (CVP), but measurements in 14 subjects while they were seated upright during parabolic flight suggested that only a slight (1.8 mmHg) increase in CVP occurs during short periods of weightlessness (Norsk *et al.*, 1987). Conversely, CVP decreased from 6.5 ± 1.3 to 5.0 ± 1.3 mmHg during parabolic flight in seven supine subjects (Foldager *et al.*, 1996), highlighting the need to clearly define whether the baseline position is seated upright or supine. When measured in one Spacelab D-2 astronaut, CVP did not change in microgravity compared to preflight measures. Peripheral venous pressure also was measured in four Spacelab 1 astronauts and assumed to be reflective of central venous pressure (Kirsch *et al.*, 1984). All four crewmembers were reported to have reductions in venous pressure, although data for only two of the astronauts were reported. One astronaut had a reduction in CVP of 2.2 and 5.1 mmHg from before flight to the first and sixth days of flight, respectively, while the second astronaut had a reduction of 6.4 and 6.0 mmHg, respectively (Kirsch *et al.*, 1984). These findings were supported by data from SLS-1, in which CVP was measured directly with a catheter placed at the level of the superior vena cava in one subject. CVP was measured before launch while the subject was seated and again while in the launch position in the orbiter, during launch, and during the initial moments upon reaching microgravity. CVP increased from 5–6 cm H_2O while seated to 10–12 cm H_2O while in the launch position, and further increased during the launch to 15–17 cm H_2O, presumably from the G_x forces, before decreasing to 0 to -3 cm H_2O upon entering microgravity. This reduction was rapid, occurring during the first minute of microgravity, and remained within 1–2 cm H_2O of this level until the catheter was removed (Buckey et al. 1993). This was one of the first reports to refute the hypothesis that CVP increased with the cephalad fluid shift experienced in microgravity. Interestingly, heart size in this astronaut increased at the same time that CVP decreased (Buckey *et al.*, 1993). Similar results were reported in two SLS-2 crewmembers (Buckey *et al.*, 1996a). Together, mean CVP (two SLS-2 crewmembers and one SLS-1 crewmember) increased from 8.4 cm H_2O before flight to 15 cm H_2O in the launch position, and fell to 2.5 cm H_2O after 10 minutes in microgravity. Despite this reduction in CVP, cardiac filling increased, suggesting that effective filling pressure was elevated because the pressure applied from the lungs and abdominal organs was reduced in microgravity.

Although direct CVP has been measured during the first days of spaceflight, CVP has never been measured during long-duration spaceflight. The long-term effects of spaceflight on CVP are unknown, and it is possible that a phenotype exists in which elevated CVP contributes to venous congestion, preventing drainage from the head. Studies currently underway in long-duration crewmembers are utilizing noninvasive technology to estimate peripheral venous pressure as a surrogate of CVP (Thalhammer *et al.*, 2007) and to correlate changes in venous pressure with ICP derived from LP or noninvasive measures.

8. Cranial Venous Drainage

In normal gravity, cranial venous blood drains primarily through the internal jugular and the vertebral veins in a posture-dependent manner (Alperin *et al.*, 2005). MRI studies suggest that over 70% of cerebral venous drainage occurs through the internal jugular veins in supine subjects. However, when seated upright, drainage through the internal jugular veins decreases to ~40%, with the remainder draining through secondary venous pathways (e.g., epidural deep cerebral and vertebral veins). Unfortunately, that study did not separate the contribution of vertebral vein outflow from the other secondary pathways. Similar data obtained in our laboratory using standard ultrasound techniques confirms a posture-dependent change in venous dynamics. We have observed a progressive increase in internal jugular cross-sectional area when tilting test subjects from 30° head up to 20° head down (Fig. 3). Additionally, a significant increase in internal jugular pressure occurs with head-down tilt (Fig. 4) (Martin *et al.*, 2015), as measured with a novel noninvasive device (Thalhammer *et al.*, 2007). Taken together, these results suggest that the cephalad fluid shift induced by head-down tilt might contribute to venous congestion in the upper body, which might inhibit cranial venous drainage. The relative shift in cranial venous drainage from vertebral veins when a person is upright to drainage from the internal jugular veins when a person is supine implies an open or complex communication between intracranial outflow vessels (Ruíz *et al.*, 2002). Additional research should be focused on defining this relationship, as alterations

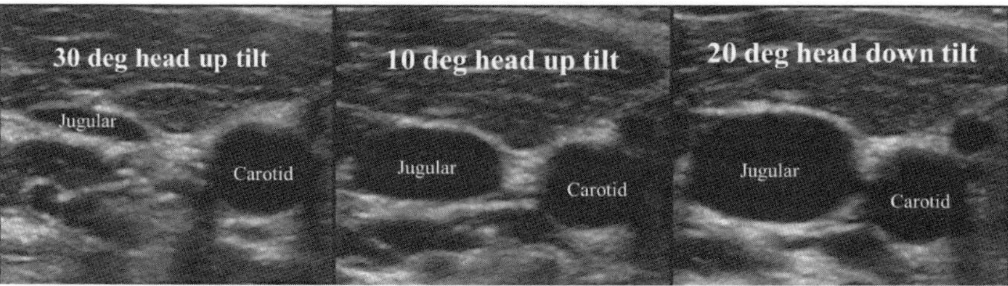

Figure 3. Jugular venous area progressively increases from head-up tilt through head-down tilt.

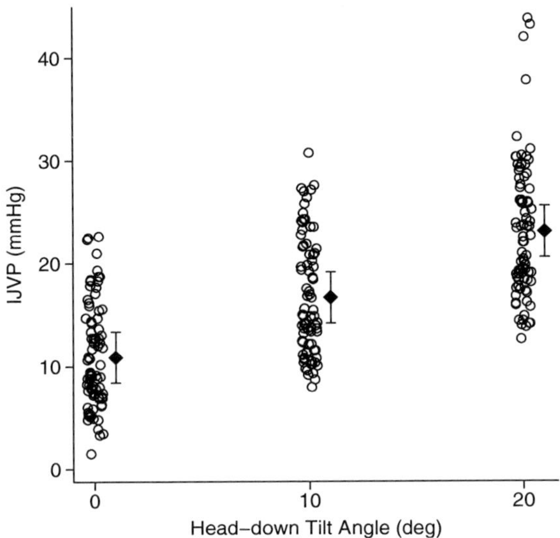

Figure 4. Noninvasive internal jugular venous pressure (IJVP) increases as head-down tilt angle increases (Martin *et al.*, 2015). Individual values are displayed as open circles, and mean values at each tilt angle are shown as the solid diamonds.

in vertebral vein blood flow are thought by some to play an important role in neurodegenerative diseases such as multiple sclerosis (Zamboni *et al.*, 2009) and could be important for our understanding of spaceflight-induced changes in ICP.

9. Intracranial Pressure and Cerebral Autoregulation

LP opening pressure provides a direct measure of cerebral spinal fluid pressure and likely reflects ICP. No direct measures of ICP have been conducted in humans during spaceflight, but during the first 20 hours of spaceflight, two Macaque monkeys demonstrated a small increase in ICP that remained within the physiologic range (Krotov *et al.*, 1994). Following prolonged spaceflight, four of five astronauts reporting VIIP symptoms had LP opening pressures ranging from 21 to 29 cm H_2O, suggesting mildly elevated ICP (normal: 10–20 cm H_2O) (Mader *et al.*, 2011). However, without ICP measures during spaceflight in astronauts, it is unknown if postflight LP measures reflect ICP in microgravity, particularly when additional spaceflight environmental factors may alter cerebrovascular reactivity and blood flow.

An elevated ICP implies that an imbalance in cerebral fluid volume regulation exists, resulting in a net inflow. Studies investigating impaired venous drainage due to the cephalad fluid shift are currently underway, but additional mechanisms that increase cerebral blood flow also might contribute to changes in cerebral volume regulation during spaceflight. Unique to the cerebral circulation, cerebral autoregulation describes the local responses of cerebral vasculature to protect a constant cerebral blood flow across a wide range of cerebral perfusion pressures, classically described to range from 60 to 150 mmHg (Lassen, 1959). However, it is possible that autoregulation operates over a more narrow plateau than previously believed (Tan, 2012), which might be further narrowed by the spaceflight environment, and therefore might be problematic in the face of a weightlessness–induced increase in cerebral arterial pressure of 20–30 mmHg (Watenpaugh and Hargens, 1996).

Just as increasing mean arterial pressure can increase cerebral blood flow (Lucas *et al.*, 2010), the cephalad fluid shift that occurs in microgravity also may increase cerebral blood flow. Subjects undergoing 30° head-down tilt for 45 minutes who had a net inflow of cerebral blood volume through their common carotid, internal carotid, and vertebral arteries had significantly greater symptoms of congestion and full-headedness than subjects who had a net outflow of cerebral blood volume, suggesting that variability in cerebral blood flow control exists between subjects (Hu *et al.*, 1999). During short periods of weightlessness induced by parabolic flight, changes in the middle cerebral artery (MCA) blood flow velocity waveform in four human subjects led authors to suggest there was an increase in ICP (Bondar *et al.*, 1990). However, data collected in unanesthetized rabbits during parabolic flight suggest that the initial increase in cerebral artery blood flow velocity during the onset of weightlessness returns to control levels within 8 seconds (Florence *et al.*, 1998).

In contrast, animals exposed to short-duration spaceflight have developed changes in cerebral vasculature that may impair cerebral autoregulation. Basilar arteries from mice flown for 13 days on a Space Shuttle showed less myogenic vasoconstriction, greater vascular distensibility, and were less stiff compared to ground-based controls animals, suggestive of lower cerebrovascular resistance and increased blood flow following short-duration spaceflight (Taylor *et al.*, 2013). Interestingly, these results contradicted data from animals undergoing tail suspension for a similar duration which suggested that cerebrovascular vasoconstriction and cerebral blood flow decreased following hindlimb unloading (Geary *et al.*, 1998; Wilkerson *et al.*, 2002; Wilkerson *et al.*, 2005). This difference between results from spaceflight and a spaceflight analog (tail suspension) further supports the idea that the physiologic changes associated with spaceflight that contribute to VIIP development are unique and may differ fundamentally from those observed in ground-based analogs. Longer exposures to spaceflight may induce cerebrovascular alterations that differ from shorter durations. Basilar arteries from mice flown for 30 days on a Bion-M1 biosatellite were found to have both impaired vasoconstriction and impaired vasodilation, which could limit the range of vascular responsiveness to changes in perfusion pressure (Sofronova *et al.*, 2014). However, species differences must also be considered when interpreting animal data for changes that may occur in humans.

Human studies of up to 42 days of bed rest or up to six months of spaceflight show little change in common carotid or MCA blood flow, suggesting that spaceflight does not change cerebral vascular control (Arbeille *et al.*, 2001). Impairment in cerebral autoregulation was initially investigated as an explanation for orthostatic intolerance following the Neurolab (STS-90) Space Shuttle mission. Measures of cerebral blood flow velocity with beat-to-beat changes in arterial pressure in four subjects after 16 days in space revealed that static autoregulation was not impaired and dynamic regulation (changes occurring during stress) was actually improved (Iwasaki *et al.*, 2007). However, none of these astronauts developed presyncope upon return to Earth, and a subsequent study suggested that only those with orthostatic intolerance demonstrated impaired cerebral autoregulation (Blaber *et al.*, 2011). Importantly, ambient environmental CO_2 was tightly controlled during flight on the Space Shuttle at <0.1% (Iwasaki *et al.*, 2007) and crewmembers did not perform resistance exercise; both of these factors have been hypothesized to contribute to VIIP in ISS astronauts.

Conversely, during long-duration spaceflight on ISS when ambient CO_2 was known to average $0.5 \pm 0.2\%$, with periodic localized spikes, especially during exercise (Law *et al.*, 2010), dynamic cerebral autoregulation was impaired (Zuj *et al.*, 2012). Whether individuals whose cerebral autoregulation was maintained or improved during short-duration spaceflight and who retained orthostatic tolerance were also protected from developing the VIIP syndrome is unknown. Combining the cerebral venous congestion that likely occurs due to loss of the hydrostatic fluid column and gravity-assisted drainage (Hu *et al.*, 1999) with poorer cerebral autoregulation due to elevated CO_2 levels (Panerai, 1998) could theoretically increase susceptibility to overperfusion of cerebral vasculature and increase the risk for elevated ICP.

10. Vascular Compliance and Remodeling

Clearly, any changes in vascular function and structure will contribute to the changes in blood flow and pressures transmitted into the upper body and head during the spaceflight-induced fluid shift. Consequently, vascular adaptations have the potential to influence the development of VIIP. While the arterial system has been well studied, less is known about venous function and compliance, particularly during and after real and simulated microgravity. It has been postulated that changes in vascular compliance in the head and neck region coupled with the cephalad fluid shift contributes to the VIIP syndrome experienced by some astronauts during and after long-duration spaceflight.

Data from animal studies (Zhang, 2001) show that arteries in the lower body and upper body differentially remodel in response to hindlimb unloading (Fig. 5); wall thickness decreases in lower body arteries while wall thickness increases in arteries of the upper body and head. We have reported similar results in normal test subjects after bed rest (Platts *et al.*, 2009); wall thickness decreased in the anterior tibial arteries in the leg, while there was no change in brachial arteries in the arm. Also, aortic compliance decreases in astronauts after spaceflight and in rodents undergoing hindlimb suspension (Tuday *et al.*, 2007). Especially interesting is that only the thoracic aorta was affected, suggesting a segmental vascular change similar to that reported in humans during bed rest (Platts *et al.*, 2009) and in rats (Zhang, 2001) after hindlimb unloading. Vascular structure and function have been studied in the arm and other vascular beds in bed rest and have shown equivocal results (Westby *et al.*, 2012). This is likely because commonly studied vessels in the arm (brachial artery and radial arteries) are close to heart level and see little or no change in hydrostatic pressure during simulated or actual micro-

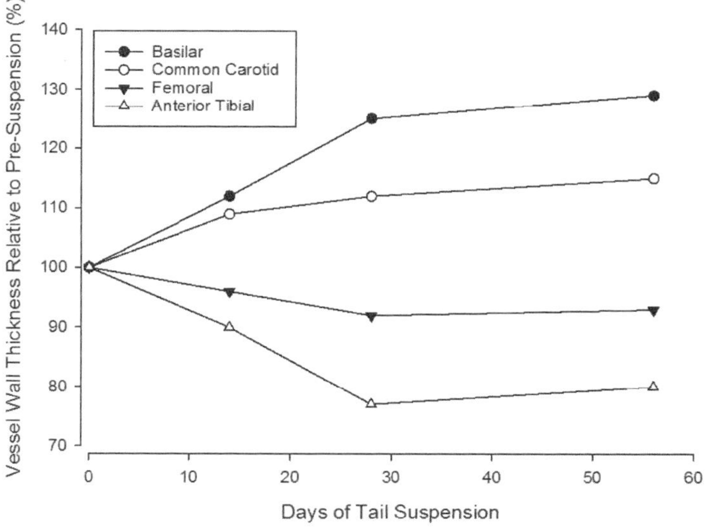

Figure 5. Changes in vessel wall thickness in response to hindlimb unloading (tail suspension). Arteries in the lower body (femoral, anterior tibial) become thinner while vessels in the upper body (basilar, common carotid) become thicker. (Redrawn from Zhang, 2001).

gravity. What remains unknown is whether remodeling also occurs in the veins and/or whether venous compliance is altered. It is possible that similar differential remodeling relative to anatomical location may occur in the venous system of astronauts in response to spaceflight.

While vascular remodeling may occur during spaceflight, astronauts may be predisposed to VIIP symptoms even before spaceflight. It is well documented that arterial stiffness increases (Vaitkevicius *et al.*, 1993; Mitchell *et al.*, 2004) and limb compliance decreases with age (Monahan *et al.*, 2001). For instance, hemodynamic characteristics of the internal jugular veins are altered in older adults (Chung *et al.*, 2010). In addition to an increased lumen area, blood flow velocity and total volume in the veins are lower, suggesting that cerebral blood outflow is impaired with aging. Impedance of outflow can result in cerebral edema, as it affects the balance between cerebral perfusion pressure and cerebral blood flow. A similar age–related decrease in jugular outflow has been shown by others (Stoquart-ElSankari *et al.*, 2007), but this also was accompanied by a decrease in arterial cerebral inflow such that a linear decline in total cerebral blood flow of ~4 ml/min per year occurred in an older subject population. With aging, the cerebrovasculature and surrounding tissues likely adapt to the reduced flow through a remodeling process (Fotenos *et al.*, 2008). One might speculate that an increase in cerebral blood flow, as might be experienced in older astronauts during spaceflight, could significantly overload the "new" baseline state causing an increase in ICP by altering cerebral perfusion pressure. However, no cerebral or neck venous compliance studies have been documented in Earth-bound subjects to demonstrate changes due to aging and none have been conducted in simulated or real microgravity.

Additionally, astronauts with a history of high-*g* exposures may have lower vascular compliance before spaceflight. Training in high-performance jet aircraft has been postulated for many years to affect tolerance to subsequent hypotensive challenges (Fritsch-Yelle *et al.*, 1996; Lee *et al.*, 1999) and has been studied in different contexts (Convertino, 1998). A number of studies have demonstrated the positive influence of high-*g* training on tolerance to orthostatic challenges (Convertino, 1998; Convertino *et al.*, 1998; Newman *et al.*, 1998) in those who were acutely or chronically trained. Mechanisms to explain an increased tolerance to hypotensive challenges in *g*-trained subjects have included higher blood volumes, increased baroreflex sensitivity, decreased venous pooling in the legs, improved venous return and maintenance of stroke volume, and increased end–organ responsiveness to sympathetic stimulation. Because of the focus of these studies was orthostatic hypotension, changes in vascular compliance in the upper body (head and neck) appear not to have been fully explored as a contributing factor to VIIP. Given that many in the US astronaut corps previously were high-performance jet aircraft pilots, participating in *g*-training during their military careers and that most maintained proficiencies through T-38 training, perhaps *g*-training results in functional and structural changes in the upper body vasculature. While it is likely that some of these adaptations would be lost while not participating in *g*-training, operating at a lower level of compliance may persist in this population of high-performance aircraft pilots and perhaps predispose them to development of the VIIP symptoms. This has yet to be fully explored in the literature.

11. Carbon Dioxide

Carbon dioxide is a potent vasodilator, and ambient CO_2 levels are 10- to 20-fold higher on ISS than on Earth, with pockets of CO_2 reported to be even higher (Law *et al.*, 2014; Law *et al.* 2010). Due in part to poor air convection, variability in CO_2 production from up to six ISS crew members, and limitations of currently available CO_2 removal hardware, ambient CO_2 levels on the ISS are ~3.5 mm Hg, or ~0.5% (Law *et al.*, 2014). Increasing the inspired CO_2 elevates the partial pressure of CO_2 (PCO_2) in arterial blood, leading to a complex interplay between cerebrovascular and ventilatory responses designed to acutely maintain central pH. Hypercapnia (high blood CO_2 levels) decreases central pH and stimulates central chemoreceptors to increase ventilation while increased cerebral blood flow "washes out" CO_2 from the brain to prevent even greater fluctuations in ventilation (Ainslie and Duffin, 2009). Wide individual variability in ventilatory and cerebrovascular sensitivity to elevated CO_2 is known to occur and may help predict or explain the variability in development of VIIP symptoms during spaceflight. For example, individuals with a strong ventilatory response to CO_2 may successfully "blow off" CO_2 and minimize elevations in arterial PCO_2, cerebral vasodilation, elevated cerebral blood flow, and ultimately changes in ICP. Alternatively, individuals with greater cerebrovascular sensitivity to CO_2 may increase cerebral vasodilation during exposure to elevated levels of CO_2 and display larger increases in cerebral blood flow than those with a blunted cerebrovascular response. While these specific hypotheses have not been tested during spaceflight, hypercapnia has been hypothesized to be a factor contributing to changes in ICP and the development of VIIP.

Negative sequelae normally associated with hypercapnia include headache, blurred vision, lethargy, irritability, and neurocognitive deficits (Law *et al.*, 2010). These symptoms typically manifest in environments with significantly higher CO_2 levels than the 24-hour averages reported on ISS, but crewmembers may experience spikes in CO_2 levels, especially during exercise or during work in confined spaces with poor air circulation, which may not be captured by wall-mounted detectors. Severe headaches have been reported by ISS astronauts 46 times

(Law *et al.*, 2014), and recent attempts to keep ambient CO_2 lower have reduced headache incidence. Because astronauts have reported symptoms related to CO_2 toxicity at levels lower than terrestrial studies predict, changes in CO_2 sensitivity during spaceflight may be occurring (Chiquet *et al.*, 2003).

Hypercapnic cerebrovascular reactivity has been extensively studied on Earth using transcranial Doppler ultrasound (Ainslie and Duffin, 2009; Willie *et al.*, 2011). Cerebral blood flow is estimated to increase 3%–4% per mm Hg increase in arterial PCO_2 (Brugniaux *et al.*, 2007). Relative to a baseline arterial PCO_2 of 40 mmHg, an iso–oxic step increase of arterial PCO_2 to 50 mm Hg increased MCA and posterior cerebral artery blood flow velocity, as well as vertebral artery and internal carotid artery blood flow, despite no increase in mean arterial pressure, indicating a direct effect of CO_2 on blood flow through these vessels (Willie *et al.*, 2012). However, hypercapnic cerebrovascular reactivity is not the same in all vessels. Cerebrovascular reactivity to hypercapnia is ~25% greater in the internal carotid artery and vertebral artery than in the MCA (Willie *et al.*, 2012), suggesting the large intracranial conducting arteries may also vasodilate in response to hypercapnia.

In addition to individual variability in the ventilatory response to CO_2 and resulting changes in arterial PCO_2, intersubject variability in cerebrovascular reactivity to CO_2 also may contribute to variable degrees of cerebral perfusion. Four subjects exposed to 0.7% and 1.2% CO_2 for 23 days had an increase in MCA blood flow velocity during the first few days of CO_2 exposure, after which the velocity decreased, yet it remained elevated relative to pre–exposure levels (Sliwka *et al.*, 1998). Because only four subjects participated in this study, it is unclear whether the increasing *variability* in cerebral blood flow velocity that occurred throughout the 23-day exposure resulted from differences in cerebrovascular reactivity or reflected the variability in resulting arterial PCO_2. Unexpectedly, cerebral blood flow velocity remained elevated for up to five days after the subjects returned to ambient air, suggesting that a chronic adaptation to increased CO_2 had in fact occurred. Despite a reduction in cerebrovascular reactivity to CO_2 *after* long-duration spaceflight (Zuj *et al.*, 2012), no measures of CO_2 sensitivity have been conducted *during* prolonged spaceflight when additional factors may be necessary to impair cerebral autoregulation and contribute to enhanced cerebral vasodilation.

If hypercapnia narrows the plateau of effective autoregulation (Meng and Gelb, 2015), the combination of increased cerebral perfusion pressure from the fluid shift of microgravity, a hypercapnic environment, and possible venous congestion may exceed autoregulatory limits and result in increased cerebral blood volume. Considering that a direct connection exists between the optic nerve sheath and cerebrospinal fluid, this combination of factors may cause the ocular structural changes indicative of VIIP, which have not developed in spaceflight analogs that do not incorporate the suite of environmental factors that may be necessary to overwhelm the system. Additionally, it is unknown whether cerebrovascular reactivity to CO_2 is altered with prolonged microgravity exposure such that cerebrovascular responses early in flight differ from responses late in flight. These hypotheses related to CO_2 and VIIP suggest that duration of spaceflight, degree of CO_2 exposure, and individual variability in CO_2 sensitivity could all contribute to variable ventilatory and cerebrovascular responses to CO_2 that could be expected during long-duration spaceflight.

12. Exercise

Another factor that has been hypothesized to contribute to elevated ICP and VIIP during spaceflight is repeated performance of heavy-load resistance exercise (Marshall-Bowman *et al.*, 2013). Intraocular pressure increases during resistance exercise on Earth (Vieira *et al.*, 2006), yet no measures of IOP or ICP have been made during or immediately after use of the ARED on ISS. Thus, it is unknown whether use of the ARED on ISS contributes to acute or prolonged changes in cerebral blood flow. Resistance exercise increases IOP, which is even greater during breath hold (Vieira *et al.*, 2006), a maneuver often employed during resistive exercise. With the increased production of CO_2 during exercise likely causing local ambient CO_2 to rise, astronauts may face enhanced cerebral vasodilation, combined with the cephalad fluid shift in microgravity, and periodic increases in cerebral perfusion during resistive exercise on ISS. Ground-based studies are currently underway to investigate the combined effects of the cephalad fluid shift with head-down tilt and resistance or aerobic exercise on changes in IOP and cerebral blood flow.

13. Intraocular Pressure

Changes in the amount and direction of the gravity vector, like the cephalad fluid shift, affect intraocular pressure (IOP). Data from short-duration bed rest studies suggest there is a transient elevation of IOP upon entering the head-down position, but this resolves as the body adapts to the altered hydrostatic pressures. The transition from the upright or seated position to the supine posture increases IOP by ~2 mmHg in healthy subjects within the first 1 min, and IOP remains relatively stable at this level for at least 10 min (Chiquet *et al.*, 2003). An increase in IOP when moving from standing to supine is consistently observed (Liu *et al.*, 2002;

Liu *et al.*, 1998; Wilson *et al.*, 1993), and IOP is further elevated in the head-down posture as the hydrostatic gradients are reversed compared to standing or sitting. In an extreme illustration, IOP almost triples when healthy volunteers move from the +90° head-up position (~12 mmHg) to -90° head-down position (~34 mmHg) (Weinreb *et al.*, 1984; Friberg and Weinreb, 1985; Draeger and Hanke, 1986). IOP increases from head-up to the supine posture, and the elevation in IOP is more dramatic once subjects progress beyond the supine posture to head-down positions. Not surprisingly, the elevated IOP is accompanied by, and is inversely related to changes in leg arterial pressures (Draeger and Hanke, 1986; Linder *et al.*, 1988).

Clearly, spaceflight is not simulated by such extreme postures as inversion, and therefore moderate head-down positions may provide more representative indications of how IOP might be expected to change with spaceflight. During 90 min of 10° head-down tilt there is an immediate increase in IOP with head-down tilt, which reaches a maximum (~24 mmHg) after 15 min (Draeger and Hanke, 1986). This rapid increase in IOP might be representative of an elevated IOP that would occur upon initial entry into weightlessness, as has been observed during brief periods of microgravity in parabolic flight (Mader *et al.*, 1993). Similarly, IOP, blood pressure, and ocular perfusion pressure are elevated upon the assumption of 7° head-down tilt and remain elevated for at least 90 min (Kergoat and Lovasik, 2005). These changes decrease choroidal pulsatile ocular blood flow and may have the potential to affect inflight visual performance. The wide range of responses to head-down tilt observed in test subjects highlights the individual variability of the response to the posture-induced cephalic fluid shift. Similarly, some but not all astronauts develop symptoms consistent with visual functional and structural changes (Mader *et al.*, 2011).

While acute changes in posture and the resulting influence on fluid shifts and IOP are not unexpected, the more chronic effects of head-down bed rest are perhaps more relevant to changes experienced by astronauts during long-duration spaceflight. Data from short-duration bed rest studies suggest that an immediate elevation of IOP occurs in the head-down position but this is reduced over the course of several days. IOP increased from seated rest to 10° head-down tilt in nine men at the start of bed rest and remained at this level for 48 hours (Mader *et al.*, 1990; Frey *et al.*, 1993). In a slightly longer bed rest study with eight women, IOP measured on the fifth and seventh days of 6° head-down tilt was significantly less than the IOP in the supine position before bed rest (Chiquet *et al.*, 2003). More recently, 16 healthy subjects, including four women, completed 14 days of 6° head-down tilt bed rest in which IOP was measured using Goldmann applanation tonometry and a handheld tonometer. Measurements were made with subjects in the seated upright position before and 3 days after bed rest and while subjects rolled onto their side during bed rest to maintain the head–down tilt position. IOP using Goldmann applanation tonometry was not significantly different after bed rest (Taibbi *et al.*, 2014). However, IOP increased early in bed rest and stabilized by day 10, similar to results from previous studies. Interestingly, the group IOP average may have masked individual variability, as three subjects had lower IOP after bed rest and two subjects had increases in IOP throughout bed rest.

In a longer bed rest study, 16 healthy subjects were studied before, during, and after 70 days of bed rest (Drozdova and Nesterenko, 1970). After 45 days, IOP reportedly decreased by 3 mmHg from a prestudy level of 20 mmHg, although how the measurement was conducted and the individual variability were not stated. The authors failed to indicate the timing of other ophthalmic examinations relative to the study timeline, but they reported that changes in visual function appeared to be coupled with structural changes within the eye. The optic disk faded and the temporal borders were indistinct, and the veins and arteries of the eye appeared to be enlarged. However, visual function and structural changes recovered upon resuming normal upright activities (Drozdova and Nesterenko, 1970). Visual acuity and the size of the visual field recovered to some extent but not fully to prestudy levels. Because no follow–up examinations were completed beyond 20 days post–bed rest, it is unclear whether the observed changes in vision and ocular structure were long lasting or permanent. While it is difficult to correlate these changes with spaceflight–induced alterations in vision with any certainty, it is relevant to note that vision and ocular structural changes among long-duration astronauts have not resolved completely in some crewmembers after long-duration spaceflight.

Only one other study has examined the effects of longer bed rest on ocular structure and function, and no changes in visual function were reported in any of the 10 subjects who participated in 35 days of horizontal bed rest (Mekjavic *et al.*, 2002). Unfortunately, IOP changes were not reported for this protocol, despite an indication that IOP was measured. Care should be taken when interpreting these results relative to other studies because the measurements were not made until the second or third day after bed rest was completed, and bed rest was conducted in the horizontal position, which acute studies have suggested does not have as dramatic an effect as head–down tilt bed rest.

The well-recognized diuresis secondary to head–down tilt might modify or attenuate IOP during the course of bed rest, although the continued hydrostatic gradient may result in filling of the choroidal vessels and increase episcleral pressures (Draeger and Hanke, 1986). It would be premature to assume that changes in IOP are not influenced by vascular adaptations during prolonged head–down tilt bed rest (Zhang, 2013). The contribution of the hydrostatic pressure gradient to the increase in IOP during bed rest is supported by the observation that IOP decreased during lower body negative pressure used to reverse the cephalad fluid shift and was restored when the decompression of the lower body was released (Draeger and Hanke, 1986). Overall, any change in IOP detected during or after bed rest falls within normal ranges, and a link between IOP and ocular structural changes in VIIP remains to be established. Further, no bed rest study that has attempted to study ocular changes in bed rest has included exercise or an elevated ambient carbon dioxide atmosphere, which are hypothesized to contribute to VIIP in spaceflight. To date, no corresponding long-term spaceflight data are available to confirm whether these observations in bed rest can be used to better understand the VIIP etiology and develop appropriate countermeasures. However, if a reduction in IOP does occur during spaceflight, it may represent the development of ocular hypotony, which Mader *et al.* note has been recognized to result in optic disk edema, global flattening, choroidal folds, and hyperopic shifts of similar magnitude to those observed in astronauts (Mader *et al.*, 2011).

14. Ocular Blood Flow

A hypothesis for the ocular structural and functional changes that characterize VIIP that has received less attention is that ocular blood flow regulation is altered by spaceflight. The anterior portion of the retina receives blood flow from the retinal artery while the posterior avascular layers are supplied through diffusion from the choroid. It is generally believed that retinal, but not choroidal, blood flow exhibits autoregulation similar to the cerebral circulation, which helps maintain constant flow across a range of perfusion pressures (Bill and Nilsson, 1985). Retinal blood vessel caliber decreased in response to HDT (Mader *et al.*, 1990; Frey *et al.*, 1993), suggesting that autoregulation maintained retinal perfusion in the face of the cephalad fluid shift (Mader *et al.*, 1990), and this was supported by fundus images during parabolic flight (Mader *et al.*, 1993). However, choroidal blood flow appears passive to changes in posture (Kaeser *et al.*, 2005; Longo *et al.*, 2004; Xu *et al.*, 2010) and increased during short periods of microgravity in parabolic flight. Furthermore, circulating factors may differentially affect these vascular beds, contributing to over- or underperfusion. Retinal blood flow, but not choroidal blood flow, appears to be vasoactively sensitive to changes in arterial CO_2 levels (Wang *et al.*, 2008), but whether the mild hypercapnic environment of ISS is sufficient to induce hyperperfusion of the retina and contribute to the VIIP syndrome is unknown. Conversely, histamine increases choroidal but not retinal blood flow (Resch *et al.*, 2005) and is known to contribute to postexercise vasodilation (Halliwill *et al.*, 2013). The role of exercise during spaceflight and changing ocular blood flow require further investigation.

15. Conclusion

That the cephalad fluid shift, which all astronauts experience, initiates the development of the VIIP syndrome remains a central hypothesis. Its influence on VIIP is likely mediated through the vasculature of the upper body, head, and eye. However, much work remains to be done to improve our understanding what roles of vascular compliance and remodeling, cerebrovascular autoregulation, intracranial and intraocular pressure, and potential modifiers, such as the elevated CO_2 environment and exercise countermeasures, play in the development of VIIP in the unique environment of space. Why not all astronauts develop the structural and functional changes that characterize VIIP remains unknown, and the variability in symptom presentation highlights the complexity of this syndrome. Determining which combination of factors leads to VIIP is further complicated by the fact that this is a spaceflight-only phenomenon that has not been replicated using ground-based analogs.

References

Ainslie, PN and J Duffin (2009). Integration of cerebrovascular CO_2 reactivity and chemoreflex control of breathing: mechanisms of regulation, measurement, and interpretation. *American Journal of Physiology–Regulatory, Integrative and Comparative Physiology*, 296, R1473–R1495.

Alfrey, CP, MM Udden, C Leach-Huntoon, T Driscoll and Pickett MH (1996). Control of red blood cell mass in spaceflight. *Journal of Applied Physiology*, 81, 98–104.

Alperin, N, SH Lee, A Sivaramakrishnan and SG Hushek (2005). Quantifying the effect of posture on intracranial physiology in humans by MRI flow studies. *Journal of Magnetic Resonance Imaging*, 22, 591–596.

Arbeille, P, G Fomina, J Roumy, I Alferova, N Tobal and S Herault (2001). Adaptation of the left heart, cerebral and femoral arteries, and jugular and femoral veins during short- and long-term head-down tilt and spaceflights. *European Journal of Applied Physiology*, 86, 157–168.

Arborelius, M Jr, UI Balldin, B Lila and CE Lundgren (1972). Regional lung function in man during immersion with the head above water. *Aerospace Medicine*, 43, 701–707.

Barr, Y, C Otto, R Brady, M Foy, S Mason, M Wear, W Tarver and M Van Baalen (2014). Differential VIIP incidence and severity among male and female astronauts. *Aviation Space Environmental Medicine*, 85, 237.

Bill, A and SF Nilsson (1985). Control of ocular blood flow. *Journal of Cardiovascular Pharmacology*, 7, (Suppl 3), S96–102.

Blaber, AP, N Goswami, RL Bondar and MS Kassam (2011). Impairment of cerebral blood flow regulation in astronauts with orthostatic intolerance after flight. *Stroke*, 42, 1844–1850.

Bondar, RL, F Stein, PJ Vaitkus, KW Johnston, LC Chadwick and JW Norris (1990). Transcranial doppler studies of flow velocity in middle cerebral artery in weightlessness. *Journal of Clinical Pharmacology*, 30, 390–395.

Brugniaux, JV, ANH Hodges, PJ Hanly and MJ Poulin (2007). Cerebrovascular responses to altitude. *Respiratory Physiology & Neurobiology*, 158, 212–223.

Buckey, JC Jr, FA Gaffney, LD Lane, BD Levine, DE Watenpaugh, SJ Wright, CW Jr Yancy, DM Meyer and CG Blomqvist (1996a). Central venous pressure in space. *Journal of Applied Physiology*, 81, 19–25.

Buckey, JC, FA Gaffney, LD Lane, BD Levine, DE Watenpaugh and CG Blomqvist (1993). Central venous pressure in space. *New England Journal of Medicine*, 328: 1853–1854.

Buckey, JC, LD Lane, BD Levine, DE Watenpaugh, SJ Wright, WE Moore, FA Gaffney and CG Blomqvist (1996b). Orthostatic intolerance after spaceflight. *Journal of Applied Physiology*, 81, 7–18.

Chiquet, C, M-A Custaud, AP Le Traon, C Millet, C Gharib and P Denis (2003). Changes in intraocular pressure during prolonged (7-day) head-down tilt bedrest. *Journal of Glaucoma*, 12, 204–208.

Christ, F, J Gamble, V Baranov, A Kotov, A Chouker, M Thiel, IB Gartside, CM Moser, J Abicht and K Messmer (2001). Changes in microvascular fluid filtration capacity during 120 days of 6 head-down tilt. *Journal of Applied Physiology*, 91, 2517–2522.

Christensen, NJ, C Drummer and P Norsk (2001). Renal and sympathoadrenal responses in space. *American Journal of Kidney Diseases Official Journal of the National Kidney Foundation*, 38, 679–683.

Chung, C-P, Y-J Lin, A-C Chao, S-J Lin, Y-Y Chen, Y-J Wang and H-H Hu (2010). Jugular venous hemodynamic changes with aging. *Ultrasound in Medicine & Biology*, 36, 1776–1782.

Convertino, VA (1998). High sustained +Gz acceleration: physiological adaptation to high-G tolerance. *Journal of Gravitational Physiology: A Journal of the International Society for Gravitational Physiology*, 5, P51–54.

Convertino, VA, LD Tripp, DA Ludwig, J Duff and TL Chelette (1998). Female exposure to high G: Chronic adaptations of cardiovascular functions. *Aviation Space and Environmental Medicine*, 69, 875–882.

Diridollou, S, AP-L Traon, A Maillet, F Bellossi, D Black, F Patat, JM Lagarde, M Berson and Y Gall (2000). Characterisation of gravity-induced facial skin oedema using biophysical measurement techniques. *Skin Research Technology*, 6, 118–127.

Draeger, J and K Hanke (1986). Postural variations of intraocular pressure — Preflight experiments for the D1-mission. *Ophthalmic Research*, 18, 55–60.

Draeger, J, R Schwartz, S Groenhoff and C Stern (1995). Self-tonometry under microgravity conditions. *Aviation Space and Environmental Medicine*, 66, 568–570.

Drozdova, NT and O Nesterenko (1970). State of the visual analyzer during hypodynamia. *Problems of Space Biology*, 13, 189–191.

Drummer, C, M Heer, RA Dressendörfer, CJ Strasburger and R Gerzer (1993). Reduced natriuresis during weightlessness. *Clinical Investigation*, 71, 678–686.

Florence, G, M Lemenn, S Desert, F Bourron, A Serra, R Bonnier, JP Blanquie, R Charbonné and J Seylaz (1998). Cerebral cortical blood flow in rabbits during parabolic flights (hypergravity and microgravity). *European Journal of Applied Physiology*, 77, 469–478.

Foldager, N, TA Andersen, FB Jessen, P Ellegaard, C Stadeager, R Videbaek and P Norsk (1996). Central venous pressure in humans during microgravity. *Journal of Applied Physiology*, 81, 408–412.

Fotenos, AF, MA Mintun, AZ Snyder, JC Morris and RL Buckner (2008). Brain volume decline in aging: Evidence for a relation between socioeconomic status, preclinical Alzheimer disease, and reserve. *Archives of Neurology*, 65, 113–120.

Frey MA, TH Mader, JP Bagian, JB Charles and RT Meehan (1993). Cerebral blood velocity and other cardiovascular responses to 2 days of head-down tilt. *Journal of Applied Physiology*, 74, 319–325.

Friberg TR and Weinreb RN (1985). Ocular manifestations of gravity inversion. *JAMA Journal of the American Medical Association*, 253, 1755–1757.

Fritsch-Yelle, JM, PA Whitson, RL Bondar and TE Brown (1996). Subnormal norepinephrine release relates to presyncope in astronauts after spaceflight. *Journal of Applied Physiology*, 81, 2134–41.

Geary, GG, DN Krause, RE Purdy and SP Duckles (1998). Simulated microgravity increases myogenic tone in rat cerebral arteries. *Journal of Applied Physiology*, 85, 1615–1621.

Halliwill, JR, TM Buck, AN Lacewell and SA Romero (2013). Postexercise hypotension and sustained postexercise vasodilatation: What happens after we exercise? *Experimental Physiology*, 98, 7–18.

Hargens, AR (1983). Fluid shifts in vascular and extravascular spaces during and after simulated weightlessness. *Medicine Science in Sports & Exercise*, 15, 421–427.

Hargens, AR and S Richardson (2009). Cardiovascular adaptations, fluid shifts, and countermeasures related to space flight. *Respiratory Physiology & Neurobiology*, 69, (Suppl 1), S30–33.

Herault, S, G Fomina, I Alferova, A Kotovskaya, V Poliakov and P Arbeille (2000). Cardiac, arterial and venous adaptation to weightlessness during 6-month MIR spaceflights with and without thigh cuffs (bracelets). *European Journal of Applied Physiology*, 81, 384–390.

Hu, Z, G Zhao, Z Xiao, X Chen, C Zhong and J Yang (1999). Different responses of cerebral vessels to -30 degrees head-down tilt in humans. *Aviation Space and Environmental Medicine*, 70, 674–680.

Iwasaki, K, BD Levine, R Zhang, JH Zuckerman, JA Pawelczyk, A Diedrich, AC Ertl, JF Cox, WH Cooke, CA Giller, CA Ray, LD Lane, JC Buckey Jr, FJ Baisch, DL Eckberg, D Robertson, I Biaggioni and CG Blomqvist (2007). Human cerebral autoregulation before, during and after spaceflight. *Journal of Physiology*, 579, 799–810.

Johnson, P, T Driscoll and A LeBlanc (1977). Blood volume changes. In: *Biomedical Results from Skylab*, Johnston RS and LF Dietlein (eds.). 235–241 pp. Washington, DC: Scientific and Technical Information Office, National Aeronautics and Space Administration.

Kaeser, P, S Orgül, C Zawinka, G Reinhard and J Flammer (2005). Influence of change in body position on choroidal blood flow in normal subjects. *British Journal of Ophthalmology*, 89, 1302–1305.

Kas'ian II, VA Talavrinov, VI Luk'ianchikov and EA Kobzev (1980). Effect of antiorthostatic hypokinesia and space flight factors on changes in crural volume. *Kosmicheskaia Biologiia Aviakosmicheskaia Meditsina*, 14, 51–55.

Keil, LC, KH McKeever, MG Skidmore, J Hines and WB Severs (1992). The effect of head-down tilt and water immersion on intracranial pressure in nonhuman primates. *Aviation Space and Environmental Medicine*, 63, 181–185.

Kergoat, H and JV Lovasik (2005). Seven-degree head-down tilt reduces choroidal pulsatile ocular blood flow. *Aviation Space and Environmental Medicine*, 76, 930–934.

Kirsch, KA, FJ Baartz, HC Gunga and L Röcker (1993). Fluid shifts into and out of superficial tissues under microgravity and terrestrial conditions. *Clinical Investigation* 71: 687–689.

Kirsch, KA, L Röcker, OH Gauer, R Krause, C Leach, HJ Wicke and R Landry (1984). Venous pressure in man during weightlessness. *Science*, 225, 218–219.

Krotov, VP, EV Trambovetskiĭ and VI Korol'kov (1994). Intracranial pressure in monkeys under microgravity. *Fiziol Zhurnal Im IM Sechenova Ross Akad Nauk*, 80, 1–8.

Lakin, WD, SA Stevens and PL Penar (2007). Modeling intracranial pressures in microgravity: The influence of the blood-brain barrier. *Aviation Space and Environmental Medicine*, 78, 932–936.

Lassen, NA (1959). Cerebral blood flow and oxygen consumption in man. *Physiological Reviews*, 39, 183–238.

Lathers, CM, JB Charles, KF Elton, TA Holt, C Mukai, BS Bennett and MW Bungo (1989). Acute hemodynamic responses to weightlessness in humans. *Journal of Clinical Pharmacology*, 29, 615–627.

Law, J, M Van Baalen, M Foy, SS Mason, C Mendez, ML Wear, VE Meyers and D Alexander (2014). Relationship between carbon dioxide levels and reported headaches on the international space station. *Journal of Occupational and Environmental Medicine American College Occupational and Environmental Medicine*, 56, 477–483.

Law, J, S Watkins and D Alexander (2010). *In-Flight Carbon Dioxide Exposures and Related Symptoms: Association, Susceptibility, and Operational Implications*. Houston, TX: NASA Johnson Space Center.

Leach, CS, CP Alfrey, WN Suki, JI Leonard, PC Rambaut, LD Inners, Smith SM, HW Lane and JM Krauhs (1996). Regulation of body fluid compartments during short-term spaceflight. *Journal of Applied Physiology*, 81, 105–116.

Leach, CS, LD Inners and JB Charles (1991). Changes in total body water during spaceflight. *Journal of Clinical Pharmacology*, 31, 1001–1006.

Lee, SM, AD Moore, JM Fritsch-Yelle, MC Greenisen and SM Schneider. (1999). Inflight exercise affects stand test responses after space flight. *Medicine Science in Sports & Exercise*, 31, 1755–62.

Linder, BJ, GL Trick and ML Wolf (1988). Altering body position affects intraocular pressure and visual function. *Investigative Ophthalmology & Visual Science*, 29, 1492–1497.

Liu, J, B Verheyden, F Beckers and AE Aubert (2012). Haemodynamic adaptation during sudden gravity transitions. *European Journal of Applied Physiology* 112, 79–89.

Liu, JH, DF Kripke, RE Hoffman, MD Twa, RT Loving, KM Rex, N Gupta and Weinreb RN (1998). Nocturnal elevation of intraocular pressure in young adults. *Investigative Ophthalmology & Visual Science*, 39, 2707–2712.

Liu, JHK, DF Kripke, MD Twa, PA Gokhale, EI Jones, E-H Park, JE Meehan and RN Weinreb (2002). Twenty-four-hour pattern of intraocular pressure in young adults with moderate to severe myopia. *Investigative Ophthalmology & Visual Science*, 43, 2351–2355.

Longo, A, MH Geiser and CE Riva (2004). Posture changes and subfoveal choroidal blood flow. *Investigative Ophthalmology & Visual Science*, 45, 546–551.

Lucas, SJE, YC Tzeng, SD Galvin, Thomas KN, S Ogoh and PN Ainslie (2010). Influence of changes in blood pressure on cerebral perfusion and oxygenation. *Hypertension*, 55, 698–705.

Mader, TH, CR Gibson, AF Pass, LA Kramer, AG Lee, J Fogarty, WJ Tarver, JP Dervay, DR Hamilton, A Sargsyan, JL Phillips, D Tran, W Lipsky, J Choi, C Stern, R Kuyumjian and JD Polk (2011). Optic disc edema, globe flattening, choroidal folds, and hyperopic shifts observed in astronauts after long-duration space flight. *Ophthalmology*, 118, 2058–2069.

Mader, TH, CR Gibson, M Caputo, N Hunter, G Taylor, J Charles and RT Meehan (1993). Intraocular pressure and retinal vascular changes during transient exposure to microgravity. *American Journal of Ophthalmology*, 115, 347–350.

Mader, TH, GR Taylor, N Hunter, M Caputo and RT Meehan (1990). Intraocular pressure, retinal vascular, and visual acuity changes during 48 hours of 10 degrees head-down tilt. *Aviation Space and Environmental Medicine*, 61, 810–813.

Marshall-Bowman, K, MR Barratt and CR Gibson (2013). Ophthalmic changes and increased intracranial pressure associated with long duration spaceflight: an emerging understanding. *Acta Astronautica*, 87, 77–87.

Martin, DS, SMC Lee, SP Stein, MB Stenger, AH Feiveson, TP Matz, TL Caine, JM Scott, CM Westby and SH Platts (2015). *Pilot Study to Evaluate a Novel Non-Invasive Technology to Measure Peripheral Venous Pressure*. Houston, TX: NASA Johnson Space Center.

Mekjavic, PJ, O Eiken and IB Mekjavic (2002). Visual function after prolonged bed rest. *Journal of Gravitational Physiology: A Journal of the International Society for Gravitational Physiology*, 9, P31–32.

Meng, L and Gelb AW (2015). Regulation of cerebral autoregulation by carbon dioxide. *Anesthesiology* 122, 196–205.

Mitchell, GF, H Parise, EJ Benjamin, MG Larson, MJ Keyes, JA Vita, RS Vasan, and D Levy (2004). Changes in arterial stiffness and wave reflection with advancing age in healthy men and women: The Framingham Heart Study. *Hypertension*, 43, 1239–1245.

Monahan, KD, FA Dinenno, DR Seals and JR Halliwill (2001). Smaller age-associated reductions in leg venous compliance in endurance exercise-trained men. *American Journal of Physiology–Heart and Circulatory Physiology*, 281, H1267–1273.

Montgomery, LD (1987). Body volume changes during simulated weightlessness: An overview. *Aviation Space and Environmental Medicine*, 58, A80–85.

Moore, TP and WE Thornton. (1987) Space shuttle inflight and postflight fluid shifts measured by leg volume changes. *Aviation Space and Environmental Medicine*, 58, A91–96.

Newman, DG, SW White and R Callister (1998). Evidence of baroreflex adaptation to repetitive +Gz in fighter pilots. *Aviation Space and Environmental Medicine*, 69, 446–451.

Nixon, JV, RG Murray, C Bryant, RL Johnson Jr, JH Mitchell, OB Holland, G-C Sanchez, P Vergne-Marini and CG Blomqvist (1979). Early cardiovascular adaptation to simulated zero gravity. *Journal of Applied Physiology*, 46, 541–548.

Norsk, P (2000). Renal adjustments to microgravity. *Pflügers Archiv European Journal of Physiology*, 441, R62–65.

Norsk, P (2005). Cardiovascular and fluid volume control in humans in space. *Current Pharmaceutical Biotechnology*, 6, 325–330.

Norsk, P, M Damgaard, L Petersen, M Gybel, B Pump, A Gabrielsen and NJ Christensen (2006). Vasorelaxation in space. *Hypertension*, 47, 69–73.

Norsk, P, N Foldager F, Bonde-Petersen, B Elmann-Larsen and TS Johansen (1987). Central venous pressure in humans during short periods of weightlessness. *Journal of Applied Physiology*, 63, 2433–2437.

Panerai, RB (1998). Assessment of cerebral pressure autoregulation in humans–A review of measurement methods. *Physiological Measurement*, 19, 305.

Parazynski, SE, AR Hargens, B Tucker, M Aratow, J Styf and A Crenshaw (1991). Transcapillary fluid shifts in tissues of the head and neck during and after simulated microgravity. *Journal of Applied Physiology*, 71, 2469–2475.

Platts, SH, DS Martin, MB Stenger, SA Perez, LC Ribeiro, R Summers and JV Meck (2009). Cardiovascular adaptations to long-duration head-down bed rest. *Aviation Space and Environmental Medicine*, 80, A29–36.

Resch, H, C Zawinka, S Lung, G Weigert, L Schmetterer and G Garhöfer (2005). Effect of histamine and cimetidine on retinal and choroidal blood flow in humans. *American Journal of Physiology – Regulatory, Integrative and Comparative Physiology*, 289, R1387–1391.

Rowell, LB (1993). *Human Cardiovascular Control*. New York: Oxford University Press.

Ruíz, DSM, P Gailloud, DA Rüfenacht, J Delavelle, F Henry and JHD Fasel (2002). The craniocervical venous system in relation to cerebral venous drainage. *American Journal of Neuroradiology*, 23, 1500–1508.

Sliwka, U, JA Krasney, SG Simon, P Schmidt and J Noth (1998). Effects of sustained low-level elevations of carbon dioxide on cerebral blood flow and autoregulation of the intracerebral arteries in humans. *Aviation Space and Environmental Medicine*, 69, 299–306.

Sofronova SI, Tarasova OS, Gaynullina D, Borzykh AA, Behnke BJ, Stabley JN, McCullough DJ, Maraj JJ, Hanna ME, Muller-Delp JM, Vinogradova OL and Delp MD (2014). Spaceflight on the Bion-M1 biosatellite alters cerebral artery vasomotor and mechanical properties in mice. *Journal of Applied Physiology*, doi: 10.1152/japplphysiol.00976.2014.

Stoquart-ElSankari, S, O Balédent, C Gondry-Jouet, M Makki, O Godefroy and M-E Meyer (2007). Aging effects on cerebral blood and cerebrospinal fluid flows. *Journal of Cerebral Blood Flow & Metabolism*, 27, 1563–1572.

Summers, RL, LH Woodward, L Jackson, DS Martin and SH Platts (2010). Ultrasound measurements of lower extremity soft tissue and interstitial fluid thickness may be used as an early indicator of dehydration. *Critical Ultrasound Journal*, 2, 43–45.

Taibbi G, Cromwell RL, Zanello SB, Yarbough PO, RJ Ploutz-Snyder, BF Godley and G Vizzeri (2014). Ocular outcomes evaluation in a 14-day head-down bed rest study. *Aviation Space and Environmental Medicine*, 85, 983–992.

Tan, CO (2012). Defining the characteristic relationship between arterial pressure and cerebral flow. *Journal of Applied Physiology*, 113, 1194–1200,

Taylor, CR, M Hanna, BJ Behnke, JN Stabley, DJ McCullough, RT Davis 3rd, P Ghosh, A Papadopoulos, JM Muller-Delp and MD Delp (2013). Spaceflight-induced alterations in cerebral artery vasoconstrictor, mechanical, and structural properties: implications for elevated cerebral perfusion and intracranial pressure. *FASEB Journal Official Publication of the Federation of American Society for Experimental Biology*, 27, 2282–2292.

Thalhammer, C, M Aschwanden, A Odermatt, UA Baumann, S Imfeld, D Bilecen, SC Marsch and KA Jaeger (2007). Noninvasive central venous pressure measurement by controlled compression sonography at the forearm. *Journal of the American College of Cardiology*, 50, 1584–1589.

Thornton, WE, GW Hoffler and J Rummel (1977). Anthropometric changes and fluid Shifts. In *Biomedical Results from Skylab*, Johnston, RS and LF Dietlein LF (eds.), pp. 330–339. Washington, DC: Scientific and Technical Information Office, National Aeronautics and Space Administration.

Thornton, WE, TP Moore and SL Pool (1987). Fluid shifts in weightlessness. *Aviation Space Environmental Medicine*, 58, A86–90.

Tuday, EC, JV Meck, D Nyhan, AA Shoukas and DE Berkowitz (2007). Microgravity-induced changes in aortic stiffness and their role in orthostatic intolerance. *Journal of Applied Physiology*, 102, 853–858.

Udden, MM, TB Driscoll, MH Pickett, CS Leach-Huntoon and CP Alfrey (1995). Decreased production of red blood cells in human subjects exposed to microgravity. *Journal of Laboratory and Clinical Medicine*, 125, 442–449.

Vaitkevicius, PV, JL Fleg, JH Engel, FC O'Connor, JG Wright, LE Lakatta, FC Yin and EG Lakatta (1993). Effects of age and aerobic capacity on arterial stiffness in healthy adults. *Circulation*, 88, 1456–1462.

Vieira, GM, HB Oliveira, DT de Andrade, M Bottaro and R Ritch (2006). Intraocular pressure variation during weight lifting. *Archives of Ophthalmology*, 124, 1251–1254.

Wang, L, C Grant, B Fortune and GA Cioffi (2008). Retinal and choroidal vasoreactivity to altered $PaCO_2$ in rat measured with a modified microsphere technique. *Experimental Eye Research*, 86, 908–913.

Watenpaugh, DE and AR Hargens (1996). The Cardiovascular System in Microgravity. In *Handbook of Physiology*, Fregly, MJ and Blatteis CM (eds.), pp. 631–674. Bethesda, MD: American Physiological Society.

Waters, WW, MG Ziegler and JV Meck (2002). Postspaceflight orthostatic hypotension occurs mostly in women and is predicted by low vascular resistance. *Journal of Applied Physiology*, 92, 586–94.

Weinreb, RN, J Cook and TR Friberg (1984). Effect of inverted body position on intraocular pressure. *American Journal of Ophthalmology*, 98, 784–787.

Westby, CM, SMC Lee, MB Stenger and SH Platts (2012). The change in lower limb venous compliance is different between women and men following 60 days of head-down bedrest but is not associated with venoconstrictor dysfunction. 2012 Experimental Biology Meeting. San Diego, CA.

Wilkerson, MK, LA Lesniewski, EM Golding, RM Bryan, A Amin, E Wilson and MD Delp (2005). Simulated microgravity enhances cerebral artery vasoconstriction and vascular resistance through endothelial nitric oxide mechanism. *American Journal of Physiology–Heart and Circulatory Physiology*, 288, H1652–H1661.

Wilkerson, MK, PN Colleran and MD Delp (2002). Acute and chronic head-down tail suspension diminishes cerebral perfusion in rats. *American Journal of Physiology–Heart and Circulatory Physiology*, 282, H328–H334.

Willie, CK, DB Macleod, AD Shaw, KJ Smith, YC Tzeng, Eves ND, Ikeda K, J Graham, NC Lewis, TA Day and PN Ainslie (2012). Regional brain blood flow in man during acute changes in arterial blood gases. *Journal of Physiology*, 590, 3261–3275.

Willie, CK, FL Colino, DM Bailey, YC Tzeng, G Binsted, LW Jones, MJ Haykowsky, J Bellapart, S Ogoh, KJ Smith, JD Smirl, TA Day, SJ Lucas, LK Eller and Ainslie PN (2011). Utility of transcranial Doppler ultrasound for the integrative assessment of cerebrovascular function. *Journal of Neuroscience Methods*, 196, 221–237.

Wilson, MR, RS Baker, P Mohammadi, NC Wheeler, DA Lee and C Scott (1993). Reproducibility of postural changes in intraocular pressure with the Tono-Pen and Pulsair tonometers. *American Journal of Ophthalmology*, 116, 479–483.

Xu, X, L Li, R Cao, Y Tao, Q Guo, J Geng, Y Li and Zhang Z (2010). Intraocular pressure and ocular perfusion pressure in myopes during 21 min head-down rest. *Aviation Space and Environmental Medicine*, 81, 418–422.

Zamboni, P, R Galeotti, E Menegatti, AM Malagoni, G Tacconi, S Dall'Ara, I Bartolomei and F Salvi (2009). Chronic cerebrospinal venous insufficiency in patients with multiple sclerosis. *Journal of Neurology, Neurosurgery & Psychiatry*, 80, 392–399.

Zhang LF (2001). Vascular adaptation to microgravity: What have we learned? *Journal of Applied Physiology*, 91, 2415–2430.

Zhang L-F (2013). Region-specific vascular remodeling and its prevention by artificial gravity in weightless environment. *European Journal of Applied Physiology*, 113, 2873–2895.

Zuj, KA, P Arbeille, JK Shoemaker, AP Blaber, DK Greaves, D Xu and RL Hughson (2012). Impaired cerebrovascular autoregulation and reduced CO_2 reactivity after long duration spaceflight. *American Journal of Physiology–Heart and Circulatory Physiology*, 302, H2592–2598.

Intracranial Pressure Physiology and VIIP   5

Sara Qvarlander, PhD and Michael A. Williams, MD, FAAN†*

**Department of Radiation Sciences — Biomedical Engineering,
Umeå University, SE-901 87, Umeå, Sweden
†Departments of Neurology and Neurological Surgery,
University of Washington Medical Center,
1959 NE Pacific St, Seattle, WA 98195, USA*

1. Introduction

The syndrome of visual impairment/intracranial pressure (VIIP) has been hypothesized to be caused by a "cephalad fluid shift" in the microgravity environment that results in elevated intracranial pressure (ICP). This chapter will review ICP physiology, the ways in which it is affected by cerebrovascular physiology and gravity, and plausible arguments for and against the fluid shift/increased ICP hypothesis.

2. Intracranial Pressure and Craniospinal Compliance

ICP is defined as the pressure of the cerebrospinal fluid (CSF) measured with reference to an anatomic landmark, typically on the head and, most commonly, the external acoustic meatus. CSF pressure was first recognized as a physiologic property when Quincke performed the first lumbar puncture (Quincke, 1891). Continuous ICP monitoring via intraventricular catheter was first described by Guillaume and Janny (Guillame and Janny, 1951), and Lundberg published the first systematic observations of ICP and its response to medical and physiologic interventions (Lundberg, 1960). ICP can become elevated as a result of either primary disorders of CSF circulation and resorption (such as hydrocephalus and idiopathic intracranial hypertension, IIH) or the presence of intracranial masses (tumor, hemorrhage, abscess, etc.). Primary disorders of CSF circulation and resorption as they may relate to VIIP will be the focus of this chapter.

2.1. *The CSF system and circulation*

CSF is secreted by the choroid plexus, which is a highly vascular tissue contained primarily within the C-shaped lateral ventricles in each hemisphere of the brain (Johanson *et al.*, 2008; Redzic and Segal, 2004; Spector *et al.*, 2015). The ventricles are cavities within the brain that contain and convey CSF from within the brain to the subarachnoid space. CSF flows from the two lateral ventricles via the foramina of Monro to the midline IIIrd ventricle, which is bounded by the thalamus and hypothalamus laterally. CSF then transits through the cerebral aqueduct in the midbrain to enter the IVth ventricle, which is bounded by the brainstem anteriorly and the cerebellum posteriorly (Fig. 1). From the IVth ventricle, CSF exits to the subarachnoid space at the level of the foramen magnum via the two lateral

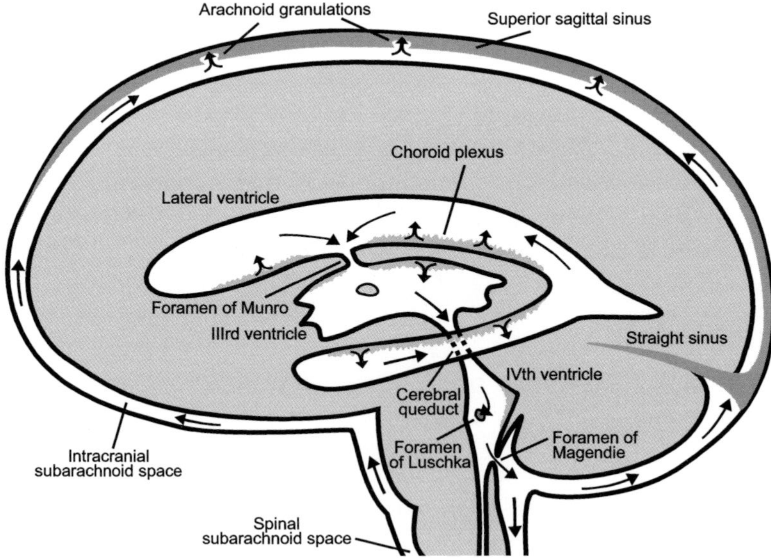

Figure 1. Schematic of the CSF system, illustrating the production of CSF in the choroid plexus, the circulation of CSF from the ventricles to the subarachnoid space, and the absorption of CSF into venous blood via the arachnoid villi.

foramina of Luschka and the inferior foramen of Magendie. The CSF circulates in the intracranial subarachnoid space, ascending through the basal cisterns, which are anterior to the brainstem, and then laterally to follow the Sylvian fissure to reach the subarachnoid space over the convexity of the brain. There, the CSF moves through the arachnoid villi into the superior sagittal sinus (SSS) and re-enters the bloodstream — a process known as CSF absorption.

The subarachnoid space also extends inferiorly through the spinal canal from the level of the foramen magnum at the base of the skull to the lowest sacral levels. The spinal subarachnoid space is distensible and can expand or be compressed (Martins *et al.*, 1972). The intracranial and intraspinal subarachnoid spaces are in direct continuity, and CSF flows freely between them via the foramen magnum.

The force thought to cause CSF flow through the ventricular system is the pulsatile expansion of the brain parenchyma from the volume of arterial blood that enters the brain with every cardiac cycle, which forces the walls of the lateral ventricles inward (Wagshul *et al.*, 2011). Although the CSF flow within the ventricles is pulsatile, meaning that it is to and fro (best seen in the cerebral aqueduct), the net bulk flow of CSF is antegrade. As a result, CSF flows into the IIIrd ventricle and eventually through the cerebral aqueduct and IVth ventricle into the subarachnoid space.

Because the rates of CSF production and absorption are normally equal, the volume of CSF throughout the craniospinal system is in steady state, or equilibrium. The CSF production rate in humans is relatively constant at ~0.34 mL/min (Edsbagge *et al.*, 2004). The CSF absorption rate, as defined by Davson's equation, is determined by the pressure gradient between the CSF space and the SSS and the resistance to absorption of CSF across the arachnoid granulations, known as the outflow resistance (R_{out}) (Eq 1) (Davson *et al.*, 1970). From this equation, an expression for equilibrium ICP can be derived (Eq 2):

$$\text{CSF absorption rate} = (\text{ICP–SSSP}) \, / \, R_{out} \qquad (1)$$

$$\text{ICP} = (R_{out} \times \text{CSF production rate}) + \text{SSSP} \qquad (2)$$

Where SSSP = superior sagittal sinus pressure.

In order for CSF to flow from the subarachnoid space into the SSS, a pressure gradient must exist, i.e., the CSF pressure must exceed the SSSP. Assuming that CSF pressure is constant, an increase in either R_{out} or SSSP will reduce the CSF absorption rate. Increased R_{out} is characteristic of hydrocephalus, which is associated with a gradual increase of the CSF volume. Increased SSSP is characteristic of IIH (also known as pseudotumor cerebri); however, because the increased SSSP also increases the cerebral venous pressure, causing cerebral venous engorgement, the CSF volume does not increase. In both instances, the ICP must rise sufficiently to drive the CSF absorption rate that balances the CSF production rate.

2.2. *Determinants of craniospinal compliance and ICP*

ICP is determined by the volume and compliance of the craniospinal system, which comprises the intracranial and intraspinal compartments and their normal contents: the brain and spinal cord, intravascular blood, CSF, and interstitial fluid. The normal adult intracranial volume of approximately 1300 mL is 87% brain, 9% CSF, and 4% blood (Rosomoff, 1961). The cerebral blood volume is ~30% arterial and ~70% capillary/venous. The CSF volume of the spinal canal in normal supine adults is 81 ± 13 mL (range 52–103 mL) (Edsbagge *et al.*, 2011).

Monro (Monro, 1783) and Kellie (Kellie, 1824) described cranial vault volume relationships, often called the Monro–Kellie doctrine, which can be summarized as follows: (1) The skull is a rigid container; (2) the normal intracranial contents are incompressible; and (3) any mass added to the cranial vault or enlargement of the volume of one of the normal contents of the cranial vault requires an equal displacement of one of the normal contents from the cranial vault (Weed and McKibben, 1919). For example, within the cranial vault, the addition of a slowly growing mass, which could include an increase in cerebral blood volume or in cerebral interstitial fluid (i.e., edema), will reduce intracranial CSF volume by displacing it into the spinal subarachnoid space via the foramen magnum. The pulsatile expansion and contraction of cerebral blood volume with every cardiac cycle is also subject to the Monro–Kellie doctrine. Movement of CSF back and forth across the foramen magnum and compression of the cerebral veins by pulsatile expansion of the brain parenchyma are the primary compliance mechanisms that accommodate the incoming arterial blood volume (Wagshul *et al.*, 2011). Because these compliance mechanisms are not instantaneous, the ICP exhibits pulsatile variation, known as the ICP pulse pressure. Slower ICP variation is seen at the respiratory frequency, presumably resulting from changes in central venous pressure (CVP) with respiration. The cerebral blood volume may change slowly because of changes in diameter of intracranial arteries and arterioles as a result of cerebral autoregulation, leading to slow waves (B-waves) in ICP. ICP pulse pressure is determined by craniospinal compliance. When compliance is high, which is the normal condition, ICP pulse pressure is low; however, when compliance is low, ICP pulse pressure is high (Avezaat and Van Eijndhoven, 1986). With each cardiac cycle, the more easily that CSF is displaced into the spinal subarachnoid space or the more easily that cerebral veins are compressed, the less ICP rises.

In pathologic conditions, the normal compliance mechanisms can be exhausted. For example, if the expansion of a mass has caused near-complete displacement of ventricular and intracranial subarachnoid CSF from the cranial vault (which can be seen on CT or MRI as effacement of the ventricles and the perimesencephalic cisterns) and if the venous blood volume has similarly been reduced by the expansion of the mass, then the effect of pulsatile arterial blood volume on ICP pulse pressure cannot be attenuated. As a result, both mean ICP and ICP pulse pressure rise. This phenomenon is illustrated by a pressure–volume curve (Fig. 2A), which describes ICP as an exponential function of volume. Because the arterial blood volume entering the brain with every cardiac cycle is generally constant, ICP pulse pressure can be an indirect indicator of intracranial compliance (Avezaat and Van Eijndhoven, 1986). The key is to examine the change in ICP (dP) in response to the constant pulsatile blood volume (dV). If ICP pulse pressure (dP) is low, then compliance is presumed normal; but if ICP pulse pressure is high, compliance is presumed low. Thus, one aspect of compliance is the steepness of the arc of the curve; another aspect is the point on the curve at which ICP is located. The arc of the curve is mathematically described by the elastance coefficient or, more commonly, the pressure volume index (PVI), which is inversely proportional to the elastance coefficient and corresponds to the volume required to raise the ICP by a factor of 10 (Marmarou *et al.*, 1975).

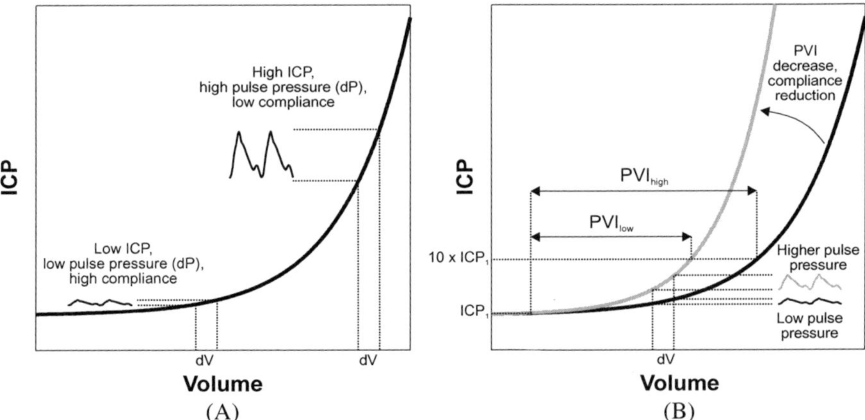

Figure 2. The pressure–volume curve, illustrating compliance and the relationship between intracranial pressure (ICP) and craniospinal volume. (A) Illustration of the change in compliance and pulse pressure that results from changes in volume, i.e., shift of ICP along the curve. (B) Illustration of how a change in the pressure volume index (PVI) alters the steepness of the curve, thereby changing the ICP, as well as the compliance and pulse pressure, at a given volume.

A compliance change may appear as a change in mean ICP and ICP pulse pressure along the curve (Fig. 2A), a shift of the curve to the left or right along the volume axis, or a change in the PVI, i.e., in the steepness of the pressure–volume curve (Fig. 2B). These changes correspond to various pathophysiologic processes. A change in location of the curve along the volume axis could be affected by a change in balance between the intracranial components, where the volume of CSF and, potentially, the venous blood are reduced (in the absence of ICP increase), meaning that less CSF and blood can be forced from the intracranial space in response to a volume increase. A change in the curvature would likely result from a change in the stiffness of intracranial veins or the walls of the spinal subarachnoid compartment, i.e., an actual physical change in the elasticity of the system.

In a normal healthy state, ICP is low and characterized by the flat part of the pressure–volume curve, with a low dP/dV (Fig 2A). Under normal physiologic conditions, the range of ICP variations also remains within the flat portion of the curve, and significant ICP elevation does not occur. However, in pathologic conditions, such as a rapidly enlarging mass, ICP rises and first approaches the upward inflection of the curve, where the dP/dV begins to increase. As ICP rises higher, it encounters the steep part of the curve, where compliance is exhausted and dP/dV is very high. The rising ICP cannot be accommodated by compliance mechanisms, and cerebral herniation may occur. However, in the case of a slowly growing tumor, secondary compliance mechanisms such as reduced volume of interstitial fluid may keep ICP on the flat part of the pressure–volume curve but closer to the inflection point than is normal. Even with slowly growing masses, eventually all compliance mechanisms are exhausted and ICP will begin to rise and become unstable, with the appearance of B-waves and plateau waves (Lundberg, 1960) (Fig. 3). In IIH, although ICP can be very high, it is rare for cerebral herniation to occur.

In the ICU setting, compliance is difficult to measure directly, and monitoring ICP and ICP pulse pressure provides reasonable estimates for clinical management, e.g., high ICP pulse pressure implies low compliance. In chronic disorders, such as hydrocephalus or IIH, compliance can be measured during an infusion investigation, in which ICP is actively increased by infusion of artificial CSF. Infusion testing in animal experiments has shown the respective contribution of the intracranial (68%) and intraspinal (32%) compartments to compliance (Marmarou *et al.*, 1975). Similarly, infusion testing combined with MR investigations of CSF flow in humans has shown that 65% of compliance is intracranial and 35% is intraspinal (Wåhlin, *et al.*, 2010).

Despite the large contribution of the intraspinal compartment to compliance, the spinal compartment has rarely been considered to play a role in disorders of CSF circulation that are associated with impaired compliance.

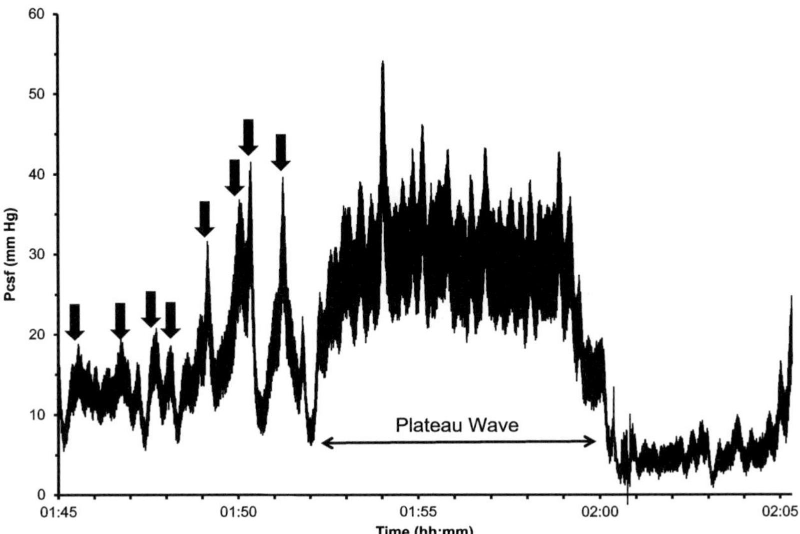

Figure 3. Illustration of CSF pressure (Pcsf) recording via a spinal catheter in a 34-year-old male with idiopathic intracranial hypertension without papilledema. Recording shows B-waves at 30–60 second intervals (arrows) and a plateau wave lasting ~8 min. Note that the B-waves persist atop the plateau wave, which terminates rapidly (<2 min) with a fall in CSF pressure from ~30 mmHg to 5 mmHg accompanied by a reduction in CSF pulse pressure and temporary loss of B-wave activity.

In theory, reduction of spinal canal volume could lower the compliance of the craniospinal system. Reduction of normal lumbosacral volume (35.8 mL) by 8.4 mL in patients with lumbar stenosis has been documented (Sullivan *et al.*, 2006), and reduction in volume of the lumbosacral compartment secondary to engorgement of the spinal epidural venous plexus has been demonstrated in pregnant women (Takiguchi *et al.*, 2006); however, no systematic analysis of this effect on craniospinal compliance has been performed.

3. Known Gravitational Effects on ICP

Most knowledge of ICP and its dynamics, including compliance, in humans is based on measurements performed with patients in the supine, or horizontal, position, in which hydrostatic pressure gradients in the fluid systems of the human body are minimal, especially along the vertical axis of the body. A similar absence of a hydrostatic pressure gradient along the vertical axis can be postulated in microgravity. However, an important difference is that humans normally spend only approximately one-third of the day in the supine position, and the remaining two-thirds in the upright position. Thus, the CSF system is normally subject to a hydrostatic gradient when persons are in the upright position, and the CSF system rapidly accommodates to changes in posture and the presence or absence of the hydrostatic gradient (see below). In microgravity, the hydrostatic gradient is always absent or minimal. It is unknown whether absence of the normal diurnal variation in the hydrostatic gradients of the CSF system during long-term spaceflight causes alterations in CSF circulation, craniospinal compliance, or ICP.

A number of studies of ICP measurements in various body positions have been published (Loman *et al.*, 1935; Magnæs, 1976a; Magnæs, 1989; Poca *et al.*, 2006), most of which focus on the effect of changes in subject position for neurosurgical procedures or in intensive-care settings (Brimioulle *et al.*, 1997; Hung *et al.*, 2000; Ledwith *et al.*, 2010; Lee, 1989; Mahfoud *et al.*, 2010; Mavrocordatos *et al.*, 2000; Ng *et al.*, 2004; Schwarz *et al.*, 2002; Winkelman, 2000) and on hydrostatically related symptomatic overdrainage in patients with CSF shunts (Bergsneider *et al.*, 2004; Chapman *et al.*, 1990; Cook and Bergsneider, 2002; Kajimoto *et al.*, 2000). Overall, these studies show the same results. With reference to the head, ICP is highest in the supine position, is gradually reduced as the torso and head are elevated, and may be negative in the upright position. Further, when measured simultaneously, the difference between lumbar and intracranial ICP corresponds to the hydrostatic gradient between them (Loman *et al.*, 1935; Magnæs, 1976a,b). In most studies the supine ICP is 8–15 mmHg higher than the upright ICP, which is usually between 0 and −4 mmHg. However, a recent Danish study using implanted intracranial telemetric ICP sensors suggested that healthy individuals might experience a slightly smaller change in ICP when they move between body positions (Andresen *et al.*, 2014).

In 1976, Magnæs presented a model for the positional/gravitational effects on ICP based on the concept of a hydrostatic indifference point (HIP), which is a point along the axis of a communicating fluid system, such as the CSF system, where pressure is independent of the orientation of the system (Magnæs, 1976b). A corresponding HIP model had previously been posited for the venous system (Gauer and Thron, 1965; Hinghofer-Szalkay, 2011). The Magnæs HIP model portrays the gravitational effect on ICP as being completely defined by the hydrostatic gradient between the HIP and the reference point for the ICP measurement. The location of the HIP depends on the distribution of compliance in the system above and below the HIP (Hinghofer-Szalkay, 2011). Based on ICP measurements in the lateral recumbent and upright seated positions, the HIP was determined by Magnæs to be at the level of the T1–T3 vertebrae for healthy individuals (Magnæs,

1976b). A limitation of the Magnæs HIP model is that it considers the CSF system in isolation and does not account for the contribution of the arterial and venous compartments that influence ICP and which themselves are influenced by gravity.

A 2013 study compared the Magnæs HIP model (Model I) to two new models that took into account the interaction between ICP and the venous system (Qvarlander *et al.*, 2013). In one of the venous models (Model II), the venous column of blood from the head to the right atrium was assumed to be continuous, regardless of postural orientation; in the second venous model (Model III), the jugular veins were presumed to collapse as posture became more upright. ICP was measured in human subjects at seven different tilt angles from supine to seated 70 degrees upright, and the results were compared to the predictions of the three models.

The Magnæs HIP model did not fully explain the positional effects on ICP. Model III, with the collapsible venous system, had the best match with observed ICP changes (Fig. 4). At higher tilt angles, the jugular veins collapse, interrupting the venous fluid column between the head and the right atrium. As a result, the upright ICP is not as low as predicted by Model II, the model without venous collapse

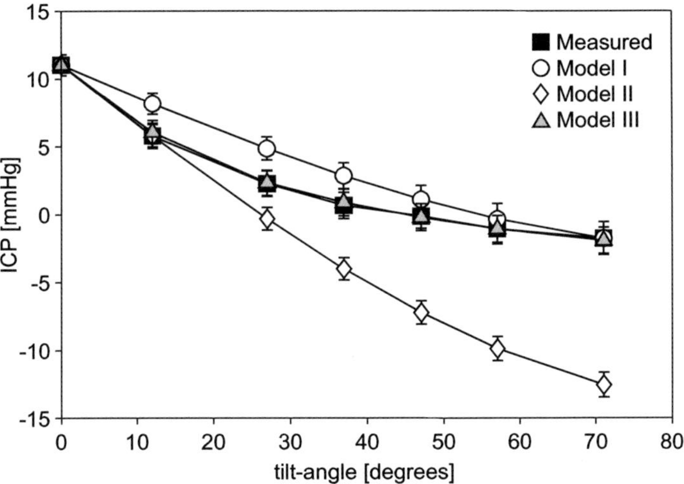

Figure 4. ICP measurements (mean with confidence interval) in 27 patients during change in tilt angle from 0 degrees (supine) to 70 degrees upright compared to ICP predicted by the Magnæs model (Model I), the model in which jugular veins are always patent (Model II), and the model in which jugular veins collapse as tilt angle increases (Model III). Model III most closely matches the measured ICP. From Qvarlander *et al.*, 2013, with permission.

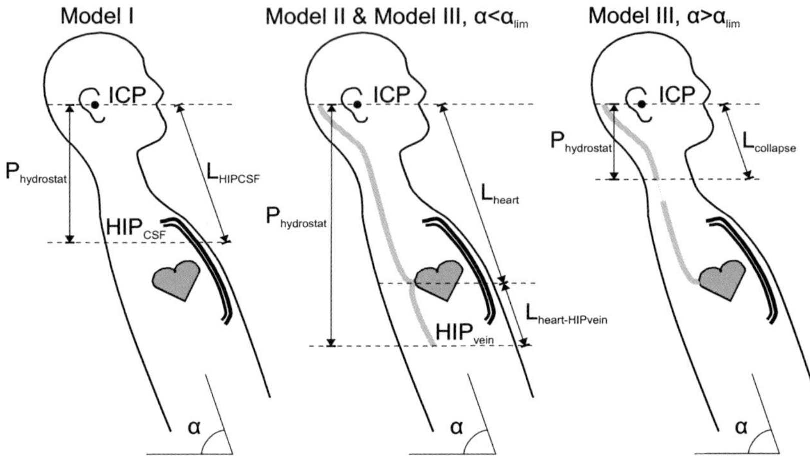

Figure 5. Illustration of the concepts of three models of postural effects on ICP.

Model I: $ICP = ICP_{supine} - P_{hydrostat} = ICP_{supine} - \rho \times g \times \sin(\alpha) \times L_{HIPCSF}$.

Model II, III before jugular vein collapse: $ICP = ICP_{supine} - P_{hydrostat} = ICP_{supine} - \rho \times g \times \sin(\alpha) \times (L_{heart} + L_{heart\text{-}HIPvein})$.

Model III after jugular vein collapse: $ICP = ICP_{supine} - P_{HIPvein} - P_{hydrostat} = ICP_{supine} - P_{HIPvein} - \rho \times g \times \sin(\alpha) \times L_{collapse}$.

From Qvarlander *et al.*, 2013, with permission.

(Qvarlander *et al.*, 2013). The venous-collapse model is consistent with earlier theories that suggested that the collapse of the venous system affects the ICP change when assuming an upright posture (von Storch *et al.*, 1937), and by Davson *et al.*, who proposed that CVP sets a "floor" for CSF pressure (Davson *et al.*, 1987).

Mathematically, the venous-collapse model, as shown in (Fig. 5), incorporates these theories by positing that:

(1) Davson's equation for CSF absorption (Davson *et al.*, 1970) and the expression for equilibrium ICP that can be derived from it are valid in any body position:

$$\text{CSF absorption rate} = (ICP - SSSP)/R_{out} \tag{1}$$
$$ICP = (R_{out} \times \text{CSF production rate}) + SSSP \tag{2}$$

(2) In supine position and positions at lower tilt angles, where the jugular veins are patent, the hydrostatic gradient affecting the SSSP is determined by the

vertical distance between the SSS and the venous HIP, which is near the top of the diaphragm (Gauer and Thron, 1965).

(3) In more upright positions, where the jugular veins collapse (Dawson *et al.*, 2004; Gisolf *et al.*, 2004; Valdueza *et al.*, 2000), the hydrostatic gradient between the SSS and the venous HIP is disrupted (Hinghofer-Szalkay, 2011), which sets a new zero level for the intracranial venous pressure, which in turn, influences ICP.

Thus, under normal gravitational conditions (1G), the venous collapse model has two different states: the upright state (where collapse of the jugular veins results in a smaller hydrostatic gradient, affecting the SSSP and thereby preventing the ICP from becoming more than a few millimeters of mercury negative) and the horizontal state (where the jugular veins are patent) (Qvarlander, *et al.*, 2013).

4. Arguments for and Against ICP Elevation in Spaceflight

Based on the known influence of gravity on the physiology of the CSF system and the arterial and venous systems, a number of hypotheses for ICP behavior in microgravity can be argued. These theories incorporate mechanisms with either direct effects on ICP, or compromise of craniospinal compliance, or both. However, until ICP is measured in humans in spaceflight, i.e., microgravity, none of these hypotheses should be considered proven or disproven.

4.1. *Cephalad fluid shift directly causes ICP elevation*

The occurrence of cephalad fluid shift in microgravity (Kas'ian *et al.*, 1980; Kirsch *et al.*, 1993; Moore and Thornton, 1987; Thornton *et al.*, 1977) is the most commonly suggested hypothesis for increased ICP in microgravity (Alexander *et al.*, 2012). Although in Earth-based experiments, cephalad fluid shift is often simulated by head-down tilt (HDT), where ICP increases in the short term (Murthy *et al.*, 1992), evidence exists that ICP may subsequently decrease during long-term HDT as a result of physiologic adaptation (Steinbach *et al.*, 2005). The implications of these results for VIIP are entirely dependent on whether HDT is a valid model for the influence of microgravity on ICP in humans.

The hydrostatic effect of HDT is probably sufficient to explain the immediate effect on ICP (Murthy *et al.*, 1992); however, an important limitation to the HDT model is that HDT creates a nonphysiologic positive hydrostatic gradient between the heart and head for the CSF, and for the venous and arterial systems that is opposite of the normal hydrostatic pressure gradient in 1G. Thus, a critical question is whether microgravity results in a pressure gradient between the heart and the head that is similar to that seen in HDT. In theory, an increase in cerebral venous blood volume or cerebral venous pressure secondary to a reversal of the normal hydrostatic pressure gradient between the head and the heart should affect ICP via reduction of craniospinal compliance or reduction of CSF absorption. In microgravity, jugular veins do not collapse and are, in fact, distended. This observation has been interpreted as a sign of elevated CVP that can cause SSSP elevation and cerebral venous congestion/stagnation (Arbeille *et al.*, 2001; Harris *et al.*, 1997; Herault *et al.*, 2000), which could lead to increased ICP. However, this line of reasoning may not be valid. Although on Earth, jugular vein distension is a sign of increased CVP (Lewis, 1930; Magder, 2005), direct measurements in microgravity show that CVP is not elevated despite visible distension of the jugular veins (Arbeille *et al.*, 1995; Buckey *et al.*, 1993; Buckey *et al.*, 1996; Foldager *et al.*, 1996; Kirsch *et al.*, 1984). The jugular vein distension is explained by change in vascular compliance secondary to lack of gravitational influence on vessels and surrounding tissues.

Given that CVP is not elevated in microgravity, there is no reason to believe that SSSP is elevated in microgravity, and therefore a normal ICP/SSSP pressure gradient should exist to permit CSF absorption. Thus, it seems unlikely that changes in venous pressure would cause ICP elevation in microgravity. Even if ICP elevation in VIIP is not dependent on resistance to CSF absorption but is more dependent on increased venous pressure, as is seen in IIH, no evidence exists to suggest increased CVP, jugular venous pressure, or SSSP in microgravity. In the absence of additional data demonstrating CVP increase in long-term microgravity, conclusive evidence that cerebral venous congestion causes increased ICP is lacking.

4.2. *ICP, SSSP, and CVP are insufficiently low in microgravity*

Even though SSSP and CVP may not be significantly elevated in microgravity, an important consideration is that they may also not be sufficiently low to match the normal gravity-influenced reduction in ICP, SSSP, and CVP in the upright position in 1G. Thus, an alternate hypothesis is that prolonged exposure to inadequately low CVP and SSSP may influence ICP — or even the eye directly — to produce signs and symptoms of VIIP. Direct, invasive CVP and ICP measurements in humans during parabolic flight for brief (<20 seconds) exposure to microgravity, and 24 hours of HDT bed rest support this hypothesis (Lawley *et al.*, 2015); however, this hypothesis has yet to be tested in long-duration spaceflight in either animal models or humans.

4.3. *Increased abdominopelvic venous volume and pressure reduces spinal canal volume and craniospinal compliance*

Although venous pressure, venous blood volume, or both seem unlikely to increase SSSP and ICP in the cranial compartment, they may play a role in altering ICP via reduction of the spinal compartmental contribution to craniospinal compliance, i.e., an increase in venous pressure and blood volume below the heart in microgravity, rather than above it. Specifically, the known reduction of venous volume in the legs during spaceflight may displace venous blood into the abdominopelvic venous plexus, which is in direct communication with the lumbosacral epidural venous plexus, often called Batson's plexus (Batson, 1940). Changes in venous return from the lower body caused by compression of the inferior vena cava during pregnancy have been demonstrated to cause expansion of the lumbosacral epidural venous plexus, with a corresponding reduction in CSF volume of the subarachnoid space (Takiguchi *et al.*, 2006). Considering that the spinal compartment is responsible for approximately one-third of craniospinal compliance, it is plausible that reduction in volume of the spinal CSF compartment would alter craniospinal compliance, in essence shifting the compliance curve to the left so that levels of ICP that would not normally be associated with increased ICP pulse pressure would be associated with increased pulse pressure; however, craniospinal compliance has not been measured in these conditions.

4.4. *Increased cerebral capillary filtration increases cerebral interstitial fluid volume and ICP*

Another aspect of a cephalad fluid shift would be increased cerebral capillary filtration, as has been demonstrated in HDT (Parazynski, *et al.*, 1991), leading to increased volume of the brain interstitial fluid, which can increase ICP, similar to interstitial edema. Some research suggests that the CSF is in communication with the interstitial fluid and, in turn, with the cerebral capillaries, and that fluid transport between these three compartments may be as important to the regulation of CSF volume as are normal CSF production and absorption pathways (Brinker *et al.*, 2014; Cserr, *et al.*, 1986; MacAulay and Zeuthen, 2010; Orešković and Klarica, 2010). However, an MRI study of water distribution of the brain suggested that HDT does not increase the amount of water in either the CSF or the interstitial fluid (Caprihan *et al.*, 1999). The validity of the HDT model, as well as the hypothesis that increased capillary filtration causes ICP increase in microgravity, is challenged by mathematical simulation of ICP in microgravity, using an established model of human hydrodynamics (Stevens *et al.*, 2005). A simulation model with no hydrostatic pressure gradients and increased capillary filtration (based on experimental results) resulted in reduced ICP in microgravity as compared to that in supine position in 1G (Stevens *et al.*, 2005). Another simulation model of HDT, incorporating hydrostatic pressure gradients (Stevens *et al.*, 2005), showed an ICP increase in the same range that was observed in actual HDT experiments in humans (Murthy *et al.*, 1992).

4.5. *Lower blood pressure causes cerebral arteriolar vasodilation and ICP elevation*

Increase in cerebral arterial blood volume, i.e., arterial/arteriolar vasodilation, could result in increased ICP in the presence of impaired craniospinal compliance. Vasodilation could occur in response to a reduction in arterial blood pressure, as cerebral autoregulation maintains constant cerebral blood flow (CBF). In fact, vasomotor reactivity is considered to be the source of slow ICP variation known as B-waves (Auer and Sayama, 1983). Some evidence suggests that cardiac output increases and arterial blood pressure decreases during spaceflight (Arbeille *et al.*, 1995; Fritsch-Yelle, *et al.* 1996; Prisk *et al.*, 1993). However, stroke volume has been reported to increase in spaceflight compared to that when standing at 1G (Prisk *et al.*, 1993) or decrease (Arbeille *et al.*, 1995). It has also been reported that CBF velocity potentially increases (Arbeille *et al.*, 1995; Kawai *et al.*, 1993), which implies cerebral arteriolar vasodilation, given the reduction in blood pressure. However, results regarding cerebral vascular resistance are conflicting (Arbeille *et al.*, 1995), and at least some of the conclusions about CBF changes are based on HDT experiments (Alexander, *et al.*, 2012; Hargens and Tipton, 1996). Thus, while an increase in cerebral arterial blood volume secondary to arteriolar vasodilation is a plausible mechanism for increased ICP in the presence of impaired intracranial compliance, no experiments in microgravity have supported this hypothesis.

4.6. *Increased CO$_2$ concentration causes cerebral arteriolar vasodilation and ICP elevation*

Another potential cause of arteriolar vasodilation and increased ICP is hypercapnia; however, this would most likely occur only in the presence of impaired craniospinal compliance. Environmental CO$_2$ concentration is known to be elevated on the ISS and in conditions of long-term spaceflight (James *et al.*, 2011;

Scully, 2014), but a TCD study in 1G suggests that sustained hypercapnia does not produce any sustained effect on CBF or vasomotor reactivity (Sliwka *et al.*, 1996), most likely due to renal acid–base buffering mechanisms that correct the respiratory acidosis associated with hypercapnia (Seifter, 2014). The influence of localized pockets of CO_2 concentration that is higher than the ambient concentration has been posited, but has not yet been demonstrated to be a chronic or frequently occurring problem on the ISS (Scully, 2014). In theory, pockets of higher CO_2 concentration during sleep around the faces of astronauts with impaired intracranial compliance could provoke ICP elevation similar to the B-waves seen in sleep apnea (Auer and Sayama, 1983; Jennum and Børgesen, 1989; Newell *et al.*, 1992), but sleep studies in astronauts before, during, and after spaceflight have shown a reduction in sleep-disordered breathing in microgravity compared to pre- or post-flight (Elliott *et al.*, 2001).

4.7. *Impaired autoregulation causes cerebral arteriolar vasodilation and ICP elevation*

Some reports suggest that cerebrovascular autoregulation can be impaired during long-duration spaceflight (Blaber *et al.*, 2011; Zuj *et al.*, 2012), which could lead to a condition of persistent arteriolar vasodilation that could impair craniospinal compliance, but other reports are conflicting (Arbeille *et al.*, 1996; Iwasaki *et al.*, 2007). It must be considered that, to date, no evidence exists to support increased CBF or cerebral arteriolar vasodilation as a cause of ICP increase in microgravity.

5. Conclusion

The hypotheses analyzed in this chapter incorporate two main proposed mechanisms for ICP alteration in microgravity. The first suggests that a cephalad fluid shift directly causes ICP elevation. The second postulates that while baseline ICP is not elevated, conditions exist that impair craniospinal compliance and that small changes in environmental conditions (e.g., localized pockets of higher CO_2 concentration) or physiologic conditions (e.g., cerebral arteriolar vasodilation) could cause the ICP to elevate intermittently because of the impaired compliance. However, as of 2016, no experiment has directly demonstrated increased ICP or impaired craniospinal compliance in microgravity or spaceflight. Furthermore, careful evaluation of the physiologic processes that underlie these mechanisms can produce strong arguments that ICP should not be elevated, nor craniospinal compliance impaired in microgravity. Although it may be tempting to argue that only one of the proposed hypotheses is a predominant reason for ICP elevation in microgravity, if such elevation exists, the more likely cause is the cumulative effects of minor perturbations in all of the physiologic processes that govern ICP and craniospinal compliance. Finally, none of the mechanisms reviewed can explain why, in the few astronauts with VIIP who have had lumbar punctures after return to Earth, ICP has remained elevated. Ultimately, the contribution of ICP elevation or impaired craniospinal compliance to VIIP will depend on accurate measurements of these variables in astronauts before, during, and after long-duration spaceflight.

References

Alexander, DJ, *et al.* (2012). Risk of spaceflight-induced intracranial hypertension and vision alterations. *Human Research Program. Human Health Countermeasures Element.* Houston, TX: National Aeronautics and Space Administration. Lyndon B. Johnson Space Center. .

Andresen, M, *et al.* (2014). Effect of postural changes on ICP in healthy and ill subjects. *Acta Neurochirurgica,* 157, 109–113.

Arbeille, P, G Fomina, J Roumy, I Alferova, N Tobal and S Herault (2001). Adaptation of the left heart, cerebral and femoral arteries, and jugular and femoral veins during short- and long-term head-down tilt and spaceflights. *European Journal of Applied Physiology,* 86, 157–168.

Arbeille, P, F Achaïbou, G Fomina, JM Pottier and M Porcher (1996). Regional blood flow in microgravity: Adaptation and deconditioning. *Medicine and Science in Sports and Exercise,* 28, S70–S79.

Arbeille, P, G Fomina, F Achaibou, J Pottier and A Kotovskaya (1995). Cardiac and vascular adaptation to 0 g with and without thigh cuffs (Antares 14 and Altair 21 day Mir spaceflights). *Acta Astronautica,* 36(8–12), 753–762.

Auer, LM and I Sayama (1983). Intracranial pressure oscillations (B–waves) caused by oscillations in cerebrovascular volume. *Acta Neurochirurgica,* 68, 93–100.

Avezaat, CJJ and JHM Van Eijndhoven (1986). Clinical observations on the relationship between cerebrospinal fluid pulse pressure and intracranial pressure. *Acta Neurochirurgica,* 79, 13–29.

Batson, OV (1940). The function of the vertebral veins and their role in the spread of metastases. *Annals of Surgery,* 112(1), 138–149.

Bergsneider, M, I Yang, X Hu, DL McArthur, SW Cook and WJ Boscardin (2004). Relationship between valve opening pressure, body position, and intracranial pressure in normal pressure hydrocephalus: Paradigm for selection of programmable valve pressure setting. *Neurosurgery,* 55(4), 851–859.

Blaber, AP, N Goswami, RL Bondar and MS Kassam (2011). Impairment of cerebral blood flow regulation in astronauts with orthostatic intolerance after flight. *Stroke,* 42(7), 1844–1850.

Brimioulle, S, JJ Moraine, D Norrenberg and RJ Kahn (1997). Effects of positioning and exercise on intracranial pressure in a neurosurgical intensive care unit. *Physical Therapy*, 77(12), 1682–1689.

Brinker, T, EG Stopa, J Morrison and PM Klinge (2014). A new look at cerebrospinal fluid circulation. *Fluids Barriers CNS*, 11(1), 10.

Buckey, JC, FA Gaffney, LD Lane, BD Levine, DE Watenpaugh and CG Blomqvist (1993). Central venous pressure in space. *The New England Journal of Medicine*, 328(25), 1853–1854.

Buckey, JC Jr, FA Gaffney, LD Lane, BD Levine, DE Watenpaugh, SJ Wright, CW Jr Yancy, DM Meyer and CG Blomqvist (1996). Central venous pressure in space. *Journal of Applied Physiology*, 81(1), 19–25.

Caprihan, A, JA Sanders, HA Cheng and JA Loeppky (1999). Effect of head–down tilt on brain water distribution. *European Journal of Applied Physiology and Occupational Physiology*, 79(4), 367–373.

Chapman, PH, ER Cosman and MA Arnold (1990). The relationship between ventricular fluid pressure and body position in normal subjects and subjects with shunts: A telemetric study. *Neurosurgery*, 26(2), 181–189.

Johanson, CE, JA Duncan, III, PM Klinge, T Brinker, EG Stopa and GD Silverberg (2008). Multiplicity of cerebrospinal fluid functions: New challenges in health and disease. *Cerebrospinal Fluid Research*, 5, 10.

Cook, SW and M Bergsneider (2002). Why valve opening pressure plays a relatively minor role in the postural ICP response to ventricular 113 shunts in normal pressure hydrocephalus: Modeling and implications. *Acta Neurochirurgica Supplement*, 81, 15–17.

Cserr, HF, M Depasquale, CS Patlak and RG Pullen (1986). Convection of cerebral interstitial fluid and its role in brain volume regulation. *Annals of New York Academy of Science*, 481, 123–134.

Davson, H, JR Hollingsworth and MB Segal (1970). The mechanism of drainage of the cerebrospinal fluid. *Brain*, 93, 665–678.

Davson, H, K Welch, Segal and MB. (1987). *The Physiology and Pathophysiology of the Cerebrospinal Fluid*, Churchill Livingstone, New York, p. 1036.

Dawson, EA, NH Secher, MK Dalsgaard, S Ogoh, CC Yoshiga, J González-Alonso, A Steensberg and PB Raven (2004). Standing up to the challenge of standing: A siphon does not support cerebral blood flow in humans. *American Journal of Physiology — Regulatory, Integrative and Comparative Physiology*, 287(4), R911–914.

Edsbagge, M, G Starck, H Zetterberg, D Ziegelitz and C Wikkelso (2011). Spinal cerebrospinal fluid volume in healthy elderly individuals. *Clinical Anatomy*, 24, 733–740.

Edsbagge, M, M Tisell, L Jacobsson and C Wikkelso (2004). Spinal CSF absorption in healthy individuals. *American Journal of Physiology–Regulatory, Integrative and Comparative Physiology*, 287(6), R1450–R1455.

Elliott, AR, SA Shea, DJ Dijk, JK Wyatt, E Riel, DF Neri, CA Czeisler, JB West and GK Prisk (2001). Microgravity reduces sleep-disordered breathing in humans. *American Journal of Respiratory and Critical Care Medicine*, 164(3), 478–485.

Foldager, N, TA Andersen, FB Jessen, P Ellegaard, C Stadeager, R Videbaek and P Norsk (1996). Central venous pressure in humans during microgravity. *Journal of Applied Physiology*, 81(1), 408–412.

Fritsch-Yelle, JM, JB Charles, MM Jones and ML Wood (1996). Microgravity decreases heart rate and arterial pressure in humans. *Journal of Applied Physiology*, 80(3), 910–914.

Gauer, OH and HL Thron (1965). Postural changes in the circulation. In *Handbook of Physiology*, WF Hamilton (ed.), Vol. III, Sect. 2, Chapter 67, pp. 2409–2440. Washington, DC: American Physiological Society.

Gisolf, J, JJ van Lieshout, K van Heusden, F Pott, WJ Stok and JM Karemaker (2004). Human cerebral venous outflow pathway depends on posture and central venous pressure. *Journal of Physiology*, 560(Pt 1), 317–327.

Guillame, J and P Janny (1951). Manometrie intracranienne continue: interet de la methode et premiers resultats. *Revue Neurologique (Paris)*, 84, 131–142.

Hargens, AR and CM Tipton (1996). Cardiovascular adaptation to spaceflight. *Medicine and Science in Sports and Exercise*, 28(8), 977–982.

Harris, BA, RD Billica, SL Bishop, T Blackwell, CS Layne, DL Harm, GR Sandoz and EC Rosenow (1997). Physical examination during space flight. *Mayo Clinic Proceedings*, 72(4), 301–308.

Herault, S, G Fomina, I Alferova, A Kotovskaya, V Poliakov and P Arbeille (2000). Cardiac, arterial and venous adaptation to weightlessness during 6-month MIR spaceflights with and without thigh cuffs (bracelets). *European Journal of Applied Physiology*, 81, 384–390.

Hinghofer-Szalkay, H (2011). Gravity, the hydrostatic indifference concept and the cardiovascular system. *European Journal of Applied Physiology*, 111(2), 163–174.

Hung, OR, GM Hare and S Brien (2000). Head elevation reduces head-rotation associated increased ICP in patients with intracranial tumours. *Canadian Journal of Anaesthesia*, 47(5), 415–420.

Iwasaki, K, BD Levine, R Zhang, JH Zuckerman, JA Pawelczyk, A Diedrich, AC Ertl, JF Cox, WH Cooke, CA Giller, CA Ray, LD Lane, JC Buckey, Jr, FJ Baisch, DL Eckberg, D Robertson, I Biaggioni and CG Blomqvist (2007). Human cerebral autoregulation before, during and after spaceflight. *Journal of Physiology*, 579(Pt 3), 799–810.

James, JT, VE Meyers, W Sipes, RR Scully and CM Matty (2011). Crew health and performance improvements with reduced carbon dioxide levels and the resource impact to accomplish those reductions. *41st International Conference on Environmental Systems*. Portland, OR.

Jennum, P and SE Borgesen (1989). Intracranial pressure and obstructive sleep apnea. *Chest*, 95(2), 279–283.

Kajimoto, Y, T Ohta, H Miyake, M Matsukawa, D Ogawa, K Nagao and T Kuroiwa (2000). Posture-related changes in the pressure environment of the ventriculoperitoneal shunt system. *Journal of Neurosurgery*, 93(4), 614–617.

Kas'ian, II, VA Talavrinov, VI Luk'ianchikov and EA Kobzev (1980). Effect of antiorthostatic hypokinesia and space flight factors on changes in crural volume. *Kosm Biol Aviakosm Med*, 14(4), 51–55.

Kawai, Y, G Murthy, D Watenpaugh, G Breit, C Deroshia and A Hargens (1993). Effects of 24 hours head-down tilt on cerebral blood flow velocity in humans. *Journal of Applied Physiology*, 74(6), 3046–3051.

Kellie, G (1824). An account of the appearances observed in the dissection of two of three individuals presumed to have perished in the storm of the 3d, and whose bodies were discovered in the vicinity of Leith on the morning of the 4th, November 1821; with some reflections of the pathology of the brain. *Transaction of the Medico-Chirurgical Society Edinburgh*, 1, 84–169.

Kirsch, KA, FJ Baartz, HC Gunga and L Rocker (1993). Fluid shifts into and out of superficial tissues under microgravity and terrestrial conditions. *Clinical Investigation*, 71(9), 687–689.

Kirsch, KA, L Röcker, OH Gauer, R Krause, C Leach, HJ Wicke and R Landry (1984). Venous pressure in man during weightlessness. *Science, 13*, 225(4658), 218–219.

Lawley, J, M Williams, L Petersen, R Zhang, T Whitworth and B Levine (2015). ICP during daily life in healthy adults: What does microgravity add to the mix? *The FASEB Journal*, 29(1), 990.10.

Ledwith, MB, S Bloom, E Maloney-Wilensky, B Coyle, RC Polomano and PD Le Roux (2010). Effect of body position on cerebral oxygenation and physiologic parameters in patients with acute neurological conditions. *Journal of Neuroscience Nursing*, 42(5), 280–287.

Lee, ST (1989). Intracranial pressure changes during positioning of patients with severe head injury. *Heart Lung*, 18(4), 411–414.

Lewis, T (1930). Remarks on early signs of cardiac failure of the congestive type. *British Medical Journal*, 1(3618), 849–852.

Loman, J, A Myerson and D Goldman (1935). Effects of alterations in posture on the cerebrospinal fluid pressure. *Archives of Neurology and Psychiatry*, 33(6), 1279–1295.

Lundberg, N (1960). Continuous recording and control of ventricular fluid pressure in neurosurgical practice. *Acta Psychiatrica Neurologica Scandinavica*, 36, 1–193.

MacAulay, N and T Zeuthen (2010). Water transport between CNS compartments: Contributions of aquaporins and cotransporters. *Neuroscience*, 168(4), 941–956.

Magder, S (2005). How to use central venous pressure measurements. *Current Opinion in Critical Care*, 11(3), 264–270.

Magnæs, B (1976a). Body position and cerebrospinal fluid pressure. Part 1: Clinical studies on the effect of rapid postural changes. *Journal of Neurosurgery*, 44(6), 687–697.

Magnæs, B (1976b). Body position and cerebrospinal fluid pressure. Part 2: Clinical studies on orthostatic pressure and the hydrostatic indifferent point. *Journal of Neurosurgery*, 44, 698–705.

Magnæs, B (1989). Clinical studies of cranial and spinal compliance and the craniospinal flow of cerebrospinal fluid. *British Journal of Neurosurgery*, 3(6), 659–668.

Mahfoud, F, J Beck and A Raabe (2010). Intracranial pressure pulse amplitude during changes in head elevation: A new parameter for determining optimum cerebral perfusion pressure? *Acta Neurochirurgica*, 152(3), 443–450.

Marmarou, A, K Shulman and J LaMorgese (1975). Compartmental analysis of compliance and outflow resistance of the cerebrospinal fluid system. *Journal of Neurosurgery*, 43(5), 523–534.

Martins, AN, JK Wiley and PW Myers (1972). Dynamics of the cerebrospinal fluid and the spinal dura mater. *Journal of Neurology, Neurosurgery & Psychiatry*, 35(4), 468–473.

Mavrocordatos, P, B Bissonnette and P Ravussin (2000). Effects of neck position and head elevation on intracranial pressure in anaesthetized neurosurgical patients: Preliminary results. *Journal of Neurosurgical Anesthesiology*, 12, 10–14.

Monro, A (1783). *Observations on the Structure and Function of the Nervous System.* Edinburgh, Scotland: Creech and Johnson.

Moore, TP and WE Thornton (1987). Space shuttle inflight and postflight fluid shifts measured by leg volume changes. *Aviation, Space and Environmental Medicine*, 58 (9 Pt 2), A91–96.

Murthy, G, J Marchbanks, DE Watenpaugh, JU Meyer, N Eliashberg and AR Hargens (1992). Increased intracranial pressure in humans during simulated microgravity. *Physiologist*, 35, S184–S185.

Newell, DW, R Aaslid, R Stooss and HJ Reulen (1992). The relationship of blood flow velocity fluctuations to intracranial pressure B waves. *Journal of Neurosurgery*, 76(3), 415–421.

Ng, I, J Lim and HB Wong (2004). Effects of head posture on cerebral hemodynamics: Its influences on intracranial pressure, cerebral perfusion pressure, and cerebral oxygenation. *Neurosurgery*, 54(3), 593–597.

Orešković, D and M Klarica (2010). The formation of cerebrospinal fluid: Nearly a hundred years of interpretations and misinterpretations. *Brain Research Review*, 64(2), 241–262.

Parazynski SE, AR Hargens, B Tucker, M Aratow, J Styf and A Crenshaw (1991). Transcapillary fluid shifts in tissues of the head and neck during and after simulated microgravity. *Journal of Applied Physiology*, 71(6), 2469–2475.

Poca, MA, J Sahuquillo, T Topczewski, R Lastra, ML Font and E Corral (2006). Posture-induced changes in intracranial pressure: A comparative study in patients with and without a cerebrospinal fluid block at the craniovertebral junction. *Neurosurgery*, 58(5), 899–906.

Prisk, GK, HJ Guy, AR Elliott, RA 3rd Deutschman and JB West (1993). Pulmonary diffusing capacity, capillary blood volume, and cardiac output during sustained microgravity. *Journal of Applied Physiology*, 75(1), 15–26.

Quincke, H (1891). Die Lumbarpunktion des Hydrocephalus. *Klinische Wochenschrift*, 28, 965–968.

Qvarlander, S, N Sundström, J Malm and A Eklund (2013). Postural effects on intracranial pressure: Modeling and clinical evaluation. *Journal of Applied Physiology*, 115(10), 1474–1480.

Redzic, ZB and MB Segal (2004). The structure of the choroid plexus and the physiology of the choroid plexus epithelium. *Advanced Drug Delivery Reviews*, 56(12), 1695–716.

Rosomoff, HL (1961). Method for simultaneous quantitative estimation of intracranial contents. *Journal of Applied Physiology*, 16, 395–396.

Schwarz, S, D Georgiadis, A Aschoff and S Schwab (2002). Effects of body position on intracranial pressure and cerebral perfusion in patients with large hemispheric stroke. *Stroke*, 33(2), 497–501.

Scully, RR (2014). NASA technical interchange meeting on carbon dioxide. Summary report, Nassau Bay, TX.

Seifter, JL (2014). Integration of acid–base and electrolyte disorders. *The New England Journal of Medicine*, 371, 1821–1831.

Sliwka, U, JA Krasney, SG Simon and P Schmidt (1996). Effects of sustained low-level elevations of carbon dioxide on cerebral blood flow and autoregulation of the intracerebral arteries in humans. *Aviation, Space and Environmental Medicine*, 69, 299–306.

Spector, R, RF Keep, S Robert Snodgrass, QR Smith and CE Johanson (2015). A balanced view of choroid plexus structure and function: Focus on adult humans. *Experimental Neurology*, 267, 78–86.

Steinbach, GC, BR Macias, K Tanaka, WT Yost and AR Hargens (2005). Intracranial pressure dynamics assessed by noninvasive ultrasound during 30 days of bed rest. *Aviation, Space and Environmental Medicine*, 76(2), 85–90.

Stevens, SA, Lakin, WD and Penar, PL (2005). Modeling steady-state intracranial pressures in supine, head-down tilt and microgravity conditions. *Aviation, Space and Environmental Medicine*, 76(4), 329–338.

Sullivan, JT, S Grouper, MT Walker, TB Parrish, RJ McCarthy and CA Wong (2006). Lumbosacral cerebrospinal fluid volume in humans using three-dimensional magnetic resonance imaging. *Anesthesia and Analgesia*, 103, 1306–1310.

Takiguchi, T, S Yamaguchi, M Tezuka, N Furukawa and T Kitajima (2006). Compression of the subarachnoid space by the engorged epidural venous plexus in pregnant women. *Anesthesiology*, 105(4), 848–851.

Thornton, WE, GW Hoffler and JA Rummel (1977). *Anthropometric Changes and Fluid Shifts*. Washington, DC: Biomedical Results from the Skylab, NASA.

Valdueza, JM, T von Münster, O Hoffman, S Schreiber and KM Einhäupl (2000). Postural dependency of the cerebral venous outflow. *Lancet*, 355, 200–201.

von Storch, TC, E Carmichael and TE Banks (1937). Factors producing lumbar cerebrospinal fluid pressure in man in the erect posture. *Archives of Neurology and Psychiatry*, 38(6), 1158–1175.

Wagshul, ME, PK Eide and JR Madsen (2011). The pulsating brain: A review of experimental and clinical studies of intracranial pulsatility. *Fluids Barriers CNS*, 8(1), 5.

Wåhlin, A, K Ambarki, R Birgander, N Alperin, J Malm and A Eklund (2010). Assessment of craniospinal pressure-volume indices. *American Journal of Neuroradiology*, 31(9), 1645–1650.

Weed, LH and PS McKibben (1919). Experimental alteration of brain bulk. *American Journal of Physiology*, 48, 531–558.

Winkelman, C. (2000). Effect of backrest position on intracranial and cerebral perfusion pressures in traumatically brain-injured adults. *American Journal of Critical Care*, 9(6), 373–380.

Zuj, KA, P Arbeille, JK Shoemaker, AP Blaber, DK Greaves, D Xu and RL Hughson (2012). Impaired cerebrovascular autoregulation and reduced CO_2 reactivity after long duration spaceflight. *American Journal of Physiology — Heart and Circulatory Physiology*, 302, H2592–H2598.

High-Altitude Illness and Intracranial Pressure   6

Mark H. Wilson, PhD, MBBChir, FRCS (SN), FIMC, MRCA, FRGS

Consultant Neurosurgeon and Pre-Hospital Care Specialist,
Imperial College, London
The Institute of Pre-Hospital Care, London's Air Ambulance,
77 Mansell Street, London, E1 8AN, United Kingdom

1. Introduction

Over the last 50 years, the availability of air transport and the increasing demand for adventurous holidays has resulted in millions of people ascending to altitude to ski, trek, and climb. Others (e.g., astronomers, miners, railway men, and guides) have to ascend to altitude for work. In such people, high-altitude illness (HAI) has become a significant and often common medical condition. The prevalence very much depends on rate of ascent; however, approximately half of the trekkers who climb up to 5000 m are affected by acute mountain sickness (AMS) (Vardy *et al.*, 2006).

There are a number of comprehensive reviews relating to the epidemiology and management of HAI (Basnyat and Murdoch, 2003; Roach and Hackett, 2001; Wilson *et al.*, 2009). This chapter explains the pathophysiology behind the spectrum of conditions that make up HAI and then relates them to intracranial pressure (ICP). The similarities with the clinical condition of idiopathic intracranial hypertension (IIH) and visual impairment intracranial pressure (VIIP) are significant.

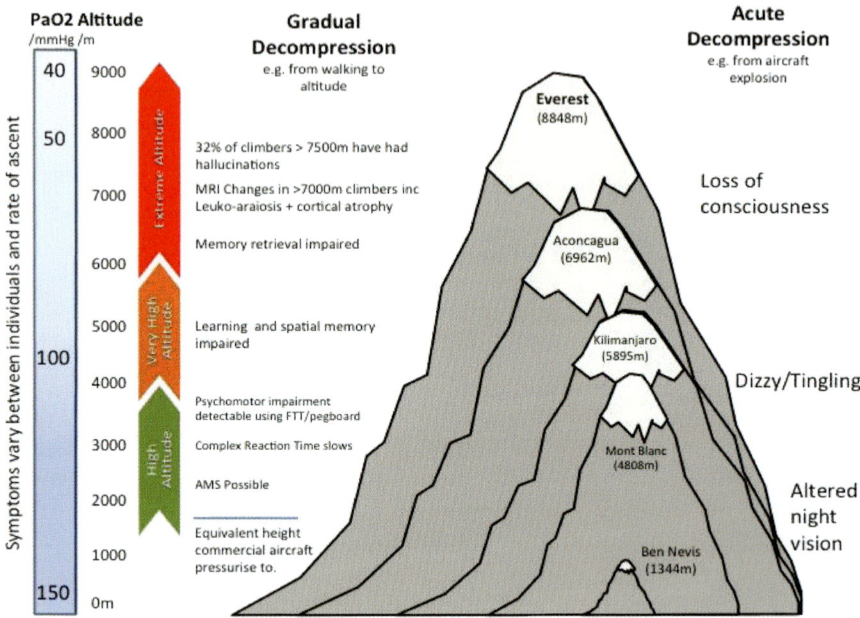

Figure 1. The relationship between altitude (classified as high [1500–3500 m], very high [3500–5500 m], and extreme [>5500 m]; Wilson *et al.*, 2009), the partial pressure of inspired oxygen (PiO$_2$), and some of the neurological consequences of acute and gradual exposure to these pressure changes.

1.1. *Changes in the atmosphere with altitude*

Although barometric pressure decreases exponentially with increasing altitude, the percentage of each gas component remains the same up to 12,000 m. The resulting reduction in partial pressure (Fig. 1) reduces the driving gradient of the oxygen cascade, which can in turn compromise oxygen delivery to the tissues.

The physiological response to compensate for this altered PiO$_2$ is to attempt to increase oxygen delivery — hyperventilation, tachycardia, erythropoietin-induced polycythemia, and increased cerebral blood flow help to maintain brain oxygenation (West *et al.*, 2007).

1.2. *Historical accounts of high-altitude hypoxia*

Plutarch (326 BC) described several features of mountain sickness during Alexander's march over India (Plutarch, 1912) as did Rustinian during Marco

Polo's exploration of Tibet (1298 AD) (Castelló-Roca, 1993); however, it wasn't until the advent of the hot air balloon that the more acute effects of high-altitude exposure were appreciated.

In 1862, Glaisher and Coxwell, two British balloonists ascended over 8800 m (Glaisher, 1862; Rodway, 2007; West, 2004), with Glaisher reporting paralysis of his arms and legs and sudden loss of vision before losing consciousness. Coxwell lost the use of his hands and had to use his teeth the pull the cord to descend the balloon. After landing they walked seven miles home with no residual neurological deficits. Thirteen years later a similar event in France resulted in the death of two balloonists.

It was, however, Thomas Ravenhill, a Birmingham medical graduate, who, in 1913 while working as a medical officer at the Collahuasi and Poderosa mines in northern Chile (at altitudes between 4690 and 4940 m), first classified HAI and described the features of both high-altitude cerebral and pulmonary edema.

1.3. *The spectrum of HAI*

Hypobaric hypoxia has a number of effects, the occurrence of which can largely be reduced by slowing the rate of ascent to allow for acclimatization. The spectrum of pathology has classically been thought of as (in increasing order of severity) — high-altitude headache (HAH); AMS and then potentially life threatening, high-altitude cerebral edema (HACE). Current recommendations are to sleep no higher than 300 m above the previous high altitude with a rest day for every 1000 m climbed — "Climb high, sleep low".

- **High-Altitude Headache**

The International Headache Society (Fischer *et al.*, 2004) defined the diagnostic criteria for HAH as (i) headache exhibiting at least two of the following character-istics: frontal or fronto-temporal, dull or pressing, mild or moderate and aggravated by exertion, movement, straining, coughing or bending, and associated with; (ii) ascent to altitude over 2500 m, and which; (iii) has developed in the last 24 h and; (iv) resolves within 8 h of descent.

HAH commonly occurs in visitor at altitude and can be difficult to distinguish from dehydration headache. It should resolve with simple analgesics/stopping ascent. If there is no improvement, descent should be advised.

- **Acute Mountain Sickness**

AMS is often considered the next stage of HAI. The Lake Louise Consensus Group defined AMS as the presence of headache in an unacclimatized person who has recently arrived at an altitude above 2500 m, plus the presence of one or more of the following: gastrointestinal symptoms; anorexia, nausea, or vomiting; insomnia; dizziness; and lassitude or fatigue (Roach *et al.*, 1993). A scoring system to quantify severity of AMS was also devised (Roach *et al.*, 1993).

Currently, it is not possible to predict from sea level data, who will develop AMS and who will not. Risk factors include: rapid ascent, exertion, past history of altitude illness, young adults, and possibly a genetic predisposition.

AMS management comprises simple analgesia and descent to a lower altitude. If this is not possible or if the severity is increasing, a physician may consider administration of acetazolamide, dexamethasone, supplemental oxygen, and if very severe then use a portable hyperbaric chamber.

● **High-Altitude Cerebral Edema**

The headache of high altitude is sometimes considered a spectrum with severity increasing through AMS to potentially life-threatening HACE. It is diagnosed clinically in people who have recently arrived at altitude, most of whom have had features of AMS or high-altitude pulmonary edema. It is characterized by psychiatric changes of varying degree, confusion, ataxia of gait, and disturbances of consciousness that may progress to deep coma (Hackett and Roach, 2004). At around 4500 m, the prevalence in trekkers is thought to be 0.5%–1% (Hackett *et al.*, 1976). Management consists of urgent descent, oxygen, dexamethasone (8–10 mg iv, im, or PO then 4 mg 6 hourly). If descent is not possible and the airway can be protected, a portable hyperbaric chamber can be used.

Note — the term edema in the title implies a pathological process although the syndrome is clinically diagnosed. Hypoxia itself, not necessarily with edema, can often cause neurological symptoms, which may be thought to be HACE.

2. Pathophysiological Theories of HAI

Other than a previous history of altitude illness, no current methods are available to determine individual susceptibility to HAI. This indiscriminate nature of AMS lead Ross in 1985 to write of "the random nature of cerebral mountain sickness" (Ross, 1985). This is based on the Monro–Kellie doctrine (Monro, 1783) of the skull being a closed box and hence if a mass (tumor/blood/edema) increases in volume in the skull something else has to be displaced or pressure will rise. This "tight fit" hypothesis proposed that interindividual variation in neuro-axis compliance accounted for the vulnerability to AMS. If correct, those with proportionally greater cerebrospinal fluid (CSF) volumes should be able to buffer cerebral swelling and be less susceptible to HAH. There is a paucity of evidence to support this (Fig. 2).

This "Tight Fit" theory (based on an anatomical/compliance model) has stood for 20 years although there is relatively little evidence (Wilson *et al.*, 2009). Hackett

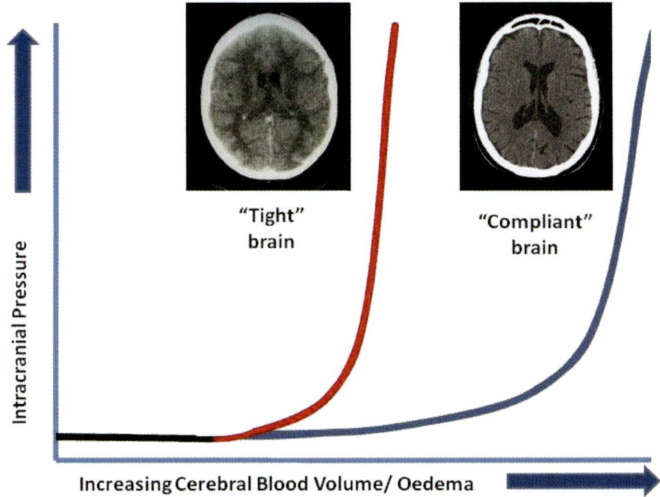

Figure 2. Hypothetical pressure: volume graphs demonstrating the pressure changes that occur with additional intracranial mass and how Ross's "Tight Fit" hypothesis may enact. A normal "tight" brain has less surrounding space to swell with edema than an atrophic "compliant" brain. The CSF is thought to act as a buffer. As the brain swells, CSF can be displaced down the spinal canal.

and Roach provided an additional physiological component to this baseline theory (Roach and Hackett, 2001). Climbers who were more prone to hypoxemia (especially with exercise) and hence edema formation would in turn have more cerebral swelling. Hence, a combination of this physiological predisposition with a lack of (anatomical predisposition) cerebral compliance could account for interindividual differences.

2.1. *Evidence for the role of ICP*

If the "tight fit" hypothesis is true, elevated ICP should underpin the development of AMS. However, studying this is difficult. Direct ICP measures are invasive. Indirect measures have inaccuracies and confounders.

2.2. *Direct invasive ICP measurement*

Brian Cummins, a neurosurgeon from Bristol, United Kingdom, is the only investigator to have directly monitored ICP in humans at altitude (Wilson and Milledge, 2008). He first investigated ICP in three climbers using a telemetric ICP monitoring device inserted prior to departure. Only the youngest subject developed AMS. All of them had normal ICPs at rest at all altitudes (ICP = <20 mmHg). However, the youngest subject suffered a dramatic rise in ICP at 4725 m during any form of mild exertion. Mild exertion and neck turning can reduce venous outflow and shift an individual from "compensating" to the "decompensating" region of cerebral compliance curve, resulting in exponential elevations in ICP (to 24 mmHg). However, this limited data set precludes definitive conclusions.

2.3. *Indirect invasive ICP measurement*

2.3.1. *Lumbar CSF pressure*

A few studies have undertaken lumbar puncture at altitude to assess lumbar CSF pressures. Schaltenbrand (1933) found a rise in lumbar CSF pressures in several subjects in normobaric hypoxia; however, the distress of the procedure may have been a confounder. Singh *et al.* (1969) demonstrated increased lumbar spinal CSF pressures in 34 Indian soldiers who were rapidly transported from sea level to 5867 m. At altitude, lumbar CSF pressures were 6–21 cm H_2O higher than sea-level baseline. However, this may reflect acute decompression effects and no relationship with AMS/HACE was shown. Hartig and Hackett demonstrated, in three subjects, that acute hypoxic gas inhalation resulted in a rise in lumbar CSF pressure. In contrast, gradual decompression to a simulated ascent of 5000 m was not associated with any change, even in those in whom AMS developed (Hartig and Hackett, 1992). Similarly, Bailey *et al.* (2006) found lumbar CSF pressures to be normal after exposure to 18 h of 12% O_2 and identified no difference in pressures between hypoxia (12.4 ± 5 cm H_2O) and normoxia (13.2 ± 5.2 cm H_2O, $n = 13$) and AMS (11.8 ± 3.7 cm H_2O $n = 8$) and non-AMS (11.8 ± 3.7 cm H_2O $n = 11$) groups.

2.4. *Noninvasive ICP measurements*

A number of noninvasive ICP measuring techniques have been used to infer ICP at altitude. Unfortunately, none are used in routine clinical practice, mainly because of concerns over accuracy.

2.4.1. *Tympanic membrane displacement*

Tympanic membrane displacement (TMD) relies on a patent cochlear aqueduct to transmit pressures from CSF to the inner ear fluids. The technique was used to study 34 subjects ascending to 5200 m (Wright *et al.*, 1995). The results suggested a rise in ICP with acute hypoxia (with rapid ascent to 3400 m), but no additional rise in those who developed mild to moderate AMS.

2.4.2. *Pulsatility index*

Transcranial Doppler is a popular noninvasive tool for monitoring cerebral blood flow noninvasively. Gosling's pulsatility index (PI) is the ratio of (systolic velocity — diastolic velocity)/mean velocity. The normal value is less than 1. A good correlation between PI and ICP has been demonstrated across a broad range of intracranial pathologies (Bellner *et al.*, 2004; Cardoso and Kupchak, 1992; Moreno *et al.*, 2000; Rainov *et al.*, 2000). Correlation appears best with ICPs greater than 20 mmHg, hence PI may be a poor measure of ICP when in the normal or mildly elevated range.

Ter Minassian used PI during a simulated ascent of Everest (Operation Everest III) in 2001 (Ter Minassian *et al.*, 2001). Eight subjects were decompressed to 5000, 6000, 7000, and 8000 m. All measurements were three days after "arrival" although at 8000 m, they were performed 4 h after arrival. They demonstrated a reduction in PI at each altitude, which conflicts with a rise in ICP being associated with a rise in PI. Of note, however, the $PaCO_2$ values also fell dramatically and this hyperventilatory response to hypobaric hypoxia may alter the interpretation of PI (a decrease in $PaCO_2$ causes cerebral vasoconstriction). Variations in $PaCO_2$ have previously been shown to alter PI independently (Czosnyka *et al.*, 1996).

2.4.3. *Optic nerve sheath diameter*

Optic nerve sheath diameter (ONSD) is largely regarded as one of the best noninvasive ICP monitoring techniques (Shevlin, 2015). Sutherland studied 13 mountaineers using ultrasound with regression analysis to explore correlation with a number of variables. ONSD was positively associated with increasing altitude (0.1 mm increase per 1000 m 95% CI 0.05–0.14) and AMS score (0.12 mm per Lake Louise Score [CI 0.06–0.18]). Associations were also found with resting heart rate and arterial oxygen saturation (0.2 mm increase per 10% SaO_2 decrease) (Sutherland *et al.*, 2008). A larger study of 287 subjects demonstrated a larger mean optic nerve sheath diameter (ONSD: 5.34 mm, 95% CI 5.18–5.51 mm) in AMS sufferers compared to nonsufferers (4.46 mm, 95% CI 4.39–4.54 mm) (Fagenholz *et al.*, 2009). However, a more recent study of 23 subjects failed to demonstrate a difference in ONSD between AMS sufferers and nonsufferers (Lawley *et al.*, 2012).

2.4.4. *Retinal imaging*

Papilledema (optic disc swelling) is a clinical sign indicative of a raised ICP. Papilledema has been seen with HACE (Wright *et al.*, 1983). Up to 55% of climbers at 6865 m have a degree of optic disc swelling (Bosch *et al.*, 2008). In addition, retinal vasculature may reflect changes in cerebral vasculature. Many studies have demonstrated both retinal arterial and venous distension with hypobaric hypoxia. Bosch *et al.* (2008) demonstrated a correlation of arterial and venous distension with headache; however, no such correlation was shown in a similar study by Willmann *et al.* (2013). This may reflect difficulties in measuring the subjective severity of headache. Wilson *et al.* (2013) demonstrated a correlation between retinal venous distension and HAH burden. While venous changes may not directly reflect ICP, they probably reflect intracranial venous pressures.

2.4.5. *Cerebral imaging*

Computed tomography scans of climbers suffering from high-altitude pulmonary edema and neurological dysfunction have demonstrated a degree of tightness (small ventricles and effaced cerebral sulci) (Koyama *et al.*, 1988). However, magnetic resonance imaging (MRI) scans demonstrating HACE are not always consistent with a "tight" brain that would cause a high ICP (Wilson *et al.*, 2009).

It has been postulated that HACE can be due to cytotoxic (intracellular) edema (Houston and Dickinson, 1975), while others have suggested it has a vasogenic origin, extracellular fluid secondary to increased blood–brain barrier permeability (Hackett *et al.*, 1998). Both should cause an increase in brain parenchymal volume hence MRI is a tool that has been used to investigate this. Diffusion weighted MRI in particular can distinguish the two forms of edema.

Unfortunately, most studies have small numbers. Morocz *et al.* demonstrated a 2.77% (36.2 mL) mean increase in brain matter volume in nine subjects with a simulated ascent to 4572 m (Morocz *et al.*, 2001). This increase was only in gray matter and did not correlate with AMS symptoms. In contrast, another study exposed 10 subjects to a simulated altitude of 4500m. Although eight developed AMS symptoms, none demonstrated cerebral edema on MRI. However, they demonstrated that ventricular CSF volume decreased in all subjects, especially those with severe AMS. This implies something other than brain parenchyma increases in volume.

Kallenberg *et al.* went further in an attempt to distinguish the nature of the edema. They exposed 22 subjects to $FiO_2 = 12\%$ (approximately equivalent to 4500 m) for 16 h. Half suffered AMS and the mean degree of cerebral swelling was 7 ± 4.8 mL (approximately 0.5% brain volume). T2 relaxation time (T2rT) was used to assess parenchymal water content and apparent diffusion coefficient (ADC) assessed the diffusibility of water. ADC distinguishes vasogenic (as water moves extracellularly it becomes more diffusible and hence ADC increases) from cytotoxic edema (as water moves intracellularly it has restricted diffusion and ADC falls). Hypoxia caused a generalized increase in T2rT implying parenchymal edema. Those with AMS had consistently lower ADC values implying an additional cytotoxic (intracellular) component to edema in this group. Additionally, those who developed AMS had a greater brain: intracellular volume ratio supporting the "tight fit" hypothesis. In a different study exposing nine subjects to N_2 enriched air (to create isobaric hypoxia) for 6 hours ADC values negatively correlated with severity of cerebral symptoms (Schoonman *et al.*, 2008) again supporting the theory that there is a general vasogenic edema with hypoxia with an additional intracellular component in AMS.

There is, however, inconsistency in studies. Dubowitz demonstrated cerebral swelling and ventricular compression with 40 min of hypoxia but did not demonstrate edema (Dubowitz *et al.*, 2009). This in contrast implies a change in intracerebral blood volume, hence it may be that the duration of hypoxia exposure is important in determining how much parenchymal volume change relates to vascular engorgement and how much relates to edema.

In a recent 22-hour normobaric 12% hypoxic model, early vascular changes were seen to precede the development of cerebral edema. There appeared to be evidence that venous outflow restriction might play a role in the formation of cerebral edema. At 22 hours, there was an increase in total brain parenchymal whole brain white and gray matter volumes, and a reduction in intracranial CSF volumes. Cumulative Lake Louise scores at 22 h correlated with the increases in total brain white matter (Sagoo *et al.*, 2016).

2.4.6. *MRI-ICP measurement*

MRI-ICP is a technique using MRI to infer ICP. It has been well validated in normoxia. The technique uses cardiac gated velocity encoding cine phase contrast imaging, a measurement of arterial inflow (internal carotid and vertebral arteries), venous outflow (internal jugular veins), and pulsatile CSF. Further details are found elsewhere in this book. Using this technique, Lawley *et al.* studied 13 subjects in 12% normobaric hypoxia. The major findings in this study were that although there was no change in ICP or cerebral perfusion pressure despite an increase in brain volume, there was a statistically significant relationship between change in ICP and AMS severity ($R^2 = 0.71$, $B = 2.3$, $P < 0.01$) after 10 hours.

In summary, most MRI studies have demonstrated an increase in parenchymal volume which may represent vascular engorgement and/or edema (which appears to be vasogenic, but can have an additional cytotoxic component in those symptomatic). Further studies are required to demonstrate if this is the contribution of vascular and edema to parenchymal swelling varies over time.

2.4.7. *Potential importance of the venous system in hypoxia and microgravity*

Extreme hypoxia dramatically increases cerebral blood flow (Wilson *et al.*, 2011a). It would appear that in some subjects, venous outflow may not be able to accommodate this increase resulting in venous engorgement, demonstrable both with MRI and retinal imaging (Wilson *et al.*, 2013). The phenotypical headaches caused by stretching of the venous structures have largely been forgotten since awake craniotomies are relatively rare (Ray and Wolff, 1940); however, the headache of high altitude has very similar properties to the headache of IIH. Patients with IIH suffer loss of peripheral vision. We now understand the IIH is commonly due to venous sinus restriction resulting in venous and then intracranial hypertension (Ball and Clarke, 2006). Because of this we proposed that relative inability to drain venous blood could underlie both headache of high altitude and VIIP (Wilson *et al.*, 2011b). In the case of hypoxia, the driver is the increase in arterial inflow. In the case of microgravity, possibly increased venous pressures secondary to the loss of gravitational pull to the legs could restrict cerebral outflow. The importance of the venous system in ICP is often forgotten. Interestingly at the turn of the last century, the venous role was much more appreciated (Hill, 1896). Figure 3 demonstrates, using a running bath analogy, how the dynamic component of in and outflow of blood can have a great effect on ICP. It is impor-

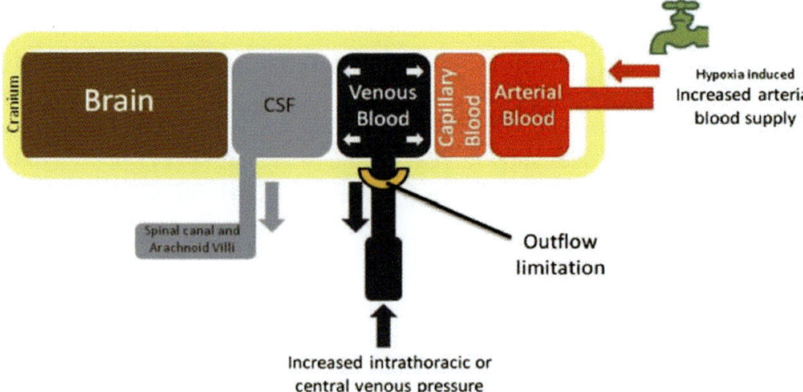

Figure 3. Modified Monro–Kellie doctrine. The CSF and venous system buffer increases in brain, arterial, or other intracranial volume, but this is a dynamic system. Small restrictions in outflow or large increases in inflow, which cannot be compensated for will cause venous engorgement.

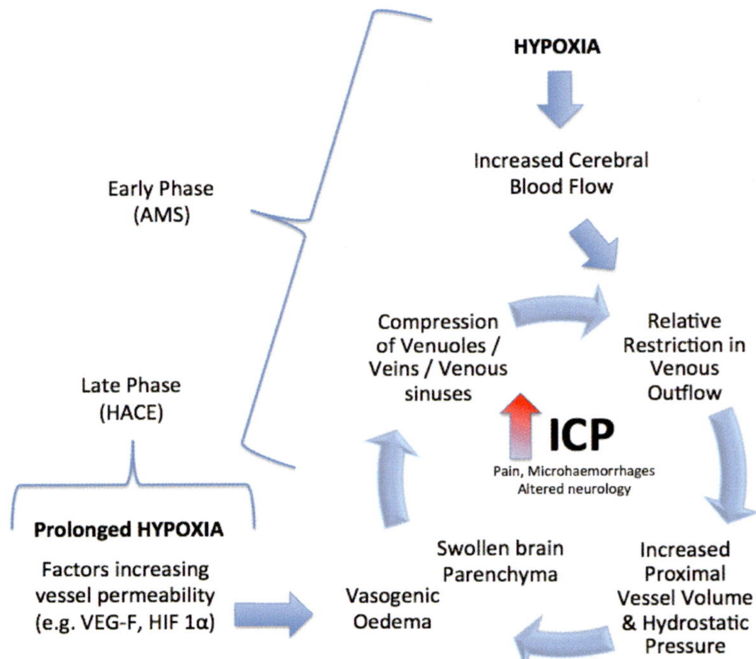

Figure 4. Hypothetical diagram demonstrating that a cycle can form where increased cerebral blood flow and relative venous outflow restriction causes hydrostatic edema formation and hence cerebral swelling. This in turn can compress and restrict further venous drainage (Wilson and Imray, 2015).

tant to remember that the volumes of flow are significant. Between 800 mL and 1 L of arterial blood enters the cranium each minute. That is a significant volume also to drain.

Figure 4 demonstrates how a cycle could theoretically develop in which cerebral swelling can compress cerebral venules further impairing cerebral venous drainage.

3. Conclusion

There has not been a study conclusively demonstrating a rise in ICP in a large number of subjects with exposure to hypoxia or with AMS/HACE. There is, however, good evidence of increased parenchymal volume with concurrent displacement/reduction of CSF. Some studies have demonstrated this occurs without edema, others have implied that edema occurs. This discrepancy may relate to the duration of hypoxia, with early parenchymal volume change relating to vascular engorgement before the formation of edema. It would appear that relative inability to drain blood from the cranium may be a primary problem both in HAH and VIIP.

References

Bailey, DM, *et al.* (2006). Free radical-mediated damage to barrier function is not associated with altered brain morphology in high-altitude headache. *Journal of Cerebral Blood Flow Metabolism*, 26(1), 99–111.

Ball, AK and CE Clarke (2006). Idiopathic intracranial hypertension. *Lancet Neurology*, 5(5), 433–442.

Basnyat, B and DR Murdoch (2003). High-altitude illness. *Lancet*, 361(9373), 1967–1974.

Bellner, J, *et al.* (2004). Transcranial Doppler sonography pulsatility index (PI) reflects intracranial pressure (ICP). *Surgical Neurology*, 62(1), 45–51, discussion 51.

Bosch, MMM, *et al.* (2008). High incidence of optic disc swelling at very high altitudes. *Archives of Ophthalmology*, 126(5), 644–650.

Cardoso, ER and JA Kupchak (1992). Evaluation of intracranial pressure gradients by means of transcranial Doppler sonography. *Acta Neurochirurgica Supplementum (Wien)*, 55, 1–5.

Castelló-Roca, A. (1993). *Hombre, Montaña y Medicina [Man, Mountains and Medicine]*. Barcelona: Editor Service.

Czosnyka, M, *et al.* (1996). Relationship between transcranial Doppler-determined pulsatility index and cerebrovascular resistance: an experimental study. *Journal of Neurosurgery*, 84(1), 79–84.

Dubowitz, DJ, *et al.* (2009). Early brain swelling in acute hypoxia. *Journal of Applied Physiology (Bethesda, MD: 1985)*, 107(1), 244–252.

Fagenholz, PJ, *et al.* (2009). Optic nerve sheath diameter correlates with the presence and severity of acute mountain sickness: Evidence for increased intracranial pressure. *Journal of Applied Physiology*, 106(4), 1207–1211.

Fischer, R, *et al.* (2004). No evidence of cerebral oedema in severe acute mountain sickness. *Cephalalgia: An International Journal of Headache*, 24(1), 66–71.

Glaisher, J (1862). Notes of effects experienced during recent balloon ascents. *Lancet*, 2, 559–560.

Hackett, PH and RC Roach (2004). High altitude cerebral edema. *High Altitude Medicine Biology*, 5(2), 136–146.

Hackett, PH, *et al.* (1998). High-altitude cerebral edema evaluated with magnetic resonance imaging: clinical correlation and pathophysiology. *JAMA: The Journal of the American Medical Association*, 280(22), 1920–1925.

Hackett, PH, D Rennie and HD Levine (1976). The incidence, importance, and prophylaxis of acute mountain sickness. *Lancet*, 2(7996), 1149–1155. Available at: http://www.ncbi.nlm.nih.gov/entrez/query.fcgi?cmd=Retrieve&db=PubMed&dopt=Citation&list_uids=62991.

Hartig, GS and P Hackett (1992). Cerebral spinal fluid pressure and cerebral blood velocity in acute mountain sickness. In *Hypoxia and Mountain Medicine*, Sutton, JR, G Coates, CS Houston (eds.), pp. 260–265. Oxford: Pergamon Press.

Hill, L (1896). *The Physiology and Pathology of the Cerebral Circulation*. London: J&A Churchill. Available at: https://ia600507.us.archive.org/2/items/physiologypathol00hill/physiologypathol00hill.pdf.

Houston, CS and J Dickinson (1975). Cerebral form of high-altitude illness. *Lancet*, 2(7938), 758–761.

Koyama, S, *et al.* (1988). The increased sympathoadrenal activity in patients with high altitude pulmonary edema is centrally mediated. *Japanese Journal of Medicine*, 27(1), 10–16.

Lawley, JS, *et al.* (2012). Optic nerve sheath diameter is not related to high altitude headache: a randomized controlled trial. *High Altitude Medicine Biology*, 13(3), 193–199.

Monro, A (1783). *Observations on the Structure and Function of the Nervous System*. Edinburgh: Creech and Johnson.

Moreno, JA, *et al.* (2000). Evaluating the outcome of severe head injury with transcranial Doppler ultrasonography. *Neurosurgical Focus*, 8(1), e8.

Morocz, IA, *et al.* (2001). Volumetric quantification of brain swelling after hypobaric hypoxia exposure. *Experimental Neurology*, 168(1), 96–104.

Plutarch (1912). *Alexander and Caesar*. London: Heinemann.

Rainov, NG, JB Weise and W Burkert (2000). Transcranial Doppler sonography in adult hydrocephalic patients. *Neurosurgical Review*, 23(1), 34–38.

Ray, BS and HG Wolff (1940). Experimental studies on headache: pain-sensitive structure of the head and their significance to headache. *Archives of Surgery*, 41(4), 813–856.

Roach, RC, P Bärtsch, O Oelz and P Hackett (1993). Lake Louise AMS Scoring Consensus Committee. The Lake Louise acute mountain sickness scoring system. In Sutton, JR, CS Houston, G Coates, (eds.), *Hypoxia and Molecular Medicine*, pp. 272–274. Burlington: Queen City Press.

Roach, RC and PH Hackett (2001). Frontiers of hypoxia research: Acute mountain sickness. *Journal of Experimental Biology*, 204(Pt 18), 3161–3170.

Rodway, GW (2007). Limb paralysis and visual changes during Glaisher and Coxwell's 1862 balloon ascent to over 8800 m. *High Altitude Medicine and Biology*, 8(3), 256–259.

Ross, RT (1985). The random nature of cerebral mountain sickness. *Lancet*, 1(8435), 990–991.

Sagoo, RS, CE Hutchinson, A Wright, C Handford, H Parsons, V Sherwood, S Wayte, S Nagaraja, E N'gandwe, M Wilson and CHE Imray, for the Birmingham Medical

Research and Expedition Society (2016). MR investigation of the potential mechanisms involved in the development of high altitude cerebral oedema. *Journal of Cerebral Blood Flow and Metabolism*, 37(1): 319–331.

Schaltenbrand, G (1933). Atmospheric pressure, circulation, respiration and cerebrospinal fluid pressure. *Acta Aerophysiol*, 1: 65–78.

Schoonman, GG, *et al.* (2008). Hypoxia-induced acute mountain sickness is associated with intracellular cerebral edema: A 3 T magnetic resonance imaging study. *Journal of Cerebral Blood Flow Metabolism*, 28(1), 198–206.

Shevlin, C (2015). Optic nerve sheath ultrasound for the bedside diagnosis of intracranial hypertension: Pitfalls and potential. *Critical Care Horizons*, 1(1), 22–30.

Singh, I, *et al.* (1969). Acute mountain sickness. *New England Journal of Medicine*, 280(4), 175–184.

Sutherland, AI, *et al.* (2008). Optic nerve sheath diameter, intracranial pressure and acute mountain sickness on Mount Everest: A longitudinal cohort study. *British Journal of Sports Medicine*, 42(3), 183–188.

Ter Minassian, A, *et al.* (2001). Doppler study of middle cerebral artery blood flow velocity and cerebral autoregulation during a simulated ascent of Mount Everest. *Wilderness Environmental Medicine*, 12(3), 175–183.

Vardy, J, J Vardy and K Judge (2006). Acute mountain sickness and ascent rates in trekkers above 2500 m in the Nepali Himalaya. *Aviation, Space, and Environmental Medicine*, 77(7), 742–744.

West, JB (2004). Paralysis and blindness during a balloon ascent to high altitude. *High Altitude Medicine and Biology*, 5(4), 453–456.

West, JB, RB Schoene and JS Milledge (2007). *High Altitude Medicine and Physiology*, 4th Ed. London: Hodder Arnold.

Willmann, G, *et al.* (2013). Missing correlation of retinal vessel diameter with high-altitude headache. *Annals of Clinical and Translational Neurology*, 1(1), 59–63.

Wilson, MH and CHE Imray (2015). The cerebral venous system and hypoxia. *Journal of Applied Physiology (Bethesda, MD: 1985)*, p.jap.00327.2015.

Wilson, MH and J Milledge (2008). Direct measurement of intracranial pressure at high altitude and correlation of ventricular size with acute mountain sickness: Brian Cummins' results from the 1985 Kishtwar expedition. *Neurosurgery*, 63(5), 970–974, discussion 974–975.

Wilson, MH, *et al.* (2013). Cerebral venous system and anatomical predisposition to high-altitude headache. *Annals of Neurology*, 73(3), 381–389.

Wilson, MH, MEG Edsell, *et al.* (2011a). Cerebral artery dilatation maintains cerebral oxygenation at extreme altitude and in acute hypoxia — an ultrasound and MRI study. *Journal of Cerebral Blood Flow Metabolism*, 31(10), 2019–2029.

Wilson, MH, CHE Imray and AR Hargens (2011b). The headache of high altitude and microgravity — similarities with clinical syndromes of cerebral venous hypertension. *High Altitude Medicine and Biology*, 12(4), 379–386.

Wilson, MH, S Newman and CH Imray (2009). The cerebral effects of ascent to high altitudes. *Lancet Neurology*, 8(2), 175–191.

Wright, AD, *et al.* (1983). Altitude-related deaths in seven trekkers in the Himalayas. *Thorax*, 38(9), 646–656.

Wright, AD, *et al.* (1995). Intracranial pressure at high altitude and acute mountain sickness. *Clinical Science (London)*, 89(2), 201–204.

Noninvasive Measurement of Intracranial Pressure with the Vittamed Absolute Value Meter

7

Eric M. Bershad, MD and Richard Dunham, MD

Baylor College of Medicine, 1 Baylor Plaza, Houston, TX 77030, USA

1. Introduction

Elevated intracranial pressure (ICP) indicates a severe disturbance of intracranial physiology and requires rapid diagnosis to avoid permanent neurological sequelae related to tissue displacement or impairment of cerebral perfusion pressure. Symptoms, such as nausea, vomiting, headache, declining levels of consciousness, or visual changes may suggest elevated ICP, but these are nonspecific. An absolute measurement of ICP is required to confirm the diagnosis so the underlying etiology can be addressed. In special relationship to the visual impairment intracranial pressure (VIIP) syndrome of long-duration astronauts, ICP has not been definitely measured to this point. A noninvasive absolute ICP measurement that can be performed multiple times in various astronauts under different conditions would be ideal to better understand the VIIP syndrome, and allow for early detection of intracranial hypertension to institute countermeasures.

ICP is traditionally measured by insertion of a catheter through the skull or lumbar thecal sac, but these procedures carry a small risk of intracranial hemorrhage, meningitis, or brain herniation. These risks are largely unacceptable on critical missions, such as spaceflight, where medical care for complications is limited, and loss of astronaut productivity may jeopardize spaceflight operations. Furthermore, there is an urgent need to develop an accurate, precise, and reliable noninvasive modality for measuring the absolute ICP value, without the need for patient specific calibration not only in outer space, but also on Earth.

2. Normal ICP Physiology

The intracranial components including the brain and spinal cord are enclosed by the skull and meninges, and remain at pressures between 5.0 mmHg and 14.7 mmHg under normal physiological conditions in the supine position (Reilly and Bullock, 2005). The bony skull and dura matter are relatively rigid, so volume is fixed within this space relatively. As described by the Monro (1783) and Kellie (1824) doctrine and subsequent iterations, an increase in one intracranial component, including blood, brain, or cerebrospinal fluid (CSF), will result in a decrease of a different component or else the ICP will rise (Reilly and Bullock, 2005). The relationship between the intracranial volume (V) and ICP is commonly described as intracranial compliance ($\Delta V / \Delta$ ICP), or more precisely, the elastance ($\Delta ICP / \Delta V$). As the elastance increases (compliance decreases) due to increased intracranial volume, ICP will increase (Bershad *et al.*, 2008). Brain tissue can be displaced as ICP increases and herniate or lead to other severe injuries from compression. Secondly, elevated ICP may impair cerebral blood flow (CBF), due to decreased cerebral perfusion pressure (i.e., CPP = Arterial Pressure – ICP). With monitoring of ICP, one may be able to detect disturbances in the intracranial physiology and implement countermeasures to prevent or attenuate permanent neurological deficits, related to chronically or periodic ICP evaluation. In astronauts, ICP measurements may help alert NASA physicians to astronauts who may be at risk for visual deficits related to impairment of the optic nerve and related structures.

3. Noninvasive ICP Monitoring

Many have hypothesized that microgravity alters cerebral hemodynamics, hydrodynamics (CSF flow), and venous drainage from the brain. However, only limited invasive ICP data are available from postlumbar puncture in selected astronauts (Mader *et al.*, 2011). The inherent risks of direct ICP measurement in space have deterred in-flight evaluations.

Noninvasive ICP assessment has been reported using a variety of methods (Kristiansson *et al.*, 2013), including fundoscopic exam (Steffen *et al.*, 1996), electroencephalogram (Chen *et al.*, 2012), optic nerve sheath diameter (Geeraerts *et al.*, 2007, 2008; Kimberly *et al.*, 2008; Nicolleto and Burkman, 2009; Rajajee *et al.*, 2011; Strumwasser *et al.*, 2011), tympanic membrane displacement (Reid *et al.*,

1989), otoacoustic emissions (Buki *et al.*, 1996, 2009), Pulsed phase lock loop technology (Steinbach *et al.*, 2005; Ueno *et al.*, 2003a, 2003b, 2005), computerized tomography (CT) scan (Toutant *et al.*, 1984; Eisenberg *et al.*, 1990; Mizutani *et al.*, 1990; Miller *et al.*, 2004; Rosenberg *et al.*, 2011), magnetic resonance imaging (MRI) (Xie *et al.*, 2013), near-infrared spectroscopy (Ghosh *et al.*, 2012), and scanning laser tomography (Heckmann *et al.*, 2004). All these approaches are based on correlation of ICP changes with some anatomical or physiological changes in the human intracranial media, skull, ear, or eye. Many of these techniques have not been validated, have not provided accurate quantitative measurements, or have other serious limitations. Correlation based methods require individual person specific calibration (Dietrich, 1991) with an invasive ICP "gold standard" measurement device, given that multiple inter-subject differences in anatomical and physiological variables exists that would preclude an absolute ICP value determination in a given person.

Absolute measurements of ICP in microgravity would enable better pathophysiologic understanding of the mechanisms and provoking factors for the VIIP syndrome. With these measurements, astronauts at risk could be identified before subsequent neurologic impairment. Early assessment has become a high priority for NASA as longer spaceflights are requiring longer exposures to microgravity. In this chapter, we will discuss a novel approach to noninvasive ICP measurement using the Vittamed two–depth Transcranial Doppler (TCD), which is based on balancing the effect of ICP on the intracranial ophthalmic artery (IOA) by applying external pressure to the orbital tissues. Similar to noninvasive arterial blood pressure measurement, patient-specific calibration is not required.

4. TCD Principles

TCD is an inexpensive and portable imaging modality used in a variety of clinical settings. Some routine clinical uses for TCD include detection of vasospasm after subarachnoid hemorrhage, intracranial vessel stenosis or occlusions in stroke patients, emboli detection, cerebral autoregulation, assessment of venous to arterial shunts, confirmation of brain death, and estimation of intracranial pressure.

All TCD devices have essentially the same components (Nicolleto and Burkman, 2009). TCD typically uses frequencies near 2 MHz ultrasound to continuously monitor intracranial arterial blood flow pulse waves. Electrical energy is transduced into ultrasonic waves, which are projected from a small probe into the skin and deeper tissues. Pulse wave technology uses pulses of ultrasound waves instead of a continuous stream. The ultrasound waves interfacing with the tissue produce echoes reflected from the moving blood inside an insonated vessel that are received by the device and transformed into blood flow velocity waveforms.

The penetrating depth of the ultrasound depends on the underlying tissue and the ultrasound frequency. Higher frequencies do not penetrate as far as lower ones, but have higher resolution. For example, a 1 MHz ultrasound penetrates up to about 4 cm in muscle and 15 cm in fat, and a 2 MHz ultrasound will only penetrate half as far as 1 MHz. Adjustments in frequency are used to change the depth of insonation. TCD devices use a lower frequency to insonate deeper arteries (Kremkau, 1995). An artery can be followed along its course through the brain by changing the depth at which the device detects the flow, and the angle of insonation. An important concept regarding TCD is that it measures cerebral blood flow velocities (CBFV), but not CBF. If the arterial diameter remains constant, one can estimate CBF, but in the setting of vasospasm or other conditions where the diameter of the arteries change, the relationship is nonlinear.

TCD power refers to the total energy delivered to the tissue. As the ultrasound waves pass through the tissue, energy is absorbed and lost as heat. When scanning through sensitive tissues, such as the orbit, the power should be minimized based on established safety standards to prevent thermal or cavitation injury. The gradual reduction of ultrasound amplitude, known as signal attenuation, relates proportionally to the distance and types of tissue the waves traverse. Increasing the gain on the device will increase the signal intensity, which can be used if the signal is too weak from deeper arteries.

Intracranial arterial waveforms have systolic peaks and diastolic troughs. If the artery is a high-resistance vessel, there may be smaller diastolic flow. The internal carotid artery, for example, is low resistance and has strong diastolic flow between the systolic peaks. The morphology can be analyzed to provide data about velocity and flow. Two common measures for evaluating a waveform are mean cerebral blood flow velocity (MCBFV)[1] and pulsatility index (PI),[2] which compares systolic flow to diastolic flow independently from the insonation angle.

Arteries can be accurately identified based on the location (cranial window) of the probe, depth and angle of insonation, vessel resistance, mean flow velocities, and arterial waveforms. The ophthalmic artery (OA) and supraclinoid internal carotid arteries are visualized through a transorbital window, which is easily obtained by placing the probe over a closed eyelid. Ideally, arteries are insonated at zero degrees, which means that the direction of the probe is parallel to the vessel as if looking into a pipe.

---

[1] MCBFV = (systolic velocity − diastolic/3) + diastolic velocity.

[2] PI = peak systolic velocity − end diastolic velocity/peak systolic velocity + end diastolic velocity.

5. OA Characteristics

Blood flow to the brain occurs primarily through three main arteries, the carotid arteries in the anterolateral neck and the posterior basilar artery. These arteries have to pass through a stiff protective covering of dura mater when entering the cranium or when exiting branches leave to supply other tissues. The OA is the first intracranial branch of the internal carotid artery, and passes through the subarachnoid space and subsequent dura mater en route to the orbit. After the intracranial ophthalmic artery (IOA) passes through the dura mater, it is referred to as the extracranial ophthalmic artery (EOA), which can be seen in (Fig. 1A). The compartmentalization of the OA between intracranial and extracranial space, allows for the determination of ICP based on the difference in blood flow characteristics between these two contiguous OA segments as will be described below (Fig. 1B).

6. Vittamed Two-Depth TCD Based NonInvasive ICP Meter

Traditional TCD imaging is limited to scanning at one depth, but flow at one arterial segment has been insufficient in quantifying ICP. TCD reliability and reproducibility may vary due to operating factors, such as the angle of insonation, location of acoustic windows to find strong pulse signals, and accurate depths of insonation. Vessels may vary considerably between individuals and these variations will lead to baseline differences in flow and arterial waveform morphology. Using one measurement in one vessel would require complex adjustments to account for these confounding variables including vessel radius, resistance, differences in autoregulation, baseline blood pressures, hematocrit, comorbidities, and other systemic differences would also provide confounding results.

There have been many approaches to correlate one-depth TCD data with ICP. The relationship between increased TCD flow velocities and increased ICP was first described using the resistance index (Klingelhofer *et al.*, 1987, 1988). The most commonly used TCD variable to correlate blood flow with ICP is PI, but the correlation coefficients comparing Doppler studies and direct ICP measurements have varied widely (Rainov *et al.*, 2000; Moreno *et al.*, 2000; Bellner *et al.*, 2004; Voulgaris *et al.*, 2005; Figaji *et al.*, 2009; Behrens *et al.*, 2010; Strumwasser *et al.*, 2011; Gura *et al.*, 2011; De Riva *et al.*, 2012).

The IOA and EOA are contiguous segments of the OA; therefore the hemodynamic variables are the same. However, given the dural border between these segments, the IOA blood flow is more directly influenced by the transmural force of ICP. As the IOA passes through the subarachnoid space, transmural pressure from the surrounding CSF modulates blood flow and the arterial waveform. The

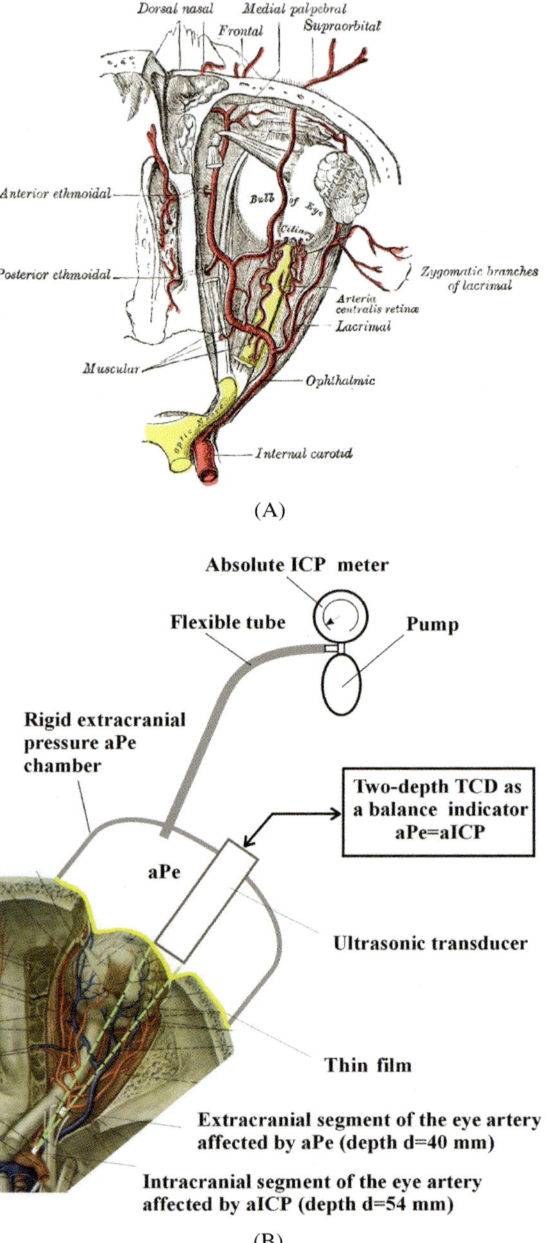

Figure 1. (A) Ophthalmic artery anatomy http://en.wikipedia.org. (B) Schematic of vittamed two–depth Transcranial Doppler (TCD) apparatus used to quantify when the extracranial pressure chamber (aPe) and intracranial Pressure (ICP) balance. (Zakelis, 2012b).

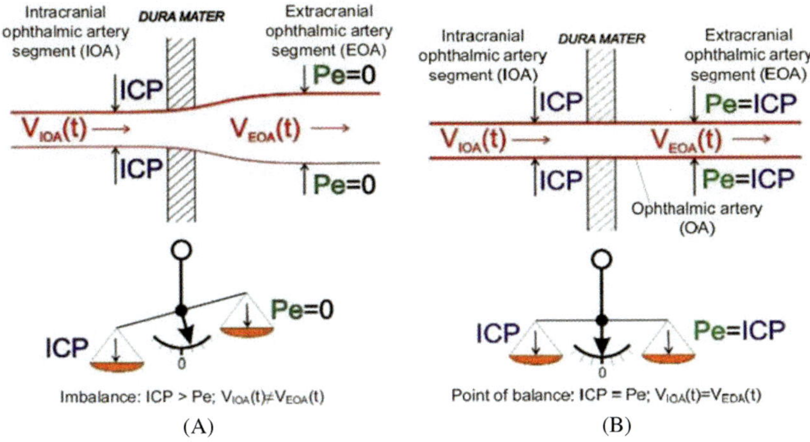

Figure 2. (A, left): Normally, the transmural pressure on the intracranial ophthalmic artery (IOA) from surrounding CSF compresses the vessel lumen and results in increased mean flow velocity (V) of blood compared to the extracranial ophthalmic artery (EOA) (Zakelis, 2012b). (B, right): When an external pressure (Pe) is applied to the extracranial portion of the OA, the velocity of flow becomes the same as the IOA and intracranial pressure (ICP) can be estimated (Zakelis, 2012a).

EOA does not have the transmural exposure to the ICP due to the dural border, and the waveform thus has slightly different characteristics. Specifically, the mean velocity of blood flow will be higher in the IOA segment as velocity is inversely related to the OA diameter and the IOA lumen decreases slightly due to a higher transmural pressure from ICP (Fig. 2A and 2B)

The Vittamed two–depth TCD based noninvasive ICP meter uses these principles to isolate ICP as the variable of measurement. By applying an external transmural pressure (Pe) to the orbital tissues, the EOA blood flow velocity morphological characteristics are matched with those of the IOA. Once the morphology of the waveforms in the IOA and EOA becomes similar, the ICP can be estimated because ICP = Pe at a given pressure level. Further technical details concerning the device are reviewed in the doctoral thesis by Rolandas Zakelis (Zakelis, 2012b).

Two–depth TCD imaging simultaneously insonates the OA at two locations (IOA and EOA) using two different depths. The subject/patient is outfitted with an open helmet that adjusts to head circumference. Underneath the helmet a deflated pressure cuff is be placed next to the eye. The transducing ultrasonic Doppler probe is inserted through the eyepiece and the opening of the pressure cuff. The probe is secured against the closed eyelid. The angle of the probe can be adjusted along six degrees of freedom to identify the proper angle that will simultaneously insonate the intracranial and extracranial ophthalmic artery segments (Fig. 3).

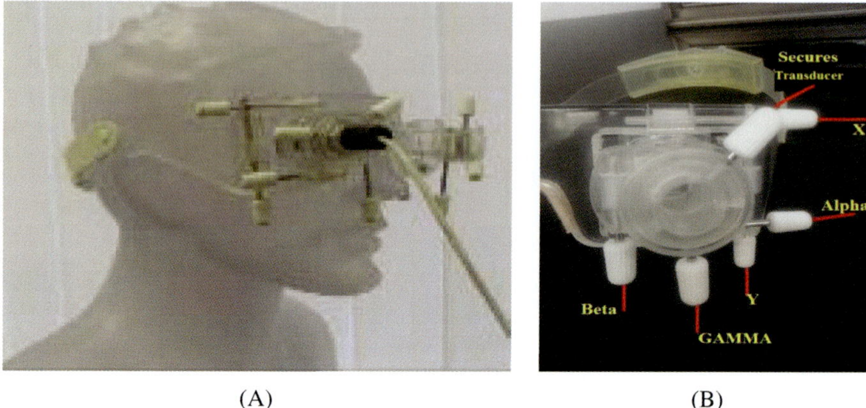

(A) (B)

Figure 3. (A) The helmet is placed around the eyes with a securing strap that connects behind the head. The black Transcranial Doppler (TCD) probe inserts through the eyepiece. (Courtesy of Arminas Ragauskas). (B) The angle of insonation is achieved by twisting knobs (X, Y, Alpha, Beta, GAMMA) that move the affixed probe in various degrees of freedom (Zakelis, 2012b).

The average depth for insonating the IOA and EOA were determined by anatomical studies of normal OA anatomy. The EOA depth ranges from 43 to 47 mm, and the IOA is usually found around 53–57 mm from the surface of the eyelid (Ragauskas *et al.*, 2012). After locating the EOA and IOA with the ultrasound probe, the automated part of the noninvasive ICP measurement begins. When the blood flow spectrograms are stable, the extraocular pressure is increased by pneumatic inflation of a small periorbital pressure cuff in stepwise increments of 2 mmHg, 3 mmHg, or 4 mmHg. Depending on the clinical scenario the range of pressure measurement can be selected. For example, if the ICP is absolutely unknown, one approach would be to start with a broad measurement from 0 to 40 mmHg using steps of 8 mmHg, and then perform a subsequent measurement with small pressure Pe increments of 4 mmHg steps in a small range to achieve a more precise measurement.

The pressure cuff increases external pressure Pe around the eye through the selected range. After the last pressure step, the cuff deflates, and an analysis of the IOA and EOA blood flow morphology at each pressure level is conducted automatically, with the best Pe match used to determine the ICP, which is automatically displayed on the screen (Fig. 4).

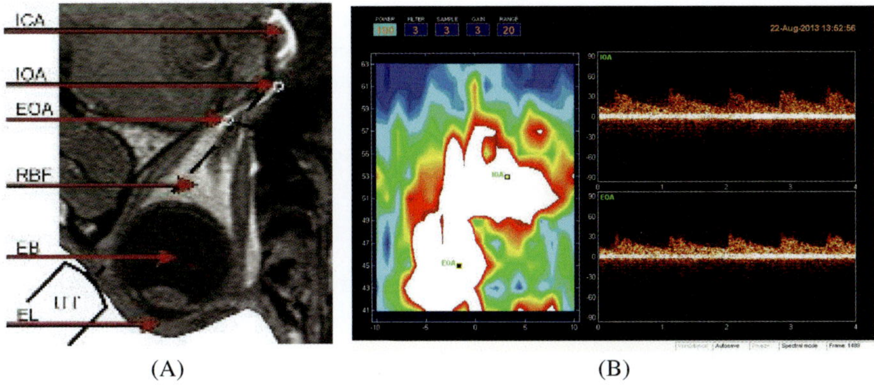

(A)　　　　　　　　　　　　　　　　(B)

Figure 4. (A) The image is an MRI view of the orbit with a schematic of an ultrasonic transducer. ICA internal carotid artery, IOA internal ophthalmic artery, EOA external ophthalmic artery, RBF retrobulbar fat, EB eyeball, EL eyelid, UT ultrasound transducer (Bartusis *et al.*, 2012). (B) Two-depth TCD monitor. The image (left) shows the color-coded signal intensity strengths, which correspond to the pulsatile IOA arterial waveforms (right) of the OA segments. (Courtesy of Eric Bershad).

7. Contraindications to Two-Depth TCD Measurement

Generally, this approach is low-risk for major adverse events given that the ultrasonic energy delivered to tissues is relatively brief and under the recommended maximum for insonation of orbital tissues (50 mW/cm^2). There is a theoretical risk for injury in some patients with uncommon ocular disorders including severe glaucoma, eye surgery with implants, corneal scarring, injury, anatomical abnormalities. However, in most cases, as long as one eye is intact, a measurement is possible. The usual maximum applied pressure to the orbital tissues (40 mmHg) is equivalent to the pressure experienced by diving under water approximately at 1.8 feet (40 mmHg).

7.1. *Previous and ongoing clinical studies*

Ragauskas and coworkers compared the noninvasive insonation of the OA using the Vittamed two-depth TCD and noninvasive absolute ICP value measurements comparing with simultaneous lumbar puncture (LP) measurements of ICP in 62 neurologic patients (Ragauskas *et al.*, 2012). The device was highly accurate with a low mean systemic error (0.12 mmHg) and precise with low SD of paired recordings (2.19 mmHg). However, the study was limited because most of the subjects had normal or mildly elevated ICP (<20 mmHg), therefore clinical validation in the higher range and by independent investigators would be ideal. Negligible systematic error in this study indicated that no systematic bias was present within the ICP range measured in this study.

8. Baylor College of Medicine and National Space Biomedical Research Institute Study

Phase 1 trial data (unpublished) at BCM Eric Bershad, principal investigator, evaluated the reproducibility and operability of the Vittamed two-depth TCD in 28 healthy subjects using 7 different operators. The subjects were Hispanic (50.0%), Caucasian (35.7%), and African American (14.3%). The operators (both novice and expert) were able to insonate both OA segments in 83.9% (141 of 168 subjects) at a median of 16 minutes. Once the arteries were located by insonation, an ICP measurement was obtained in 68% of the studies at a median of 8 min.

The repeatability of measurements was good and was estimated using 17 pairs of consecutive measures, Pearson correlation coefficient 0.577 ($P = 0.015$). We note that repeatability measurements in a human subject without invasive ICP monitoring are limited by the normal physiological variability of ICP and uncertainty of the true ICP. Using 10 pairs of measures, there was good inter-eye agreement, Pearson correlation coefficient 0.711 ($P = 0.021$). This study is ongoing in order to collect more data in healthy volunteers for reproducibility measurements (two consecutive trained operators in the same subject).

Twenty-four paired measurements of Vittamed versus lumbar CSF pressure (lumbar puncture) were made in 24 different subjects, mostly with idiopathic intracranial hypertension. The average difference between non-invasive and invasive ICP was 4.5 mmHg (SD 3.1). Bland Altman analysis showed that the 95% limits of agreement were −10.5 to +11.0 mmHg. There was negligible systematic bias between the invasive and non-invasive methods (0.25 mmHg). Technical factors precluded measurement in about 50% of enrolled patients. Further versions of the device have been developed and undergoing evaluation.

8.1. *Potential limitations*

One of the limitations of this approach is anatomic variation. The OA appears to have an intradural origin in 88%–95% of people (Erdogmus and Govsa, 2006), but this may account for some cases of insonation failure since the OA may have extradural origin in a small percentage of people. In our early experience, we have encountered several other obstacles, but we have found possible solutions. First, eye movements can change the location of the OA segments and lead to difficulty with insonation due to the small size of the artery. In this case, we found that providing a target for visual fixation with intermittent pausing for relaxation minimizes this problem. Second, the helmet should be tightly secured. Otherwise, the helmet may shift when the pressure cuff inflates, and the angle of insonation can be lost. Third, the ICP may not be calculated if the preselected pressure range measured does not include the balance point where IOA and EOA averaged pulse wave spectrograms match. Finding the appropriate range can be ensured by a prescreening measurement that includes a wide range of ICP (for example, 0–40 mmHg) with pressure steps of 8 mmHg, and then performing a subsequent measurement using a closer spaced pressure step interval of 4 mmHg. Future software development will include automatic analysis of the required pressure range to measure. Lastly, the operator requires significant training in insonation and maintaining the signals throughout the study. This limitation is being addressed with development of automated robotic scanning with the ultrasonic transducer, and improvements that will reduce some of the manual scanning currently required.

8.2. *Safety measures*

The device was determined to be nonsignificant risk status by the FDA, as long as specific exclusion criteria were applied for preexisting ophthalmological conditions. These included conditions would theoretically increase the risk for ocular injury if excessive pressure was applied to the orbital tissues. For the purposes of our research study, we chose to be conservative, and included many conditions that will likely be relative rather than absolute contraindications.

Our Phase 1 study evaluated several safety parameters. There was a trend toward decreasing intraocular pressure from pre- to postmeasurement, which is likely related to increased outflow of aqueous humor due to transorbital pressure. No significant hemodynamic changes systolic pressure or pulse rate were seen. The diastolic pressure decreased by 2.3 mmHg postmeasurement, but this is not clinically significant.

9. Future Aims

There are several modifications to the current version of the device which are being developed that will improve the portability of the hardware and reduce the

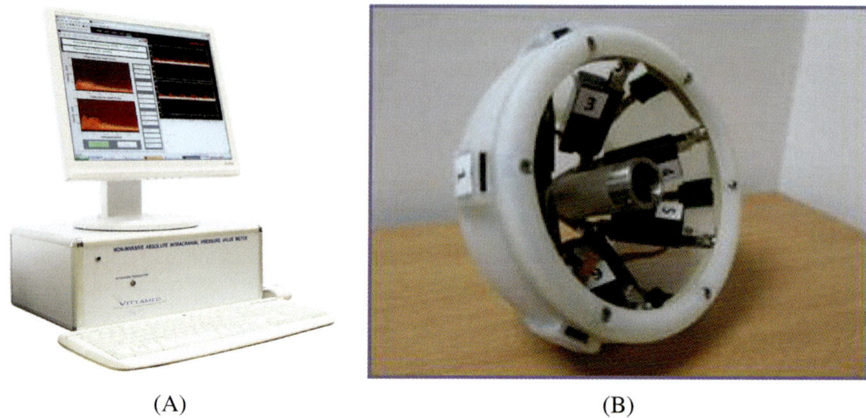

(A)   (B)

Figure 5. (A, left) Hardware components including Doppler, pressure chamber, computer integrated in one box (Courtesy of Arminas Ragauskas). (B, right) Robotic probe prototype for automatic scanning of TCD (Courtesy of Arminas Ragauskas).

need for operator expertise to identify and measure the OA signals. These include automated detection of the OA blood flow velocities, hardware integration of the Doppler, computer and pressure chambers components into one box, improved helmet design, quicker measurement time, and automated determination of the measuring range (Figs. 5A and 5B).

There is a significant population both in space (astronauts) and globally on Earth at risk for increased ICP, including those with intracerebral hemorrhages, subarachnoid hemorrhages, and traumatic brain injury hydrocephalus, pseudotumor cerebri (idiopathic intracranial pressure), anoxic brain injury, concussion, who need frequent monitoring of ICP. This device represents a unique and promising means for noninvasive monitoring of ICP, and further study and development of this device is needed.

Acknowledgments

We thank Arminas Ragauskas, ScD, Rolandas Zakelis, PhD, Laimonas Bartusis, MS, and Vytautas Petkas for providing technical support for the Vittamed device and training, and providing some of the figures in this chapter. We thank the National Space Biomedical Research Institute for funding our study.

References

Bartusis, L, R Zakelis, G Daubaris, A Ragauskas, S Rutkauskas, V Matijosaitis and A Preiksaitis (2012). Ophthalmic artery as a sensor for non-invasive intracranial pressure measurement electronic system. *Electronics and Electrical Engineering Kaunas: Technologija*, 122, 45–48.

Behrens, A, N Lenfeldt, K Ambarki, J Malm, A Eklund and L Koskinen (2010). Transcranial Doppler pulsatility index: Not an accurate method to assess intracranial pressure. *Neurosurgery*, 66, 1050–1057.

Bellner, J, B Romner, P Reinstrup, K Kristiansson, E Ryding and L Brandt (2004). Transcranial Doppler sonography pulsatility index (PI) reflects intracranial pressure (ICP). *Surgical Neurology*, 62, 45–51.

Bershad, E, W Humphreis and J Suarez (2008). Intracranial hypertension. *Seminars in Neurology*, 28, 690–702.

Buki, B, P Avan, J Lemaire, M Dordain, J Chazal and O Ribari (1996). Otoacoustic emissions: A new tool for monitoring intracranial pressure changes through stapes displacements. *Hearing Research*, 94, 125–139.

Buki, B, F Giraudet and P Avan (2009). Non-invasive measurements of intralabyrinthine pressure changes by electrocochleography and otoacoustic emissions. *Hearing Research*, 251, 51–59.

Chen, H, J Wang, S Mao, W Dong and H Yang (2012). A new method of intracranial pressure monitoring by EEG power spectrum analysis. *Canadian Journal of Neurological Science*, 39, 483–487.

De Riva, N, K Budohoski, P Smielewski, M Kasprowicz, CZ weifel, L Steiner, M Reinhard, N Fábregas, J Pickard and M Czosnyka (2012). Transcranial Doppler Pulsatility Index: what it is and what it isn't. *Neurocritical Care*, 17, 58–66.

Dietrich, C (1991). *Uncertainty, Calibration and Probability: The Statistics of Scientific and Industrial Measurement*. Boca Raton: CRC Press.

Eisenberg, H, HJ Gary, E Aldrich, C Saydjari, B Turner, M Foulkes, J Jane, A Marmarou, L Marshall and H Young (1990). Initial CT findings in 753 patients with severe head injury. A report from the NIH Traumatic Coma Data Bank. *Journal of Neurosurgery*, 73, 688–698.

Erdogmus, S and F Govsa (2006). Anatomic features of the intracranial and intracanalicular portions of ophthalmic artery: For the surgical procedures. *Neurosurgical Review*, 29, 213–218.

Figaji, A, E Zwane, A Fieggen, P Siesjo and J Peter (2009). Trancranial Doppler pulsatility index is not a reliable indicator of intracranial pressure in children with severe traumatic brain injury. *Surgical Neurology*, 72, 389–394.

Geeraerts, T, Y Launey, L Marin, J Pottecher, B Vigue, J Duranteau and D Benhamou (2007). Ultrasonography of the optic nerve sheath may be useful for detecting raised intracranial pressure after severe brain injury. *Intensive Care Medicine*, 33, 1704–1711.

Geeraerts, T, S Merceron, D Benhamou, B Vigue and J Duranteau (2008). Non-invasive assessment of intracranial pressure using ocular sonography in neurocritical care patients. *Intensive Care Medicine*, 34, 2062–2067.

Ghosh, A, C Elwell and M Smith (2012). Review article: Cerebral near-infrared spectroscopy in adults: A work in progress. *Anesthesia & Analgesia*, 115, 1373–1383.

Gura, M, I Elmaci, R Sari and N Coskun (2011). Correlation of pulsatility index with intracranial pressure in traumatic brain injury. *Turkish Neurosurgery*, 21, 210–215.

Heckmann, J, M Weber, A Junemann, B Neundorfer and C Mardin (2004). Laser scanning tomography of the optic nerve vs CSF opening pressure in idiopathic intracranial hypertension. *Neurology*, 13;62, 1221–1223.

Homburg, A, M Jakobsen and E Enevoldsen (1993). Transcranial Doppler recordings in raised intracranial pressure. *Acta Neurologica Scandinavica*, 87, 488–493.

Kimberly, HH, S Shah, K Marill and V Noble (2008). Correlation of optic nerve sheath diameter with direct measurement of intracranial pressure. *Acadamic Emergency Medicine*, 15, 201–204.

Klingelhofer, J, B Conrad, R Benecke and D Sander (1987). Intracranial flow patterns at increasing intracranial pressure. *Klinische Wochenschrift*, 65, 542–545.

Klingelhofer, J, B Conrad, R Benecke, D Sander and E Markakis (1988). Evaluation of intracranial pressure from transcranial Doppler studies in cerebral disease. *Journal of Neurology*, 235, 159–162.

Kremkau, F (1995). *Doppler Ultrasound: Principles and Instruments.* Philadelphia: WB Saunders Company.

Kristiansson, H, E Nissborg, JJ Bartek, M Andresen, P Reinstrup and B Romner (2013). Measuring elevated intracranial pressure through noninvasive methods: A review of the literature. *Journal of Neurosurgical Anesthesiology*, 25, 372–385.

Mader, TH, CR Gibson, AF Pass, LA Kramer, A GLee, J Fogarty, WJ Tarver, JP Dervay, DR Hamilton, A Sargsyan, JL Phillips, D Tran, W Lipsky, J Choi, C Stern, R Kuyamjian and JD Polk. (2011). Optic disc edema, globe flattening, choroidal folds, and hyperopic shifts observed in astronauts after long-duration space flight. *Ophthalmology*, 118, 2058–2069.

Miller, M, M Pasquale, S Kurek, J White, P Martin, K Bannon, T Wasser and M Li (2004). Initial head computed tomographic scan characteristics have a linear relationship with initial intracranial pressure after trauma. *Journal of Trauma*, 54, 972–963.

Mizutani, T, S Manaka and H Tsutsumi (1990). Estimation of intracranial pressure using computed tomography scan findings in patients with severe head injury. *Surgical Neurology*, 33, 178–184.

Moreno, JA, E Mesalles, J Gener, A Tomasa, A Ley, J Roca and J Fernandez-Llamazares (2000). Evaluating the outcome of severe head injury with transcranial Doppler ultra-sonography. *Neurosurgical Focus*, 8, e8.

Nicolleto, H and M Burkman (2009). Transcranial Doppler series Part II: Performing a transcranial Doppler. *American Journal of Electroneurodiagnostic Technology*, 49, 14–27.

Ragauskas, A, V Matijosaitis, R Zakelis, K Petrikonis, D Rastenyte, I Piper and G Daubaris (2012). Clinical assessment of noninvasive intracranial pressure absolute value measurement method. *Neurology*, 78 1684–1691.

Rainov, N, J Weise and W Burkert (2000). Transcranial Doppler sonography in adult hydrocephalic patients. *Neurosurgical Review*, 23, 34–38.

Rajajee, V, M Vanaman, JJ Fletcher and TL Jacobs (2011). Optic nerve ultrasound for the detection of raised intracranial pressure. *Neurocritical Care*, 15, 506–515.

Reid, A, R Marchbanks, D Bateman, A Martin, A Brightwel and J Pickard (1989). Mean intracranial pressure monitoring by a non-invasive audiological technique: a pilot study. *Journal of Neurology, Neurosurgery & Psychiatry*, 52, 610–612.

Reilly, P and R Bullock (2005). *Head Injury. Pathophysiology and Management*. Boca Raton: CRC Press.

Rosenberg, J, A Shiloh, R Savel and L Eisen (2011). Non-invasive methods of estimating intracranial pressure. *Neurocritical Care*, 15, 599–608.

Steffen, H, B Eifert, A Aschoff, G Kolling and H Volcker. (1996). The diagnostic value of optic disc evaluation in acute elevated intracranial pressure. *Ophthalmology*, 103, 1229–1232.

Steinbach, G, B Macias, T Ueno, W Yost and A Hargens (2005). Intracranial pressure dynamics assessed by noninvasive ultrasound during 30 days of bed rest. *Aviation, Space, and Environmental Medicine*, 76, 85–90.

Strumwasser, A, RO Kwan, L Yeung, E Miraflor, A Ereso, F Castro-Moure, A Patel, J Sadjadi and GP Victorino (2011). Sonographic optic nerve sheath diameter as an estimate of intracranial pressure in adult trauma. *Journal of Surgical Research*, 170, 265–271.

Toutant, S, M Klauber, L Marsha, B Toole, S Bowers, L Seelig and J Varnell (1984). Absent or compressed basal cisterns on first CT scan: Ominous predictors of outcome in severe head injury. *Journal of Neurosurgery*, 61, 691–694.

Ueno, T, R Ballard, B Macias, W Yost and A Hargens (2003a). Cranial diameter pulsations measured by noninvasive ultrasound decrease with tilt. *Aviation, Space, and Environmental Medicine*, 74, 882–885.

Ueno, T, B Macias, W Yost and A Hargens (2003b). Pulsed phase lock loop device for monitoring intracranial pressure during space flight. *Journal of Gravitational Physiology*, 10, 117–118.

Ueno, T, B Macias, W Yost and A Hargens (2005). Noninvasive assessment of intracranial pressure waveforms by using pulsed phase lock loop technology. *Journal of Neurosurgery*, 103, 361–367.

Voulgaris, SG, M Partheni, H Kaliora, N Haftouras, IS Pessach and KS Polyzoidis (2005). Early cerebral monitoring using the transcranial Doppler pulsatility index in patients with severe brain trauma. *Medical Science Monitor*, 11, CR49–CR52.

Xie, X, X Zhang, J Fu, H Wang, J Jonas, X Peng, G Tian, J Xian, R Rich, L Li, Z Kang, S Zhang, D Yang, N Wang and Beijing iCOP Study Group (2013). Noninvasive ICP estimation by orbital subarachnoid space measurement: the Beijing Intracranial and Intraocular Pressure (iCOP) studies. *Critical Care*, 17, R162.

Zakelis, R (2012a). Analysis of the Electronic System for Human Intracranial Pressure Non-Invasive Monitoring, Kaunas, Lithuania: Kaunas University of Technology.

Zakelis, R (2012b). Summary of doctoral dissertation: Analysis of the electronic systemic for human intracranial pressure non-invasive monitoring, Kaunas: University of Technology.

NASA's Research Approach to the Visual Impairment Intracranial Pressure Risk

8

Christian Otto, MD

Universities Space Research Association, University of Houston-Clear Lake, 3600 Bay Area Blvd, Houston, TX 77058, USA

1. Introduction to the Problem

The visual impairment intracranial pressure (VIIP) syndrome is currently one of NASA's top human spaceflight risks (Alexander *et al.*, 2012). The syndrome, which is related to microgravity exposure, manifests with changes in visual acuity (hyperopic shifts) and in eye structure (optic disc edema, choroidal folds, globe flattening, and distended optic nerve sheaths). In some cases, elevated cerebrospinal fluid (CSF) pressure has been documented postflight, reflecting increased intracranial pressure (ICP). While the eye appears to be the main affected organ of this syndrome, the ocular manifestations are thought to be caused by the combined interaction of the ocular, cardiovascular, and the central nervous system (CNS).

Current U.S. astronaut data indicate that after approximately 6 months of spaceflight, 22 of 33 crew members show a range of signs and symptoms of the VIIP syndrome. Returning crew members are currently graded according to criteria in the Spaceflight-Induced Intracranial Hypertension Clinical Practice Guideline adapted for research (Fig. 1). The symptom criteria include refractive change, presence of globe flattening, optic nerve sheath distension (ONSD), choroidal folds, cotton wool spots (CWS), increased retinal nerve fiber layer (RNFL) thickness, and severity of optic disc edema (using the Frisen Scale). Prevalence to

Class 1
≥.50 diopter cycloplegic refractive change and/or CWS

Class 2
≥.50 diopter cycloplegic refractive changes or CWS
Choroidal folds and/or (ONSD) and/or globe flattening and/or scotoma

Class 3
≥.50 diopter cycloplegic refractive changes and/or CWS
ONSD, and/or globe flattening and/or choroidal folds and/or scotoma
Papilledema of Grade 1–2.

Class 4
≥.50 diopter cycloplegic refractive changes and/or CWS
ONSD, and/or globe flattening and/or choroidal folds and/or scotoma
Papilledema Grade 2 or above.
Presenting symptoms of new headache, pulsatile tinnitus and/or transient visual obscurations
CSF opening pressure ≥ 25 cm H_2O

Figure 1. VIIP research case definition.

date has shown a rate of 66.7% of those tested, of those, 21.2% demonstrate the more severe finding of clinical grade optic disc edema (classes 3 and 4).

The leading hypotheses for the development of VIIP involves microgravity-induced headward fluid shifts, CO_2–induced vasodilation, altered cranial nerve lymphatic drainage of cerebral spinal fluid, and loss of gravity-assisted drainage of venous blood from the brain, leading to cephalic venous congestion and increased ICP. The degree of cephalad fluid shift (and cerebral venous drainage) is hypothe-sized to vary based on individual levels of vascular compliance, which can be influenced by environmental and/or individual risk factors. Six of the seven crew members with clinical grade disc edema underwent postflight lumbar puncture (LP) at various time points (Table 1). Resting ICP in normal adults in the supine position is <10 mmHg (13.6 cm H_2O) (Schwartz *et al.*, 2013; American College of Surgeons, 2012; Eklund *et al.*, 2016; Marini *et al.*, 2005). Opening pressure in all six crew members who underwent postflight LP demonstrated an elevated CSF opening pressure ranging from 18 to 28.5 cm H_2O. Moreover, these elevated pressures were present from 6 days to over 2 months postflight. Since, 66.7% of tested crew members have manifested clinical signs of the VIIP syndrome; it is suspected that the majority of astronauts exposed to microgravity have some degree of ICP elevation in flight. Consistent with this hypothesis, is the finding of elevated ONSD in-flight which has been associated with the finding of increased ICP when studied terrestrially

Table 1. Postflight CSF opening pressures in U.S. astronauts.

Case	CSF opening pressure (cm H_2O)	Days after flight LP performed
A	28.5	57
B	28.0	12
C	22.0	66
D	21.5	6
E	21.0	19
F	18.0	8

Normal (<13.6 cm H_2O, <10 mmHg). (Schwartz *et al.*, 2013; American College of Surgeons, 2012; Eklund *et al.*, 2016; Marini *et al.*, 2005).

(Geeraerts *et al.*, 2008). For example, when ICP increases in patients with head trauma, a greater volume of CSF is forced into the optic nerve sheath subarachnoid space causing the nerve sheath to distend. Therefore, increasing ONSD has been used as a qualitative indicator of increasing ICP. Prolonged elevations of ICP can cause long-term reduced visual acuity and affect the peripheral vision in clinical patient populations. It has also been reported to cause mild cognitive impairment in a subset of patients in the analog terrestrial population of idiopathic intracranial hypertension (IIH) (Sørensen *et al.*, 1986; Kharkar *et al.*, 2011; Yri *et al.*, 2014). These potentially irreversible health consequences underscore the importance of identifying and mitigating the factors that lead to this syndrome.

The operational space medicine and human research communities at NASA are working collaboratively to understand the mechanisms of the VIIP syndrome and to provide mitigation and countermeasure strategies. The Medical Operations Group has implemented a clinical monitoring program to observe and record changes in ocular health measures. In addition, they have developed a clinical classification guideline (Clinical Practice Guideline for Spaceflight-Induced Intracranial Hypertension). The spectrum of VIIP signs and symptoms spans a range from mild (choroidal folds, globe flattening, and change in refraction) to more clinically significant findings (optic disc edema, scotomas, and visual field changes such as an enlarged blind spot). These observations suggest that VIIP signs and symptoms develop along a clinical continuum, and if discovered early could be mitigated with the application of suitable countermeasures to minimize long-term health concerns. Successful countermeasure development will be dependent on a thorough understanding of the cause and progression of this syndrome, including the identification of the most prevalent environmental and individual risk factors that contribute to its onset. The primary research goal is to understand the cause and progression of the VIIP syndrome and the risk factors that most significantly influence the development of VIIP.

NASA's Human Research Program, which established the VIIP Research Project, has developed an integrated research plan covering four identified gaps (etiology, technology, analogs, and countermeasures), encompassing more than 70 studies. Five projects have been completed, 25 are currently in progress, and the remaining are planned.

2. VIIP Etiology

What are the etiological mechanisms and contributing risk factors for ocular structural and functional changes associated with spaceflight? Limited data are available to definitively establish the underlying etiological mechanisms and contributing risk factors for the VIIP syndrome. Understanding the mechanisms and contributing risk factors for the ocular structural and functional changes seen in-flight and postflight in astronauts is currently considered the highest research priority. Consequently, several new research projects are focused in this area. Several investigations are being conducted in-flight. These studies provide valuable data through the assessment of astronaut subjects in the environment that the condition manifests. However, the operational and financial cost of these investigations is high. Conducting experiments on the International Space Station (ISS) requires years of preparation and typically 2–3 years of data collection with currently only six crew members on ISS. Although ground research cannot replicate the conditions on the ISS with complete accuracy, several analogs have been adopted for spaceflight research. "Zero Gravity" flights do recreate weightlessness but only for very short periods lasting approximately 20 s. These experiments are housed inside of large jet aircraft that fly a series of parabolas creating "weightlessness" when the aircraft noses over and enters a dive. However, this is followed by hypergravity when the aircraft pulls out of the dive and enters a climb to repeat the process. In this manner, short intervals of weightlessness are provided for data collection. In addition, 6° head-down tilt (HDT) bed rest is a common ground analog for spaceflight and has traditionally been used for human cardiovascular and musculoskeletal studies. Bed rest with HDT aims to recreate a fluid shift, and the deconditioning associated with loss of gravity in space. Investigations are underway to determine if 6° HDT is adequate for studying the VIIP spaceflight risk. Similarly, the "hind limb suspension" (HLS) analog is used for rodent experiments and induces a cephalad fluid shift. Animals are suspended by their tail so that their hind quarters and torso remain above the head while the animal can move about using their forelimbs. Animal hind limb suspension experiments offer the advantage of incorporating multiple variables and invasive techniques. This animal model was established and validated at NASA Ames Research Center (Morey-Holton *et al.*, 1998). Finally, mathematical computer modeling is an analog that has the advantage of incorporating multiple parameters such as environmental conditions, subject characteristics, existing clinical data, and an assessment of variable interaction. Currently, all of these experimental methods are being utilized by NASA's VIIP research program.

The VIIP research program is divided into key areas of investigation; cardiovascular, CNS, ocular, and genetic. Several investigations focus on a single area, while others examine a combination of key areas. A current summary of project tasks addressing gaps for the, "Risk of Spaceflight-Induced Intracranial Hypertension/Vision Alterations," can be found online (https://humanresearch roadmap.nasa.gov/Risks).

3. Cardiovascular

Work done in the 1990s on postflight orthostatic hypotension revealed two general groups of responders; those who demonstrated greater resistance to postflight orthostatic hypotension and those who did not (Waters *et al.*, 2002).

The subjects who displayed greater resistance tended to have higher blood pressure and a more mesomorphic body habitus in comparison to those who quickly became hypotensive who were either female or tended to have lower blood pressure and a more ectomorphic body habitus. This data suggest that vascular compliance may play a role in long-duration spaceflight-induced VIIP syndrome. One of the contributing factors may be the compliance of the major capacitance vessels in the splanchnic and thoracic vasculature which may affect right heart preload and resistance to cerebral venous drainage in the setting of a cephalad fluid shift.

To determine if cardiovascular status is related to the VIIP risk, an occupational data mining effort (Phase I) was undertaken between the VIIP research project and the NASA Medical Operations Division utilizing the Lifetime Surveillance of Astronaut Health database. The goal is to analyze baseline crew member data collected prior to flight to determine whether trends are present, which contribute to underlying risk factors for developing the VIIP syndrome, and provide evidence for potential mechanisms. Data from annual crew health exams were analyzed, including biochemistry, body composition, cardiac, and aerobic capacity. Ten of 13 parameters revealed significant correlation with classification of VIIP severity. Phase II of this analysis is underway and will correlate baseline measures of cardiovascular health with postflight ocular outcomes.

The *Cardiovascular Data Mining for VIIP study* analyzed existing multisystem data obtained from astronauts who participated in the cardiovascular Medical Operation tilt/stand test evaluations before and after both short- and long-duration space missions. Data were compiled on 20 crew members (3 females and 17 males) who averaged 5207 (3447–8934) flight hours across both long- (MIR-23 through ISS Expedition-16) and short- (STS-27 through STS-101) duration missions between 1988 and 2008. Crew members in the highest tertile for both systolic and diastolic blood pressure demonstrated less variability in pulse pressure. This reduction is due in part to lower levels of compliance as indicated by similar or higher levels of total peripheral resistance postflight compared with preflight levels. Whether there is a relation between blood pressure regulation and total peripheral resistance in crew presenting with reductions of visual acuity remains to be determined. However, a higher total peripheral resistance combined with lower vascular compliance is generally associated with greater pathological changes to the cardiovascular system and potentially to the surrounding tissues.

An upcoming prospective study led by the NASA JSC Cardiovascular and Vision Laboratory will quantify upper body (head and neck) arterial and venous vascular compliance during HDT bed rest and determine measured variable contributions to the VIIP syndrome. The study will determine whether noninvasive measures of venous and arterial compliance are altered by bed rest and whether these changes are related to the development of the VIIP syndrome. The study will also determine whether previous spaceflight experience or training in high-performance jet aircraft predispose astronauts to lower venous compliance and/or the development of the VIIP syndrome. The third component of the study will utilize 14 days of 6° HDT bed rest as a model of spaceflight to evaluate the effect of aging on vascular compliance using a subject population similar to younger (25–35 years) and older (45–55 years) astronaut cohorts.

4. Central Nervous System

Preliminary evidence from astronauts, classified as VIIP cases, may suggest raised ICP as the precipitant. The primary mechanism believed to be at play is cerebral venous congestion and altered CSF homeostasis. Five imaging studies focusing on the brain have been initiated to date; four of these studies are currently ongoing. These magnetic resonance imaging (MRI) studies have or will be conducted on astronauts pre- and postflight. Since elevated CSF pressure is hypothesized to play a role in the VIIP syndrome, two studies are planned to assess CSF pressure invasively, one of them will also analyze CSF constituents.

4.1. *Venous sinus evaluation*

Intracranial hypertension (IH) can alter the configuration of anatomic structures within the cranial vault. In many cases of IH, an increased cerebral venous pressure inhibits CSF resorption and raises the intracranial pressure causing venous sinus compression (Rohr *et al.*, 2011).

Neuroimaging shows secondary narrowing of the sinus lumen by compression (Karahalios *et al.*, 1996; King *et al.*, 2002; Farb *et al.*, 2003; Higgins *et al.*, 2003; Higgins and Pickard, 2004) as a consequence of raised ICP. Rohr and coworkers (Rohr *et al.*, 2007) demonstrated that this phenomena could be reversed by LP or shunt surgery procedures (King *et al.*, 2002; Baryshnik and Farb, 2004; Higgins and Pickard, 2004). The *Pre and Postflight Magnetic Resonance Venography (MRV) Review for Central Venous Congestion* is a retrospective study, led by Dr. Roy Riascos, MD, of preflight and postflight scans from 19 astronauts, 10 short-duration (Shuttle) and 9 long-duration (ISS) crew, to determine if changes in the caliber of the cerebral venous sinuses occur following flight. This study utilizes a unique technique of measuring the cross-sectional area of the sagittal, transverse, and sigmoid venous sinus from 3.0 Tesla T1-weighted images.

4.2. *CSF production and outflow*

Animal data from multiple space shuttle flights indicate that CSF secretory processes are dramatically altered upon exposure to microgravity from a structural and regulatory perspective (Herbute *et al.*, 1994; Gabrion *et al.*, 1996; Davet *et al.*, 1998; Masseguin *et al.*, 2000). These findings have been replicated in HLS experiments on the ground and suggest a vigorous response to elevated ICP (Davet *et al.*, 1998). Similar processes may be occurring in astronauts during microgravity exposure. In a recent retrospective analysis of 14 astronauts (seven short duration and seven long duration), changes in CSF production rate and peak velocity were examined before and after exposure to microgravity (Kramer *et al.*, 2015). Qualitative analysis was performed on T2-weighted axial images through the orbits for degree of flattening of the posterior globe. CSF production rate and peak velocity was calculated from cine phase-contrast MRI and compared to seven healthy controls. Six astronauts with significant posterior globe flattening demonstrated a 70% increase in CSF production rate postflight compared to baseline ($P = 0.01$). There was a significant increase in CSF peak velocity in the subgroup without posterior globe flattening ($P = 0.01$). Increased postflight CSF production rate in astronauts is compatible with the hypothesis of microgravity-induced IH inferring downregulation in CSF production in microgravity that is upregulated upon sudden return to normal gravity. Increased postflight CSF peak velocity in astronauts with negative flattening suggests acquired increased craniospinal compliance during spaceflight that could infer reduced susceptibility to microgravity-induced IH with additional exposure.

If ICP is elevated in microgravity, multiple CSF outflow routes may be impaired due to the cephalad fluid shift. These include drainage via cranial nerve lymphatics (Yoffey *et al.*, 1939), an altered pressure gradient across the arachnoid granulations (Bateman and Siddique, 2014) and impaired caudal displacement of CSF into the spinal canal (Martins *et al.*, 1972). An animal investigation is planned to examine cranial lymphatic drainage, hormonal regulation of CSF and aquaporin expression, cellular junction proteins, and cellular permeability in the arachnoid granulations and choroid plexus ("CSF Production and Outflow", 2016). The aims are to investigate the role of cranial lymphatic drainage in a hind limb suspended animal model and to determine whether HLS induces structural and functional changes in choroid plexus (where CSF is produced) and arachnoid granulations (where CSF is absorbed). This study will determine whether HLS induces structural and functional changes in choroid plexus and arachnoid granulations, including evidence of inflammation or fibrosis, changes in aquaporin expression, and changes in cell–cell adhesion protein expression. These changes are hypothesized to occur concomitantly with fluid shift caused by a positional change, which may affect the production and paracellular/transcellular CSF outflow and thus, CSF homeostasis. Supraphysiologic pressures in the *in vitro* model also simulates this fluid shift and allows for direct measurement of changes in paracellular/transcellular CSF outflow through the arachnoid cell layer (Holman *et al.*, 2010).

4.3. *CSF dynamics pre and post-flight*

Understanding the influence of intracranial compliance on development of the VIIP syndrome, and having a noninvasive means of measuring ICP preflight and postflight are important steps forward. The *Retrospective Pre and Postflight Measurement of Cerebrospinal Fluid (CSF) Dynamics*, led by Noam Alperin, PhD, will analyze previously collected pre- and postflight specialized MRI sequences, known as MRICP, and assess the dynamics of blood and CSF flow into and out of the cranium, and evaluate the CSF pulsation between the cranium and the spinal canal. The well-defined closed cranio-spinal system enables derivation of the pressure inside from these inputs and outputs (Alperin *et al.*, 2000). These sequences are currently available for 25 crew members (15 long duration and 10 short duration). This study quantifies baseline and postflight total cerebral blood flow, venous drainage, intracranial compliance, intracranial pressure, and cranio–spinal compliance distribution. These MRI variables will be correlated with alterations observed in eye function and morphology and will also be correlated with spinal elongation, which may affect distribution of CSF. These analyses will inform the role of headward CSF shift in the etiology of VIIP, will define hydrodynamic measures that may predict susceptibility to VIIP, and may lead to the identification of new countermeasures. From analysis of the collected data, an estimate of intracranial pressure and other parameters will be calculated and correlated with available clinical data.

4.4. *Cerebral vascular autoregulation*

Cerebral autoregulation is controlled by metabolic, myogenic, and neurovascular factors to maintain sufficient cerebral blood flow over a wide range of systemic blood pressure. Blaber and coworkers reported impairments in cerebral blood flow velocity regulation in astronauts with orthostatic intolerance (Blaber *et al.*, 2011). This orthostatic intolerance may be the result of changes in autoregulation within the preflight blood pressure range. It was determined that the orthostatic intolerant group in a postflight orthostatic tolerance test had a mean cerebral blood flow velocity that was much higher both supine and standing compared to the group that completed the tilt test. This indicated that the orthostatic intolerant group may have been operating at a higher cerebral vasodilation for a given blood pressure. Furthermore, the nonfinishers had a greater decrease in the landing day mean blood flow velocity (MFV) with standing compared to preflight than that of the finishers. This was additional evidence of impaired cerebral autoregulation, which may have precipitated presyncope in the nonfinisher astronauts. Female astronauts have also been reported to have greater impairments in cerebral autoregulation following flight in comparison to males (Blaber *et al.*, 2011). Interestingly, Taylor and coworkers also reported evidence of cerebral vasodilation in mice following spaceflight (Taylor *et al.*, 2013). Understanding the contribution of cerebral vascular autoregulation to the VIIP syndrome will aid in defining the etiology and those who are most susceptible. The study *Human Cerebral Vascular Autoregulation and Venous Outflow in Response to Microgravity-Induced Cephalad Fluid Redistribution*, led by Donna Roberts, MD, will characterize intracranial adaptation to long-term microgravity, using MRI to allow functional characterization of the intracranial contents. A suite of MRI sequences will be employed in conjunction with gadolinium contrast and a CO_2 challenge to characterize weightlessness-induced intracranial compartmental fluid volume changes at the macroscopic (brain, CSF), microscopic (brain tissue water), and vascular (venous) levels following adaptation to long-term spaceflight. Secondly, an assessment for potential hemodynamic changes (cerebral perfusion) in the brain following spaceflight will be conducted. This study will characterize intracranial compartmental fluid and hemodynamic changes induced by long-term microgravity.

4.5. *White matter microstructure*

In grey matter, water molecules diffuse in different directions; however, in white matter they diffuse along the length of axons, since the hydrophobic myelin restricts movement. Diffusion tensor imaging (DTI) is an MRI technique that enables the measurement of the restricted diffusion of water molecules to produce images of the neural tracts. Diffusion is termed isotropic if the motion is equal in all directions; in the case of white matter, where water molecules diffuse asymmetrically, it is referred to as anisotropy. Using this property, directional information is obtained in a particular voxel, a unit of graphic information that defines a point in three-dimensional (3-D) space. Therefore, DTI allows direct in vivo examination of the white matter microstructure, enabling mapping of the orientation of the white matter tracts.

The study *Association of Diffusion Tensor Imaging Parameters of Optic Tracts and Cerebral White Matter Tracts with Visual Impairment and Structural Changes of the Eyes and Optic Nerves in Long-Duration Microgravity Exposure,* led by Roy Riascos, MD, aims to investigate alterations in nerve structure in correlation with intracranial pressure and compliance measures in astronauts during pre- and postflight microgravity exposure. The examination of brain microstructure has not been investigated in this context before and may reveal alterations to the brains of crew members. The degree of alteration in diffusion tensor (DT) metrics, including fractional anisotropy (FA) and mean diffusivity (MD), in cerebral optic and corticospinal (CST) tracts in astronauts may correlate with the presence, severity, and duration of symptoms. Pre- and postflight DT metrics will be quantified in the optic and CST of approximately 10 short-duration (space shuttle) crew members, and approximately 10 long-duration crew members (ISS missions). The data will be analyzed for significant alterations in DTI metrics in those with and without in-flight and postflight signs and/or symptoms of the VIIP syndrome. Severity of VIIP syndrome and duration of exposure will also be correlated.

4.6. *Biomarker analysis and LP*

Microgravity-induced IH has long been suspected from anecdotal spaceflight accounts and terrestrial analogs (Jennings, 1990; Lakin *et al.*, 2007). However, ICP has never been directly measured in humans during microgravity exposures. In-flight elevation of ICP is currently the leading hypothesis explaining the signs and symptoms of the (VIIP) syndrome. Terrestrially, CSF manometry via LP is the gold standard and most common technique for obtaining a CSF pressure measurement indicative of ICP in ambulatory patients. Currently, LPs are not conducted during medical testing of astronauts before, during, or after spaceflight. To date, postflight LPs have been performed on six astronauts who had postflight optic disc edema. In all six astronauts, the opening pressure was found to be elevated (range 18–28.5 cm H_2O). Preflight measurements were not collected for these crew members to allow comparison. The study *Zero G and ICP: Invasive and Noninvasive ICP Monitoring of Astronauts on the ISS*, led by Michael Williams, MD, aims to assess the role of ICP in the development of VIIP by measuring LP opening pressure in-flight. The study will also evaluate biomarkers in CSF and blood, via preflight and postflight LP, which may indicate structural and functional integrity of the CNS, whether levels of metabolites normally found in the CSF vary in VIIP and whether neural markers indicative of cellular damage escape from the CSF into the systemic blood. Several CSF constituents have been associated with elevated ICP: vasopressin (Sørensen *et al.*, 1984), atrial natriuretic peptide (Skau *et al.*, 2010), and inflammatory markers: IL-6, IL-23, and FoxP3 (Hannerz *et al.*, 2011). Comparison of pre- and postflight astronaut CSF samples may reveal biochemical evidence for elevated ICP. In addition, chronic elevations in ICP have been associated with downregulation of CSF production (Herbute *et al.*, 1994; Masseguin *et al.*, 2000) and impaired CSF circulation (Silverberg *et al.*, 2002; Wostyn, 2004). This sequence of events may lead to decreased clearance of CNS toxins, in particular, beta amyloid and tau proteins, which are implicated in dementing diseases. Analysis for these and other CNS toxins from pre- to postflight would be suggestive of disturbed CSF circulation in microgravity. The aim of the *VIIP Biomarker Analysis Study*, led by Susanna Zanello, PhD, is to perform prospective biochemical and cytological analyses of pre- and postflight CSF, blood, and urine to identify biomarkers unique to (1) elevated ICP, (2) choroid plexus damage, and (3) white or gray matter damage. In addition, stored samples from prior astronaut CSF sampling will be evaluated.

A funded ground analog study aims to investigate the novel use of vesicles carrying genetic encoding information. Exosomes contains various molecular constituents from their cell of origin, including proteins, RNA, and micro RNA, which are small noncoding RNA molecules that have a central role in physiological and pathological responses to stress. Exosomes can be thought of as "genetic biopsies" from the cells of various tissues throughout the body, allowing access to transcriptome information. Accordingly, exosomes may be used as biomarkers of disease processes. The *Brain Gene Expression Signatures from Cerebrospinal Fluid Exosome RNA Profiling* study, also led by Susanna Zanello, PhD, will investigate changes in brain gene expression via exosome analysis in IIH patients suffering from elevated ICP. The target population will be individuals with moderate ICP increase since their condition resembles more closely that of the astronauts exposed to microgravity in long-duration spaceflight.

4.7. *Direct ambulatory intracranial pressure measurement: invasive ICP*

Direct measurement of ICP during spaceflight would provide the most convincing evidence for elevated ICP. If ambulatory indwelling intracranial pressure measurements are feasible, this study will utilize miniaturized ICP transducers that will be implanted prior to flight in the crania of several long-duration crew members, in a subdural or intraparenchymal location, providing continuous long-term monitoring of ICP. Intracranial pressure will be measured in all phases of flight, during a variety of in-flight activities, postures, and with and without countermeasure use. These devices are fully implantable (no extension outside the skin), interrogation is done via radiofrequency, there is no battery in the implantable device (the power is external). Moreover, these devices have been verified to be free of measurement drift over many months. Risks associated with implantation of the device under controlled conditions (hospital environment, implanted by experienced neurosurgeons) are anticipated to be lower than the risks of performing an LP test in the uncontrolled environment of spaceflight by medically trained but nonexpert operators. Due to the dynamic nature of ICP, continuous or intermittent long-term monitoring during spaceflight will provide superior results compared with sporadic (once or twice in a space mission) measurement of LP opening pressures, advancing the understanding of the pathophysiology of the VIIP syndrome. One of the key concerns regarding ICP is the 24-h mean pressure in-flight compared with the terrestrial mean 24-h pressure. Knowledge of ICP dynamics in-flight, and the effects of provocative activities, is key to identifying susceptible individuals and in the development of effective countermeasures.

5. Ocular

Several ocular specific studies are currently planned or underway. Two are aimed at understanding the impact of ocular biomechanics in the onset of VIIP, and the individual susceptibility to VIIP. The principal load-bearing tissue of the eye is the sclera, primarily in the peripapillary area. In the posterior pole of the eye, both the geometry and material properties of the sclera and lamina cribrosa (LC) contribute to their structural stiffness, and determine the ability of the optic nerve head (ONH) and peripapillary sclera to withstand strain when exposed to translaminar pressure shifts (IOP-ICP). The ONH biomechanics are therefore determined by the geometry (size and shape of the scleral canal, scleral thickness, regional laminar density, and collagen beam orientation) and the material properties (stiffness) of the LC and sclera. As a consequence, eyes with identical IOPs may exhibit very different strain fields due to differences in their structural stiffness (Bellezza *et al.*, 2000). When mechanical failure of the load-bearing connective tissues of the ONH occurs, then progressive damage to the adjacent axons (with eventual retinal ganglion cell death) ensues from a combination of both compressive and ischemic mechanisms. Interindividual variation in peripapillary scleral thickness can result in significantly different biomechanical responses to IOP. In a prior study, five input factors that had the largest influence across all outcome measures were in ranked order: stiffness of the sclera, radius of the eye, stiffness of the LC, IOP, and thickness of the scleral shell (Sigal *et al.*, 2005). Modeling predictions indicate that scleral properties have the largest effect when the sclera is more compliant. Increased scleral compliance occurs, for example, in myopia, either because of scleral thinning or due to alterations to the scleral extracellular matrix, which could help explain the higher incidence of glaucomatous optic nerve damage in highly myopic eyes at a given IOP. The study "Data Mining — Ocular Structure and Biomechanics in Relation to the VIIP Syndrome" ("Ocular Structure", 2016) aims to evaluate the changes in ocular structure and biomechanics during spaceflight, such as crowded disc, posterior eye radius, degree of refraction, intraocular pressure (IOP), retinal pigmented epithelial angle (RPE), and translaminar pressure gradient (TLPG), in addition to preflight characteristics associated with significant VIIP-related findings in-flight.

A recently completed study "Phase I: SD-OCT Analysis of the Optic Nerve Head and Surrounding Structures in Long Duration ISS Crew Members Compared to Terrestrial Bound Normals" led by Nimesh Patel, OD, PhD, examined morphological ocular changes measured with spectral domain optical coherence tomography (SD-OCT) in the ONH, peripapillary structures (retinal pigmented epithelium and choroid), and general choroidal thickness seen in ISS crew members exposed to long-duration zero gravity and compared them to age matched controls. OCT allows the assessment of the RNFL, the neural retinal rim (NRR), and integrity of the retinal layers in the posterior 30° of the eye. However, little is known about the changes in the presentation of the structures around the optic nerve and the vascular supply layer (choroid) of the eye in the affected ISS crew and how they may compare to terrestrial normals.

Data from 43 controls and 19 crew members were analyzed. Global and quadrant RNFL measures were calculated for regions 250, 500, 1000, and 1500 μm from the Bruch's membrane opening (BMO). Patel and colleagues found that the average total retinal thickness within the BMO was significantly larger in astronauts compared with the controls (Patel *et al.*, 2014). Similarly, RNFL was significantly larger in crew members. The BMO angle was significantly lower in the astronauts postflight. For circumpapillary scans, the average RNFL thickness for crew members was significantly larger than normals. The average circumpapillary choroidal thickness was also significantly larger than the controls. These findings may indicate that spaceflight exposure may be contributory to these changes. Using the same postflight crew cohort, 15 of the 19 subjects had both preflight and postflight scans available. Analysis revealed a significant postflight increase in global RNFL in 21 of 30 eyes, the inferior quadrant demonstrating a statistically significant RNFL difference. There was also a significant decrease in BMO height postflight in 20 eyes, compared to preflight.

Disc edema in seven U.S. crew members, along with cases of CWS, indicates that vascular flow to optic nerve and retina may be compromised. In addition, OCT evidence indicates that the choroid becomes engorged in-flight in astronauts. Thus, it is highly probable that blood flow to the retina is compromised. The "Retinal Vascular Remodeling study" led by Patricia Parsons, PhD, will examine alterations in the vascular patterning of the human retina in response to fluid shift during spaceflight. Alterations will be mapped and quantified by analyzing existing pre- and postflight OCT images. The goal of the study is to investigate potential changes in the branching patterns of the retinal arterial and venous trees following microgravity exposure. The investigators hypothesize that transfer of fluids is a major microvascular regulatory function. Furthermore, retinal blood vessels, especially the fragile, actively remodeling smaller vessels, adapt and remodel to accommodate fluid shift in microgravity. It is proposed that healthy retinal vascular adaptations will return to normal after returning to Earth; however, more pathological, irreversible adaptations contributing to ocular and visual impairments will not. To study vascular remodeling directly, VESsel GENeration Analysis (VESGEN) Software (Parsons-Wingerter *et al.*, 2000a,b; Parsons-Wingerter *et al.*,

2006) will be used to map and quantify arterial and venous trees extracted from pre- and postflight crew clinical images obtained by fundoscopy. "The VESGEN computer program analyzes major vascular branching parameters in a binary (black/white) image of a vascular tree, vascular network, or a tree-network composite. Mapping and quantification by VESGEN analysis automatically segments vessels within a tree into branching generations ($G1$, $G2$, …, Gx) according to coordinate change in vessel diameter and branching" (Parsons-Wingerter *et al.*, 2010). It is possible that angiogenesis, neovascularization, and/or possibly vascular dropout may occur as a result of hypoxic conditions at the tissue level.

6. Genetic

Both genetic predisposition and alterations in gene expression may play a role in VIIP. The study "Spaceflight Effects on the Mouse Retina: Histological, and Gene Expression after Flight on STS-133" (Zanello *et al.*, 2013) examined histological and genetic changes in female 10–12 week-old BALB/cJ mice flown on a 12-day shuttle mission, STS-133. Eyes were collected at one, five, and seven days after landing and were fixed for histological sectioning. The contralateral eye was used for gene expression profiling by quantitative reverse transcription polymerase chain reaction (RT-qPCR). Thin sections were visualized by hematoxylin/eosin stain and processed for 8-hydroxy-2′-deoxyguanosine (8-OHdG), caspase-3, and glial fibrillary acidic protein (GFAP) and β-amyloid double-staining (Zanello *et al.*, 2013). 8-OHdG and caspase-3 immunoreactivity was increased in the retina in-flight samples at return from flight compared to ground controls, indicating oxidative stress-induced DNA damage and increased apoptosis, respectively. Both were decreased at day seven postflight. β-amyloid was seen in the nerve fibers at the postlaminar region of the optic nerve in the flight samples and it was only in these mice that there was an increase in GFAP staining adjacent to LC in the optic nerve, indicating that the astrocytes and oligodendrocytes were activated in this region possibly due to mechanical trauma. It was suspected that long-term damage in the optic nerve was evident after spaceflight because there was no resolution following seven days on Earth. Inflammatory response genes Nfkb1 and Tgfb1 were elevated after flight. Correspondingly, genes coding for the antioxidant enzymes heme-oxygenase-1, peroxiredoxin, and catalase, were elevated after flight. The results of this study indicate that the microgravity environment may lead to oxidative and cellular changes in the retina, which were partially reversible upon return to Earth. Fluid shift related ICP increase, and elevated radiation effects may both be contributing factors. Future study will be required to determine their respective impacts on VIIP.

A second retinal gene expression study, led by Susanna Zanello, PhD, will perform histological and gene expression analysis of retinas collected from C57BL/6 mice flown in STS-135 (and from their ground control counterparts) and compare these results to similar analyses performed on BALB mice from STS-133. Histological and gene expression outcomes will be focused on cellular stress, oxidative stress, DNA damage, and cellular death and survival, but will also investigate genome-wide changes by expression microarray analysis. Retinal gene expression differences between STS-135-flown mice and their ground counterparts may have an epigenetic basis, by analyzing DNA methylation in specific target genes. Using the same methodological approach as outlined in the STS-133 investigation, the STS-135 experiment will also determine the utility of the mouse model in spaceflight to study degenerative processes in the retina due to microgravity and radiation to better assess and characterize the risk and define outcomes for future countermeasure testing.

Another ongoing genetic study is the *Risk of Visual Impairment and Intracranial Hypertension After Space Flight: Evaluation of the Role of Polymorphism of Enzymes Involved in One-Carbon Metabolism*, led by Scott Smith, PhD. In evaluating data collected from the Nutritional Status Assessment Supplemental Medical Objective (SMO), elevations in four metabolites of the one-carbon metabolism pathway has been identified in affected crew members studied to date (Zwart *et al.*, 2012; Zwart *et al.*, 2016). These elevations and related data strongly suggest that polymorphism(s) of one or more of the enzymes in this pathway exist(s) in the affected crew members. The incidence of such polymorphisms in the general population is relatively high, and they have been with increased risk of stroke, cardiovascular events, and specifically cerebrovascular events. Therefore, it is within the realm of plausibility, given the number and ethnic background of the affected astronauts that these polymorphisms could be contributing to the cerebrovascular and optical medical issues of astronauts. The proposed study will assess the one-carbon pathway for polymorphisms in astronauts.

7. Combined System Studies

7.1. *Analog*

The current understanding of VIIP pathophysiology is based on an interaction of the cardiovascular, CNS, and ocular system. Several studies are underway to define the interactions among these systems in the development of VIIP pathology. The study "Effects of Microgravity on Intracranial Pressure" led by Ben Levine, MD, aims to directly measure ICP and cerebral hemodynamics, and structure of the visual apparatus during parabolic flight that mimics microgravity for brief periods, in addition to ground-based HDT experiments (Lawley *et al.*, 2017). One of the primary hypotheses of the study is that the location of the intracranial hydrostatic indifference point determines the magnitude of the increase in ICP during changes in posture and in microgravity; if so, this characteristic could be a testable risk factor for visual impairment in space. The second hypothesis suggests that microgravity-induced changes (via parabolic flight) in ICP and CSF flow will be greater than those observed during bed rest.

To test these two hypotheses, adult patients with direct access to the intracranial compartment via an implanted Ommaya reservoir will be recruited. These subjects will have been previously treated for a hematologic malignancy and received prophylactic brain chemotherapy. These subjects allow direct measurement of ICP with little risk. Simultaneous measurement of right atrial pressure will be conducted. In addition, intra-arterial pressure, echo–Doppler ultrasound of the middle cerebral artery, carotid and jugular vessel size, blood velocity, and flow will be obtained. Moreover, ocular ultrasound for axial length, and optic sheath diameter, plus near infrared spectroscopy to assess oxygen delivery/utilization will provide a comprehensive assessment of cerebrovascular hemodynamics during parabolic flight, positional change, and 24 h of HDT bed rest. The hydrostatic indifference point will be determined in each subject. Other interventions will include exposure to elevated $PaCO_2$, and resistance exercise maneuvers to determine the additive effects of these two parameters.

7.2. *In-flight*

The Prospective Observational Study of Ocular Health in International Space Station (ISS) Crews, initiated by Christian Otto, MD, aims to systematically gather physiological data to characterize the risk of developing the VIIP syndrome in crew members assigned to a 6-month ISS mission. The data collected will mirror NASA's Medical Requirements Integration Documents (MRID) requirements and testing performed during space missions and annual medical exams. The study will result in a greater frequency of in-flight and postflight testing; increasing the number of sessions from five during a 2-year period, to 13 sessions over a 3-year period. This enhanced frequency of testing will provide greater accuracy in assessing changes that may be occurring in the visual, vascular, and central nervous systems upon exposure to microgravity. The primary focus of this protocol is to monitor in-flight changes and postflight recovery once the baseline has been established. The enhanced data collection will aid in; defining the temporal sequence for the appearance of VIIP signs and symptoms, delineate the interaction between duration of weightlessness and the severity of symptoms, establish the postflight time course for recovery and identify the presence of prolonged changes in crew health, define the interaction between individual susceptibility and severity of symptoms, and aid in understanding the mechanism for the development of the VIIP syndrome. Data from this study will also guide the development of countermeasures and targeted treatments to prevent VIIP and its complications. Preflight, in-flight, and postflight measures include: tonometry, ocular ultrasound, fundoscopy, visual acuity, and OCT; while MRI and bio-microscopy will be captured preflight and postflight exclusively. Three additional, non-MRID measures will be collected preflight, in-flight, and postflight, including blood pressure and cardiac output to assess arterial vascular compliance, and transcranial Doppler (TCD) of the middle cerebral artery to assess for changes in cerebral hemodynamics. During the preflight and postflight portions of the TCD collection, subjects will be tilted at four different angles during TCD data collection: 85°, 0°, –15°, and –25°. Data collection will begin 1 year prior to flight, continue in-flight approximately once per 30 days, and continue through to the end of the first postflight year with data collections the first week of return to Earth, and at 30, 90, 180, and 365 days (Fig. 2). In circumstances where abnormalities may persist beyond one year, postflight data

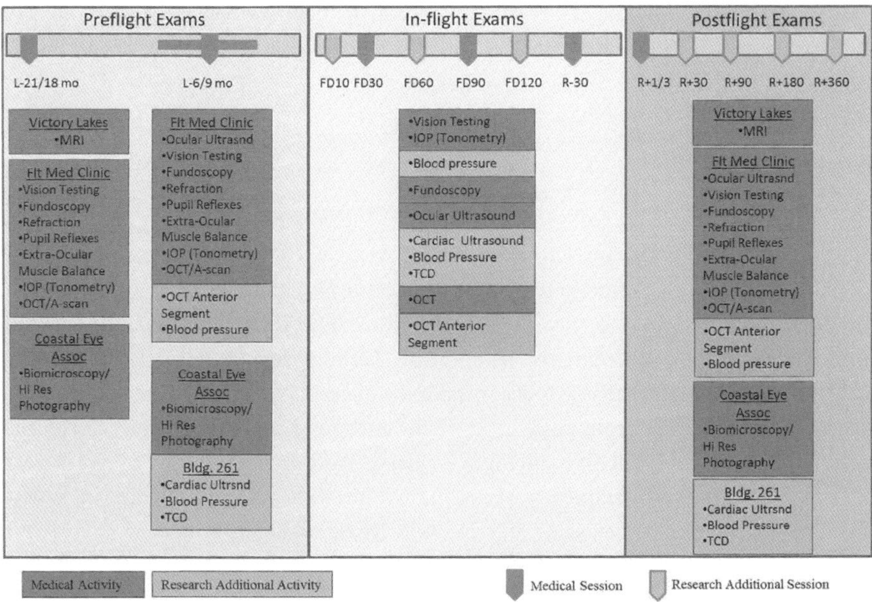

Figure 2. Prospective observational study of ocular health in International Space Station (ISS) crew data collection preflight, in-flight and postflight.

will continue to be collected, but as per the MRID requirements (MedB 1.10) and Visual Impairment/Intracranial Pressure (VIIP) clinical practice guidelines.

The *Fluid Shifts* study, led by Alan Hargens, PhD, Michael Stenger, PhD, and Scott Dulchavsky, MD, PhD, is designed to understand the impact of long-duration spaceflight on fluid shift and subsequent compartmentalization. The redistribution of fluid, particularly in the upper body, is hypothesized to be predictive of changes in intracranial pressure and vision disturbance, which will differ from the effect of the cephalad shift seen during bed rest studies, a weightlessness analog. This mechanistic study will include the direct manipulation of volume and fluid shift using tilt, and lower body negative pressure; with simultaneous measurement of changes in the ocular, cardiovascular, and central nervous system. The specific aims are: (1) to characterize fluid distribution and compartmentalization before, during, and after long-duration spaceflight. (2) To correlate in-flight alterations of eye structure, ocular vascular parameters, and vision with headward fluid shifts, vascular dimensions, and flow patterns. (3) To determine systemic and ocular factors of individual susceptibility to the development of ICP elevation and/or vision alterations.

Astronauts will be studied before, during, and after spaceflight missions consisting of approximately 180 days of flight. Data collection for total body water and extracellular fluid volume will occur concurrently with existing Medical Requirement sample collections. One baseline data collection at or before 90 days before launch (L-90); once early (flight day 45), and late (R-45) during flight; once in the week after landing (R+1/3) and two more times after flight to track recovery (R+30 and R+180) (Fig. 3). Pre- and postflight measures will be performed seated, supine and 15° HDT.

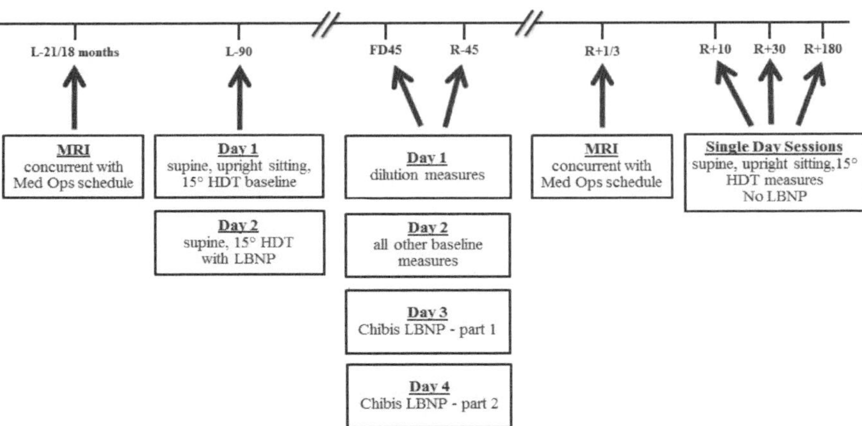

Figure 3. Fluid Shifts Study preflight, in-flight and postflight data collection.

This study will evaluate the individual differences in the time course and magnitude of spaceflight-induced cephalad fluid shift, as well as the subsequent compartmentalization of fluid. Fluid status of lower body tissues and swelling of upper body tissues will be assessed via ultrasound measurement of venous diameters and interstitial thickness before launch, early and late in flight, and postflight to track venous volume shift and subsequent filtration or absorption of body fluid.

Responses to the fluid shift are expected to recover within the first month upon return to Earth gravity. Therefore, indicators of fluid distribution will be correlated to changes in eye structure and severity of visual impairment. For example, the degree of facial edema, upper body vein engorgement, and optic nerve sheath distention will be compared.

Peripheral venous pressure (PVP) will be measured before, during, and after spaceflight using a noninvasive ultrasound pressure transducer device (Baumann *et al.*, 2005; Thalhammer *et al.*, 2007, 2009).

During the preflight and in-flight phases, lower body negative pressure (LBNP) will be applied to subjects to impart a caudal fluid shift to determine the impact on vascular, CNS, and ocular structures and determine whether LBNP during HDT or microgravity results in reversal of fluid distribution toward a more typical 1G orientation.

Prior to spaceflight, cardiovascular, ocular, and CNS responses during acute seated, supine, and 15° HDT will be measured. It is anticipated that the responses to this acute HDT will be predictive of the magnitude of the response in spaceflight and after long-duration spaceflight.

In addition, data will be shared from testing performed by the Flight Medicine Clinic. For example, tonometry will be performed on the right and left eye using a commercial tonometer to obtain IOP. Subjects will be tested for near and far visual acuity for each eye, independently with and without corrective lenses.

At the conclusion of the study, it is anticipated that characterization of the effects of long-duration spaceflight on the magnitude of the fluid shift and subsequent compartmentalization will be realized. This redistribution of fluid, especially in the upper body, will be predictive of changes in intraocular/intracranial pressure and vision disturbance, which will differ from the effect of the cephalad shift seen during bed rest analogs.

7.3. *Modeling*

The Digital Astronaut Project (DAP) "Visual Impairment Intracranial Pressure Modelling" is a collaborative effort between Glenn Research Center, Johnson Space Center, and external scientists. The goal is the development of a VIIP model to use for further identification of risk factors and countermeasure development.

While the observed physiologic changes are likely caused by both biomechanical and biochemical pathways, the DAP aims to investigate the biomechanical responses to the microgravity environment that could result in VIIP syndrome.

The aim of the VIIP DAP is to implement computational models to inform ground and flight studies to quantify:

(1) The role of compliance (vascular, ocular, and cranial) ICP, IOP, and measures of visual acuity, and ONH or foveal displacement
(2) The role of microgravity-induced cephalad fluid shift on ICP, IOP, and measures of visual acuity
(3) The role of chronic and multiple exposures to microgravity on ICP, IOP, and measures of visual acuity

To address microgravity-induced visual impairment and intracranial pressure changes a computational modeling and simulation approach will be adopted. Integration of lumped-parameter models for both whole body and the eye will be used to study ICP and IOP in microgravity. A detailed model of the eye and surrounding tissues will be developed to investigate biomechanical stress and anatomical changes due to long-term microgravity exposure. Key factors will include cephalad fluid shift, hydrodynamic forces governed by ICP and blood/CSF flow in the intracranial space, quasi-static and dynamic biomechanical responses of the corneo–retino–scleral shell, choroid layer and retina, retrobulbar subarachnoid space, the ONH and its surrounding tissues to changes in ICP, IOP, and fluid flow, and tissue properties such as scleral deformation and remodeling characteristics.

Lumped-parameter modeling will be beneficial in assessing the impact of cephalad fluid shift on VIIP. A lumped-parameter, whole-body and eye model for time-dependent pressure/flow of blood and CSF in the CVS, CNS, the eye, and subarachnoid space posterior to the eye will integrate the impacts of cephalad fluid shift. The model will take into account mean ICP and IOP after fluid redistribution has stabilized in space, in addition to heartbeat-dependent fluctuations for peak ICP after fluid redistribution, and the effects due to exercise and Valsalva maneuvers (VMs) (Fig. 4).

It is predicted that gravitational unloading causes ophthalmic changes, and modeling provides insight into plausible biomechanical pathways for these changes. Guidelines will be developed to apply these models independently or in an integrated fashion to inform research.

Modeling studies will make important contributions to the research effort by integrating environmental and physiological inputs from multiple body systems to provide a better understanding of how they may interact to cause VIIP signs and

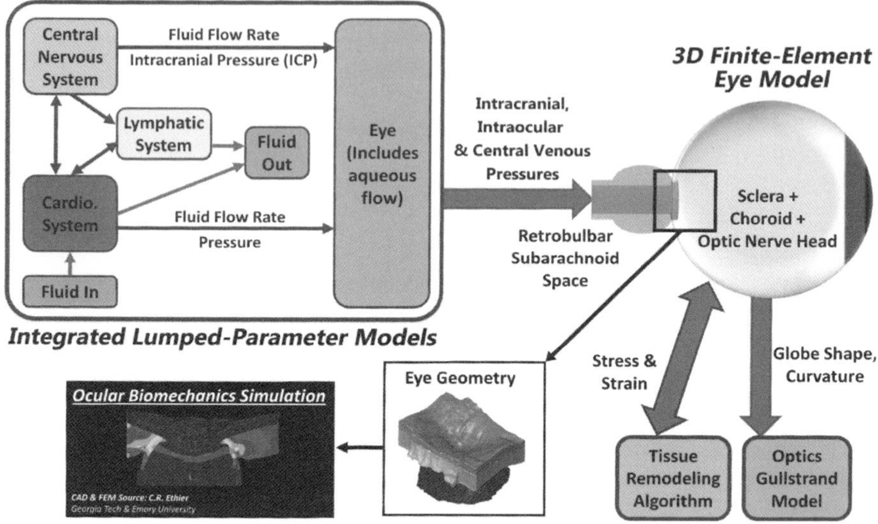

Figure 4. Graphical representation of the integrated LP and finite element computational models being implemented to further understand the causal mechanisms of VIIP syndrome (Courtesy of NASA's Digital Astronaut Project and C. R. Ethier of Georgia Institute of Technology and Emory University).

symptoms. The gradual onset of VIIP, its chronicity, and the similarity of clinical findings to those seen in patients with elevated ICP indicate that biomechanical forces are involved in the etiology of VIIP, and that connective tissue remodeling must be evaluated to understand the pathophysiology of VIIP (Ethier *et al.*, 2015). The "Microgravity-driven Optic Nerve/Sheath Remodelling Study", led by Ross Ethier, PhD, will develop validated tools for computing IOP and ICP in microgravity. These tools will be based on modeling of fluid shifts between the eye and compartments in the cardiovascular, cerebrospinal, and lymphatic systems. Three integrated computer models will be developed (Ethier *et al.*, 2015). First, a set of linked lumped-parameter sub-models to predict fluid transport within and among the cardiovascular system, CNS, lymphatic system, and the eye. Second, a spatially resolved finite-element model (FEM) of the eye and retrobulbar subarachnoid space that will allow computation of tissue biomechanics for important ocular structures. "This FEM is coupled to a tissue remodeling algorithm that predicts temporal changes in tissue properties and geometry in response to the local biomechanical state. The third is an optical eye model that uses computed changes in eye shape to predict alterations in visual acuity in VIIP. An integrated model will result in a unified, open and extensible software package that can predict ocular biomechanics and ocular connective tissue remodeling under microgravity conditions.

The integrated model will allow study and examination of clinically observable attributes and determine the role they may play in the development of VIIP" (Ethier *et al.*, 2015).

A third modeling effort, "The Role of Cranial Venous Circulation in Microgravity Associated Visual Changes", led by Jay Buckey, MD, and Scott Phillips, PhD, at Creare LLC, is developing two primary mathematical models: a structural model of the eye and a fluid model of the cranial vascular system. The vascular system model estimates changes in intracranial vascular flow, volume, compliance, and pressure in response to fluid shifts and changes in hydrostatic gradients. The vascular model predicts the pressures around the eye in response to these changes, and the structural model shows the effects of the new pressure environment on the eye. The resulting tissue stresses are calculated to understand the environment from which remodeling may occur. The unique features of these models are that they include the effects of gravity on both hydrostatic gradients and tissue weight.

Model validation is underway by collecting physiological data in ground-based tests using interventions that changes both the direction of the gravitational vector (supine vs. prone measurements) and the direction and magnitude of the fluid shift (lower body negative pressure and lower body positive pressure). These ground-based data will be used with the model to generate hypotheses about how changes in hydrostatic gradients, fluid redistribution, and cranial venous anatomy can influence microgravity-induced visual changes (Phillips *et al.*, 2014). The structural eye model was also compared with data collected in parabolic flight — a microgravity analog that simulates weightlessness. The investigators evaluated the effects of short-term microgravity exposure on the eye by measuring IOP, axial length, aqueous depth, and choroidal volume in subjects before, during, and after short-term microgravity exposure. The results from these studies show that hydrostatic gradients within both the eye and cranial vascular system are important to consider when interpreting microgravity effects (Anderson *et al.*, 2016).

The cranial vascular model validation includes acquiring MRI of the head to measure changes in venous flow, venous volume, venous pressure, intracranial compliance, CSF volume, and flow pulsatility during fluid shifts and changes in body position. These data reflect the effects of changes in the direction of the gravitational vector (supine vs. prone) and the effects of fluid shifts. These data are essential to refine the mathematical models of the eye and cranial vascular system and to use them to extrapolate the effects of microgravity exposure. The models can also be used to estimate effects on parameters that cannot be easily measured, such as episcleral venous pressure and intracranial pressure. The study team hypothesizes that by incorporating the effects of hydrostatic gradients and tissue weight within the models, and validating them with ground-based measures, new hypotheses can be generated about how microgravity affects the eye and cranial venous circulation.

The modeling effort may also be useful for generating hypotheses about why not all astronauts develop serious ocular changes in space. Some astronauts may be predisposed to developing visual changes as a result of microgravity exposure, and this may be related to their vascular anatomy. This study will identify individuals with common intracranial venous variants and assess them using the described protocols. This modeling effort and the data from these studies will allow hypothesis testing to determine which tissue and vascular parameters have the greatest impact on vision and provide estimates of changes in intracranial pressure and venous pressure in space (Figs. 5 and 6). The hope is that this may offer predictions about future visual changes in an individual (Phillips *et al.*, 2014).

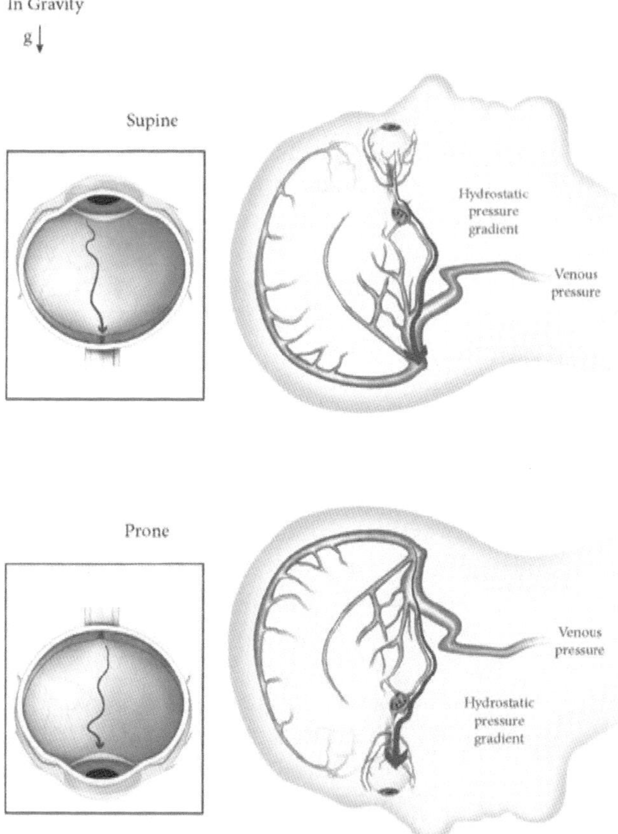

Figure 5. Hydrostatic pressure (arrow), as well as gravitational induced mechanical forces, alter the eye in the supine and prone posture. Image credit: Caroline O'Driscoll, Cobalt Studios (Phillips *et al.*, 2014).

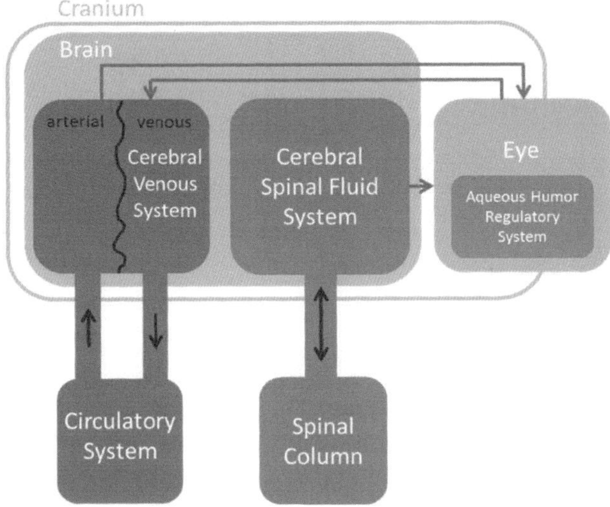

Figure 6. Schematic of the Cerebral/Cranial Venous Physiology Model (Phillips *et al.*, 2014).

7.4. *Animal studies*

Using an animal model, the "Head-down Tilt in Rats as a Model for Intracranial and Intraocular Pressures, and Retinal Changes During Spaceflight" experiment, led by Charles Fuller, PhD, will help understand if the cephalic fluid shift during microgravity exposure is a causative factor leading to the ocular changes seen in astronauts after long-term spaceflight. The HLS rat model will allow a systems approach to these questions and potentially fulfill multiple objectives. A 90-day extended HLS experiment will be conducted, roughly the equivalent of a 2.5-year exploration class mission in human subjects based on lifespans, followed by a 90-day recovery period (Fuller *et al.*, 2014). The study is designed to assess the influence of age and sex on the development of the VIIP syndrome, since both factors influence endovascular health, which is believed to play a critical role (Otto *et al.*, 2015). In addition, hypercapneic exposure will aid in understanding the influence of a chronically elevated CO_2 environment upon ICP given that CO_2 is a potent cerebrovascular vasodilator. This animal experiment provides several advantages, namely; chronic instrumentation, a high number of subjects, induced cephalad fluid shift, and the ability to alter the ambient CO_2 environment.

Simultaneous measurement of ICP and IOP will be conducted allowing determination of the TLPG, the pressure across the LC, which is thought to be altered in microgravity (Otto, 2013). The rat does have an LC, which separates the intraocular compartment from the subarachnoid space, and has been reported to develop papilledema with elevated ICP (Griffith *et al.*, 1938). Ocular coherence tomography will be conducted to assess the changes in the retina as a result of HLS.

Approximately 276 rats will be studied over a 3-year period. The animals will be divided into four groups of 66 subjects each. Two of the cohorts will be males 3 months of age, another will be females 3 months of age, and the fourth group will be males 9 months of age. Since the rat has a short lifespan, the 6-month age difference between cohorts will allow the comparison of responses between young and old animals. One of the 3-month-old male cohorts will be exposed to a hypercapneic environment for the duration of their HLS (1% CO_2 in air). This will mimic the highest average peak concentrations of CO_2 on the ISS, which is 10 times nominal terrestrial levels.

All animals will receive an ophthalmic examination on days 7, 14, 28, and 90 for both the HLS and recovery periods. This will include a slit lamp biomicroscope assessment, indirect and direct ophthalmoscopy to survey optic nerve morphology. Cycloplegic refraction to assess refractive change and possible hyperopic shift, corneal and lens curvature will be measured; in addition, A-scan ultrasound will be used to measure globe axial length. Ocular coherence tomography of the ONH and fundus will provide data on retinal cell layers. Assessment of inner retinal and central visual pathway function will be measured using a pupillometer. Seven Tesla MRI T1-weighted imaging will be conducted to monitor for changes in the lens, retina, and optic nerve.

Each cohort will have 12 animals instrumented with biotelemetry (BTS) to allow the collection of ICP and electroencephalogram (EEG) for visual evoked potentials. Six of the BTS animals will serve as controls, while the other six animals will undergo HLS. Recordings will be made during the first 2 weeks of both the HLS and recovery phase, and for 2 weeks preceding days 28 and 90 of the HLS and recovery phase. A total of 8 weeks of biotelemetry data will be collected. In addition, IOP will be recorded at baseline, and daily for the first 2 weeks of HLS and then once weekly. The same schedule will be followed during the 90-day recovery phase. Control animals will have the same data collection schedule over the 180 days. Twelve animals will undergo MRI imaging of their eyes and optic nerves, six of these will be exposed to HLS, and six will serve as controls. MRI imaging will occur at baseline and at 30, 60, and 90 days in both the HLS and recovery periods. The balance of each cohort will undergo histological examination, 24 of these as HLS animals and 18 as controls (Table 2).

Three animals in the experimental group and two in the control group will be sacrificed after 7, 14, 28, and 90 days HLS and recovery for analysis of the retina.

Table 2. Cohort interventions and experimental data collection.

Young Male Long-Evans	Telemetry (ICP)	MRI	Histology
Hindlimb suspended	EBY; n = 6	EMY; n = 6	EHY; n = 24
Control	CBY; n = 6	CMY; n = 6	CHY; n = 18

Table Key: Y = Young Male; E = HLS Experimental; C = non-HLS Control;
B = Biotelemetry Subgroup; M = MRI subgroup; H = Histology Subgroup

Retinal histology will center on morphological analysis of the retina, including immunohistochemical staining of retinal cell types.

It is anticipated that ICP and IOP will increase during HLS. Comparison of ICP data between the HLS and control group will allow determination of changes in ICP as a result of HLS. The biotelemetry data will allow an assessment of any change in ICP and IOP during HLS and recovery and thus the translaminar pressure gradient (TLP). The effects of significant alterations in the TLP will be readily quantified by OCT measurement and histological analysis of the retina. It is anticipated that HLS will precipitate optic disc edema, choroidal folds, ONSD, retinal nerve fiber thickening, and retinal histological changes consistent with optic disc edema. Such changes will result in altered visual evoked potentials (VEP).

Male rats are expected to be more affected than female rats of the same age due to higher vascular compliance among the females. Correspondingly, older male rats are expected to be more affected than younger male rats due to lower vascular compliance among older rats. The addition of CO_2 is expected to result in greater changes indicative of the VIIP syndrome, compared to rats of the same age not exposed to CO_2.

Another aspect of this study involves assessment of retinal microvascular changes, and markers of oxidative stress, hypoxia, and cellular death studied by gene expression analysis and immunohistochemistry as a result of HLS-induced optic disc edema (Theriot *et al.*, 2014). It is hypothesized that cephalad fluid shift precipitates vascular engorgement, venous stasis, and therefore hypoxia, microvascular remodeling, and cellular degeneration. The study investigators' believe that this is mediated by hypoxia inducible factor (HIF) signaling pathway upregulating vascular endothelial growth factor (VEGF) to induce angiogenesis and vascular permeability.

It is hypothesized that small retinal blood vessels adapt and remodel to accommodate fluid shift in microgravity. It is proposed that alterations in the vascular patterning of the retina in response to fluid shift during HLS will contribute to ocular and visual impairments. VESGEN software (Parsons-Wingerter *et al.*, 2000a,b; Parsons-Wingerter *et al.*, 2006) will be used to map and quantify arterial and venous trees. Alterations in retinal vasculature branching patterns will be mapped and quantified following administration of fluorescein dextran and preparation of retinal section flat-mounts. The investigators hypothesize that transfer of fluids is a major microvascular regulatory function. Furthermore, retinal blood vessels, especially the fragile, actively remodeling smaller vessels, adapt and remodel to accommodate fluid shift in microgravity. VESGEN analysis will be conducted on 15 animals per cohort. Plasma volume will be measured before and after HLS, using the Evans Blue method (Kutscher, 1971; Probst *et al.*, 2006), to determine whether HLS induces a change in plasma volume.

Markers for oxidative damage in the retina will be evaluated including 8-hydroxydeoxyguanosine (8-OHdG) and 4-hydroxy-2-nonenal histidine adduct, Müller cell, and astrocytic expression of GFAP (Lieth *et al.*, 1998; Bringmann *et al.*, 2006). In addition, apoptosis of retinal cells will be monitored via caspase-3 labeling (Singh *et al.*, 2001), and inflammatory marker detection will be measured using NFκB nuclear translocation (Kubota *et al.*, 2009). Histological evaluation of the inner nuclear layers and ganglion cell layer will also be performed to detect the presence of inflammatory cells and edema.

Gene expression profiling will be performed using microarray analysis. Genes that display significantly different expression following HLS in comparison to controls will receive additional evaluation with real-time PCR. The changes in gene expression will provide insights into the mechanisms causing ocular pathology associated with the VIIP syndrome. Total RNA will be isolated form the whole retina. The yield and integrity of the isolated RNA will be evaluated. Microarray analysis will be performed on total RNA pooled from three eyes each from the HLS and the control group. The research teams involved in this study have identified genes that may be affected by HLS, and primarily involve pathways involving cellular stress response, oxidative stress, hypoxia response, cellular death, and glial activation.

8. *Environmental Impacts*

8.1. *CO_2*

Carbon dioxide levels on the ISS have ranged from 2.3 mmHg to 5.3 mmHg, which represent 7.7–17.7 times the typical atmospheric partial pressure of 0.3 mmHg (Law *et al.*, 2014). Carbon dioxide is a known potent stimulator of cerebrovascular dilation mediated through changes in H+ concentration and its effects on blood pH. Vascular dilation results in increased blood volume, and within the rigid cranial vault, this increases intracranial pressure. The impacts of CO_2 on ICP are so potent that patients with life threatening increases in ICP can be saved by rapid reduction of CO_2 levels through hyperventilation. The NASA Medical Operations Branch has been conducting a data mining effort to evaluate the in-flight CO_2 levels during flight with the time course of identified visual changes experienced by crew members to determine if increase CO_2 levels could be a contributing factor to the VIIP syndrome. ISS crew members have been noted to report with greater frequency the presence of headache, fatigue, irritability, and sleep difficulties, when CO_2 levels rose above 4 mmHg. Coincidentally, crews would report symptom relief when CO_2 levels were reduced below 2 mmHg, and during extravehicular prebreath of 100% oxygen (Law *et al.*, 2014). On the ISS, CO_2 levels are controlled by regenerable absorber technology that requires electrical power, approximately 900 W, and 200–1000 W of heat load rejection to the ISS thermal control system (James *et al.*, 2011). Electrical power and thermal unloading are limited resources on the ISS and must be taken from other systems and therefore have operational impacts. As a result it is not practical to limit CO_2 to below 3 mmHg when six crew members are onboard the ISS (James *et al.*, 2011).

In a recent retrospective review of the onboard CO_2 data, the Medical Operations Group and the NASA Longitudinal Surveillance of Astronaut Health group examined the relationship of CO_2 with sex, VIIP pathology, and incidence of headache. A statistically significant association was found between higher CO_2 levels and an increased incidence of reported headaches in otherwise healthy astronauts. In addition, based on data modeling, to maintain a risk of headache below 1%, the average 7-day CO_2 level had to be below 2.5 mmHg. When sex was included in the model there were no differences in associations with CO_2. Similarly, there were no associations found between CO_2 levels and VIIP-related vision or ocular changes. However, these findings cannot be considered conclusive, therefore this evaluation continues.

A prospective study evaluating the combined effects of cephalad fluid shift and elevated CO_2 is warranted based on the VIIP findings to date, the known impacts of elevated CO_2 on cerebrovascular dilation and ICP, and the association of headaches with elevated levels of CO_2 on the ISS. To clearly delineate the impacts of CO_2 and cephalad fluid shift on ICP and the associated ocular changes seen with the VIIP syndrome, the study "Does 30 Days of Head-Down Bed Rest in Humans Combined with Ambient 0.5% CO_2 Induce Changes Related to the Spaceflight Associated Vision Impairment Intracranial Pressure (VIIP) Syndrome?" ("Integrative Physiology", 2016) will be conducted. This study will take place at envihab, the German Aerospace Center (DLR) Institute of Aerospace Medicine research facility in Cologne, Germany. Among the eight modules that comprise the facility is the baro lab which is capable of enriching the atmosphere with CO_2 up to 4%. Subjects will undergo 30 days of 6° HDT bed rest while exposed to 0.5% CO_2. Pressure locks allow staff and supplies to enter the facility while maintaining the altered atmosphere. Onsite MRI and positron emission tomography (PET) scanning facilities allow for imaging of subjects with minimal transfer and interruption of experimental conditions.

8.2. *Radiation*

In terms of eye-specific studies examining environmental effects on the retina, radiation and dietary iron are two environmental factors that may act synergistically causing damage to retinal cells of the eye. During spaceflight, astronauts experience iron overload due to the consumption of iron-fortified foods on the space station, at times consuming three to six times the recommended daily allowance. In addition, astronauts are exposed to several forms of radiation. Gamma rays, produced by various astronomical processes, are a form of ionizing radiation, and therefore biologically hazardous. Typically, these rays are screened by the Earth's atmosphere, but a higher percentage reaches the ISS given its orbit high above the Earth's surface. It is known that radiation exposure and high dietary iron loads promote oxidative stress therefore increasing the sensitivity to radiation due to decreased scavenging of cellular free radicals. The recently completed study, *Combined Effects of Gamma Radiation and High Dietary Iron on Oxidative Damage and Antioxidant Status in Rat Eyes*, (Theriot *et al.*, 2015) found that a high iron diet altered the normal iron status of the rats which affected the physiological response to fractionated low doses of ionizing radiation. The study included four separate experimental groups of eight 12 week-old Sprague–Dawley rats. Two groups received no radiation; the control group received 45 mg iron/kg diet, and a high iron group was fed a 650 mg iron/kg diet. The two radiation groups were fed the same as the nonradiation groups; the first a 45 mg iron/kg diet, the second a 650 mg iron/kg diet, and both received a 3 Gy dose, fractionated at 37.5 cGy/d every other day for eight fractions.

The investigators characterized the cellular responses in the retina and identified potential components related to vascular remodeling that provide insight into the pathophysiology of spaceflight-related changes in visual impairment. Cellular protection mechanisms appear to be overwhelmed due to the combination of increased iron loads and radiation exposure evidenced by increases in expression of the oxidative stress-related genes, specifically Hmox1, Nrf2, and SOD2. With regard to vascular health, "collagen molecules were downregulated after radiation independent of diet and several matrix proteases were differentially expressed with the combined treatment of high iron diet and radiation. Of particular interest are matrix metallopeptidases (MMP) 8, 10, and 11 which were all statistically down-regulated when treated with the high iron diet or radiation" (Theriot *et al.*, 2015).

To quantify oxidative DNA damage in the eye, densitometric quantification of 8-OHdG immunohistochemistry was performed on the retinal sections. In the iron, radiation and, iron and radiation group, 8-OHdG was present in the retina with increased levels compared to the control group. There was a significant interaction between radiation exposure and dietary iron on 8-OHdG levels in all retinal cell layers, potentially triggering cytoprotective mechanisms in the eyes exposed to both iron and radiation. In addition, gene expression analysis showed altered profiles in retinal samples suggesting increased sensitivity to radiation with the high iron diet. This study indicates that gamma radiation exposure combined with high dietary iron adversely affect retinal and vascular health by inducing a state of oxidative stress thereby causing damage to intracellular molecules resulting in cell death, inflammatory responses, and fibrosis and tissue remodeling.

8.3. *Exercise*

The effects of exercise on VIIP symptoms are unknown, however, two forms of exercise are believed to have opposite effects on in-flight ICP and hence exacerbation of VIIP signs and symptoms. Continuous aerobic exercise on the ISS is required to maintain cardiorespiratory fitness and involves the T2 running treadmill, or the cycle ergometer with vibration isolation and stabilization system (CEVIS). Crew members conduct approximately 3.5 h per week of continuous exercise. Both devices activate and engage large lower limb musculature thereby drawing increased blood volume into the lower limbs. Theoretically, this would have a beneficial effect on reducing ICP as some of the cephalad shifted volume would move caudally during the duration of exercise. In contrast, resistance exercise using the advanced resistive exercise device (ARED), unlike continuous aerobic exercise, is known to elevate ICP and was initially thought by some to possibly be a causative factor in development of the VIIP syndrome. Crew members perform approximately 6 h of resistance training per week to maintain bone and muscle strength (Haykowsky *et al.*, 2003). Haykowsky *et al.* demonstrated that upright resistive exercise without a VM increased ICP by 3 mmHg and by 18 mmHg with a VM. Available data indicate that ARED resistance exercise may exacerbate VIIP signs and symptoms by increasing ICP transiently, but it is unlikely "the" causative agent. Given that relatively little is known about the effects of continuous and resistance exercise on ICP in the presence of cephalad fluid shift, a greater understanding is required to mitigate individual crew member risk. The *Influence of Exercise Modality on Cerebral-Ocular Hemodynamics and Pressures* study, led by Jessica Scott, PhD, will characterize the effects of acute resistance, continuous moderate-intensity aerobic, and high-intensity aerobic exercise on cerebral-ocular hemodynamics.

Following instrumentation, subjects will be positioned in a 15° HDT orientation to rest quietly for 10 min. They will then complete the exercise session and rest for 20 min.

All exercise protocols will be based on sessions currently performed by long-duration astronauts. The HDT/resistance exercise session will consist of a 5-min warm up and four sets of 12 repetition maximum leg press exercise conducted with a brief VM, replicating the technique used in-flight by astronauts. The HDT/continuous session will consist of 30 min of cycling at 60% VO_2 max, and the HDT/interval session will consist of a 5-min warm up at ~50% VO_2 max, followed by 4 × 4 min intervals of exercise at 85% VO_2 max with 3-min active rest periods (Scott *et al.*, 2016).

During each HDT session, blood flow in extracranial arteries (common carotid, internal carotid, external carotid, and vertebral artery) and veins (internal jugular and vertebral vein) will be measured using color-coded duplex ultrasonography. Due to the technical challenges of simultaneously evaluating blood flow in ipsilateral cerebral arteries, measurement of vessels will be alternated with each interval or resistance set and continuous time points. Internal jugular vein and vertebral vein flow will be acquired at the same time as IOP. This sequence will be repeated throughout rest and exercise.

To acquire a surrogate measure of ICP, the pulsatility index will be calculated from TCD. The PI is calculated as: PI = systolic flow velocity−diastolic flow velocity/mean flow velocity, and has been shown to provide a noninvasive estimate of ICP (Bellner *et al.*, 2004; Moreno *et al.*, 2000). IOP will be measured using an applanation rebound tonometer. Measurements will be taken during rest periods on resistance and interval sessions; for the continuous session subjects will be asked to briefly stop exercising for approximately 1 min while IOP is acquired (Fig. 8).

Blood pressure and heart rate will be recorded and cardiac output (Q) will be calculated from the blood pressure waveform using the Modelflow method that incorporates age, sex, height, and weight. Total peripheral resistance will be estimated by dividing mean arterial pressure (MAP) by Q, and cerebral vascular conductance will be calculated by the equation middle cerebral artery (MCA) × cerebral blood flow (CBF) velocity/MAP (Scott *et al.*, 2016).

This study promises to provide a clearer understanding of the impact of exercise modality and cephalad fluid shift upon crew member ICP and the TLPG, the two components believed to be central to the development of the VIIP syndrome.

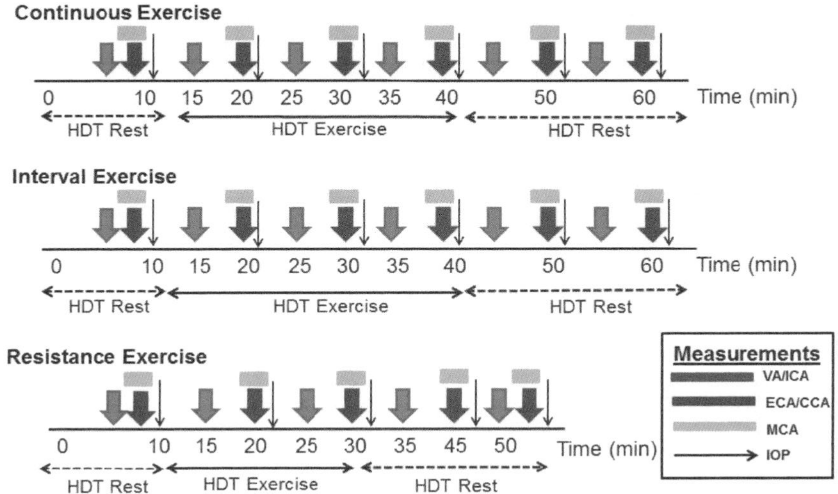

Figure 8. Experimental protocol and target time points. Subjects will be positioned in 15° head-down-tilt (HDT) during rest and exercise and the vertebral artery (VA), internal carotid artery (ICA), external carotid artery (ECA), common carotid artery (CCA), middle cerebral artery (MCA), and intraocular pressure (IOP) will be measured.

9. *Diagnostic tools*

Several diagnostic tools are used to evaluate astronauts for the presence of VIIP-related signs. All U.S. astronauts undergo specific medically required testing preflight, in-flight, and postflight. These tests are outlined in NASA's Medical Operations MRID. The tests relating to eye health are the MRID requirements MedB 1.10 ("MedB 1.10 Pre and Postflight Physical", 2011) and VIIP Clinical Practice Guidelines (unpublished).

A suite of tests provide information on eye and brain health for flight qualification, prior to a mission, to aid in monitoring astronauts for the development of VIIP-related signs and symptoms during flight, and to monitor their recovery after flight.

Twenty-one to 18 months before a mission, and within the first three days of returning from space, a three Tesla MRI of the brain and orbits is performed. The brain anatomy is evaluated against standard clinical criteria for the presence of abnormalities in the white and grey matter, CSF spaces, and vasculature; with particular attention paid to signs of elevated ICP such as enlarged ventricles, compression of the pituitary gland, or changes in the configuration of the sella turcica. Orbital images are assessed for optic nerve sheath diameter, optic disc elevation, globe flattening, and optic nerve tortuosity, all findings that may indicate the onset of VIIP.

Ocular ultrasound can document globe flattening, ONSD, and optic nerve sheath tortuosity, cardinal signs of VIIP. The test is conducted 9–6 months before flight and during the first 3 days postflight. For ground testing, subjects are seated and the sonographer positions the ultrasound probe, with ultrasound echo gel, over the closed eyelid to collect ocular ultrasound images. During flight, measurements are made on flight days 30, 90, and R–30 (30 days before returning to Earth). In-flight sessions are remotely guided by sonographers in mission control via real-time cabin video and ultrasound feed from the ISS. The astronauts onboard the ISS acquire the images on one another while receiving expert guidance from mission control.

Vision testing is performed twice before flight first between 21 and 9 months before launch, and again between 6 and 9 months prior to launch. In the postflight period, testing is completed during the first 3 days upon return to Earth. The ground portion of vision testing consists of:

Vision Questionnaire
Visual Acuity (distance and near)
Refraction (manifest and cycloplegic)
Amsler Grid
Contrast Sensitivity
Pupil Reflexes
Extraocular Muscle Balance
Biomicroscopy (slit lamp)
Dilated Fundoscopic Examination
Applanation Tonometry
Handheld Tonometry
OCT (high resolution)
Threshold Visual Fields
High Resolution Retinal Photography
Optical Biometry
Magnetic Resonance Imaging (brain and orbits)

Far visual acuity is tested for each eye with and without corrective a lens using a software application loaded onto the OCT Laptop that provides a screenshot of a standard Snellen chart. The astronaut is positioned 15 ft away from the OCT Laptop. Ground support will control the software application by accessing the OCT Laptop remotely and will guide the astronaut taking the test and record the results. Amsler grid testing will also be administered during each session, for both the right and left eye, using the software. The astronaut sits at 16 in. from the grid and focuses on the dot in the center of the grid while slowly bringing the grid toward the uncovered eye until one of the red ovals disappears. Any changes to the appearance of the grid (wavy, blurred, or missing lines) indicate a positive for this test. Near visual acuity will be tested for each eye with and without a corrective lens using a paper-based eye chart located 16 in. from the astronaut on the wall of the laboratory module. Contrast sensitivity testing assesses the ability to differentiate between light and dark (contrast), an important measure of visual function. The contrast sensitivity chart consists of a horizontal line of capital letters. The contrast of the letters (relative to the chart background) decreases with each screen.

OCT is a diagnostic imaging technique that is based on analysis of the reflection of low-coherence light from the tissue under examination. It involves measurements of retinal thickness, volume, and RNFL thickness using a method of quantitative cross-sectional analysis. The OCT software is able to identify and "trace" two key layers of the retina, the nerve fiber layer and the retinal pigment epithelium. OCT is conducted preflight, in-flight, and postflight to detect changes in the RNFL of the ONH. The OCT scans are performed with the subject placing their chin on a chin rest while the device performs a scan of the eyes.

Direct fundoscopy is performed on the right and left eye to obtain images of the retinal surface. All in-flight exams will be remotely guided using the current fundoscope and desktop streaming software technology. Astronauts will set up the fundoscope hardware, OCT Laptop, video camera, and then perform dilation, and complete the exam. Still images and short cine clips will be recorded and downlinked.

The in-flight vision questionnaire asks if the crew member has noticed any change in his or her vision since launch or the last in-flight exam. Respondents rate any change as mild — does not affect daily activities, moderate — crew member had to make changes to accommodate which resulted in completion of all activities, and severe — changes significantly affected or interfered with completion of daily activities. The vision change questions include: distortion, vision in dim light, fluctuation in visual acuity, depth perception, double vision, transient visual loss, and change in near, intermediate, and distance vision. Additional questions include use of trifocal or superfocus adjustable eyewear, use of any additional eyewear. If yes, the crew member is asked if for reading or distance? Also the crew member is asked about the presence of the following symptoms: headaches, tinnitus, nausea, or impairment in cognition? If present, he or she is asked to rate the intensity as mild, moderate, or severe.

Refractive error is an error in focusing light by the eye and may affect visual acuity. Two types of refraction tests are utilized to measure refractive error, manifest, and cycloplegic. In manifest refraction, refractive errors are measured while the eyes own crystalline lens is able to accommodate. During manifest refraction, subjects may "over-use" their accommodative ability while trying to read a line of letters. This must be controlled in order to properly determine the refractive error and prescribe the appropriate correction. Cycloplegic refraction allows determination of the total refractive error by temporarily paralyzing the muscles that aid in focusing the eye. Cycloplegic eye drops are used to temporarily relax the ciliary body, a focusing muscle of the lens.

Threshold peripheral visual field testing is conducted preflight and postflight. It is used for screening and follow-up of peripheral vision. Humphrey's automated static threshold perimetry tests different locations throughout the visual field one at a time. In a SITA standard 30-2 protocol, the central 30° of the near peripheral visual field is tested. A dim light is presented at a particular location. If the patient does not visualize the light, it is made gradually brighter until it is seen. The minimum brightness required for the detection of a light stimulus is the "threshold" sensitivity level for that location. This procedure is then repeated at several other locations, until the entire visual field is tested. When the 30° test is employed, 76 individual points are assessed, each point is separated by 6°.

Additional testing conducted pre- and postflight includes pupillary reflexes, extraocular muscle balance, biomicroscopy, and optical biometry. Retinal photography is conducted during all three mission phases.

9.1. *Diagnostic tools under development*

Several diagnostic tools are under development to help characterize physiological changes occurring with VIIP during the various phases of flight. The *Pilot Study to Evaluate a Novel Non-Invasive Technology to Measure Peripheral Venous Pressure,* led by David Martin, MS, aimed to evaluate a noninvasive means of measuring PVP. It is hypothesized that central venous pressure (CVP) is elevated in spaceflight (Alexander *et al.*, 2012; Hamilton *et al.*, 2012). A noninvasive means of measuring deviations in CVP would provide insight into the role of cephalic venous congestion in spaceflight. Compression sonography visualizes a vein via ultrasound and upon compression, when the two walls of the vein touch, the occlusion pressure is recorded via an integrated pressure transducer (Vein Press 2010, Vein Press GmbH, Switzerland) (Fig. 9) and is assumed to be equal to the vessel pressure according to Laplace's law. Ten subjects participated (five male and five female) and noninvasive measures of PVP were made in four veins: the supratrochlear vein in the forehead, the jugular vein in the neck, the cephalic vein in the arm, and the greater saphenous vein in the leg. In addition, noninvasive measurements

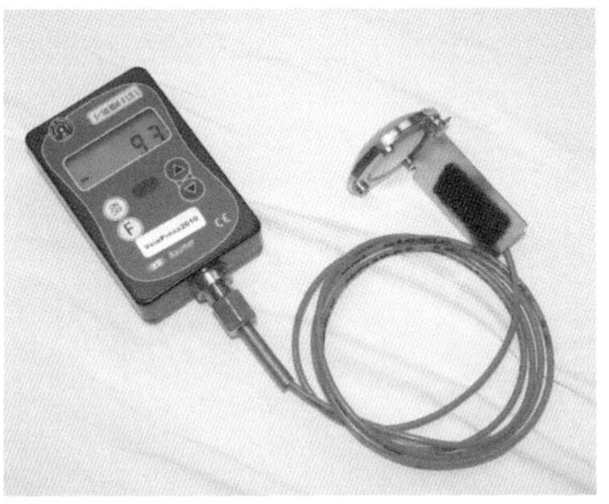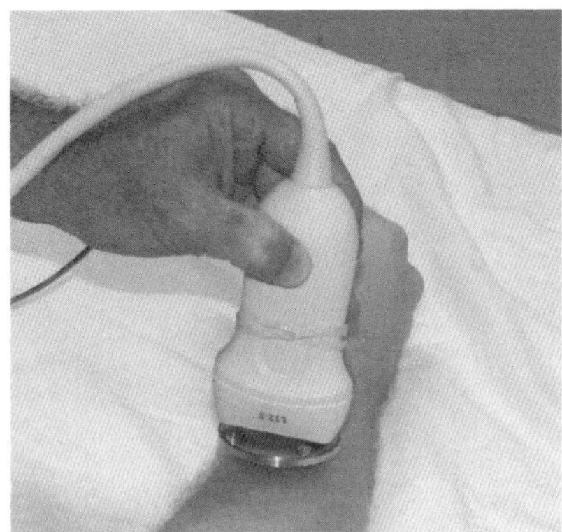

Figure 9. VeinPress (left) and ultrasound probe during vein pressure measurements on arm (right) (Martin *et al.*, 2015).

for the greater saphenous and cephalic vein were compared to invasive measurements collected using a Draeger Infinity Delta XL (Draeger Medical Systems, Inc., Danvers, MA).

The noninvasive NIPVP measures increased from the baseline condition with increasing levels of venous occlusion or HDT angle. However, the noninvasive measures were significantly different than the invasive measures (Fig. 10).

The vein compression device may be a low-risk, noninvasive method of evaluating trends in venous pressures in response to simulated or real microgravity.

Accurate measurement of ICP in-flight would provide a clearer understanding of the exact role that cerebral volume changes may play in the VIIP risk. Invasive measurement in-flight is currently deemed too risky, including measurement of LP opening CSF pressure. Therefore, it is highly desirable to acquire a reliable noninvasive measure of ICP that has a lower associated risk. Aaron Dentinger of General Electric Global Research leads the study on *Non-Invasive Monitoring of Intracranial Pressure with Volumetric Ultrasound* whose objective is to build a 3-D ophthalmic ultrasound imaging capability that will integrate with the current onboard GE Vivid q Ultrasound platform. Volumetric imaging will improve the reliability of in-flight ocular measurements, and provide a means of noninvasively monitoring ICP based on 3-D optic nerve sheath volume changes, and posterior globe flattening. Volumetric ultrasound also promises to reduce image acquisition time and the degree of remote guidance required from the ground (Dentinger and Patwardhan, 2014). The current ultrasound does not support 3-D imaging, and the probe for acquiring ocular images is a linear array, 14 mm × 47 mm probe making it cumbersome for ocular ultrasound. The new volumetric probe will have a smaller footprint

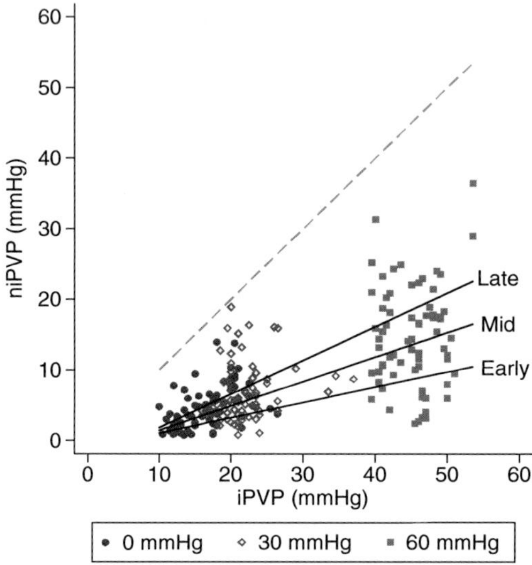

Figure 10.   Noninvasive peripheral venous pressure (niPVP) vs. invasive PVP (iPVP) for the cephalic vein. Early to late indicates accumulated operator experience, as compared to the line of equality (dashed line). (Martin *et al.*, 2015).

of 12 mm × 30 mm, and will be capable of sweeping a 60° volume that corresponds to 30 mm × 30 mm area × 20 mm depth. The 3–D probe will connect to the current ultrasound via an external control unit that drives the probe motor without modification to the current hardware and minor changes to the software. Evaluation of the new 3–D probe will include in vivo measurements of ONSD and globe flattening during tilt table experiments and mild increases in ICP, in addition to animal experiments where higher ICPs will be induced (Dentinger *et al.*, 2014).

The Vittamed two–depth TCD device has shown promise in providing a noninvasive quantitative measure of ICP (Bershad *et al.*, 2015). Drs. Bershad and Dunham provided a detailed overview of this technology in the chapter "Noninvasive Measurements of Intracranial Pressure with the Vittamed Absolute Value Meter". The technology is based on simultaneously measuring the blood flow velocity waveform in the intracranial and extracranial portions of the ophthalmic artery (OA) before, during, and after, discrete increases in pressure applied to the closed eye (Ragauskas *et al.*, 2012).

10. VIIP Mechanical Countermeasures

Mechanical devices that counteract cephalad fluid shift have the potential to decrease cephalad venous congestion and lower ICP. The Braslet-M thigh cuff is a tourniquet-like device developed by the Russian space agency for use in cosmonauts for the first few days in flight to mitigate the head fullness and congestion caused by cephalad fluid shift in microgravity. A cuff is worn proximally on each thigh and is individually calibrated per subject on the ground during HDT. The device decreases venous flow velocity in the vascular bed of the lower extremities distal to the cuff causing a sequestration of fluid in the extremities thereby limiting the circulating volume. In a study involving nine crew members onboard the ISS, Hamilton *et al.* (2012) found that 10–30 min following application of the Braslet-M the following significant changes resulted: femoral vein area increased by 89%, cardiac output fell 19%, and stroke volume was lowered 12%, compared to no Braslet-M in microgravity. There was a corresponding 23.4% decrease in internal jugular vein area; however, it was not statistically significant. However, Herault *et al.* (2000), in studying cosmonauts during a 6-month stay on the Mir space station, found that cardiac output and stroke volume declined 14% and 15%, respectively, after 5 h of daily use for 1 month. This effect diminished, however, by 3 months into the flight. It is possible that combining Braslet-M with other mechanical devices could prolong its effect.

10.1. *Lower body negative pressure*

Lower body negative pressure is another mechanical option which has been shown to reduce cerebral venous volume (see Chapter 11). This technology exists on the ISS in the Russian segment and is used by Russian crew members as a prelanding countermeasure to stress the cardiovascular system. The Chibis lower body negative pressure device is a pantsuit that covers the lower extremities to the top of the iliac crest where a rubberized pressure seal is formed. A motorized pump and microprocessor creates a variable vacuum on the lower body contained within the suit. Pressures of −35 to −45 mmHg can be applied. The hydrostatic stress pulls fluid volume toward the lower limbs creating a hydrostatic posture that more closely resembles what exists in 1G. Creating negative pressure in a body compartment has been found to be effective in altering hemodynamics in clinical ground studies. Valenza *et al.* (2003) applied negative abdominal pressure to 30 hemodynamically monitored stable ICU patients. A pressure of −5 cm H_2O decreased intra-abdominal pressure (IAP) 4.4 mmHg with an associated significant fall in CVP from 9.2 ± 3.4 mmHg to 7.5 ± 3.5 mmHg. In a second clinical study, Sugerman *et al.* (2001) applied negative abdominal pressure to seven patients with IIH who had a mean CSF opening pressure of 32.9 cm H_2O ± 9.2. There was a mean decrease in urinary bladder pressure (a measure of IAP) of 6.6 cm H_2O (4.85 mmHg). This resulted in a 22.5% reduction in internal jugular vein cross-sectional area ($P = 0.06$), and a significant reduction in headache severity and pulsatile tinnitus after only 1 h of use. After using the device for 10 h per night over 3 days, 4/5 subjects reported complete cessation of headache and pulsatile tinnitus, whereas previously, they had reported persistent severe headache. Decreasing IAP may decrease central venous and jugular venous pressure thereby relieving cerebral venous congestion and decrease ICP.

10.2. *Alter the translaminar pressure gradient by increasing IOP*

Another mechanical countermeasure involves increasing IOP to alter the TLPG across the ONH. Unlike classic glaucoma, VIIP may involve a lower IOP compared to retro-orbital subarachnoid space CSF pressure. Increasing the IOP within the clinical range, even a few mmHg, can alter the gradient favorably and decrease the likelihood of papilledema developing. Morgan and coworkers (2008) examined at a simple method of raising IOP using swimming goggles. Tension from the head-band causes a compressive force on the footprint of the goggle thereby compressing the orbital vasculature causing an increase in IOP. Fifteen Caucasian subjects were studied, eight males, using various swim goggle designs. The mean baseline IOP was 14.9 ± 3.9 mmHg, with a mean corneal thickness of 536 µm (± 32 um). Measurements of IOP were made in the seated position through cutouts in the goggle lens after 2 min, and 20 min of wear. There was a significant rise in mean IOP with all goggles of 4.5 mmHg (± 3.7 mmHg). Selecting the goggle based on the area of the eye piece impacted IOP rise due to force per unit area; smaller areas caused higher IOP compared with larger google footprints. Hence, use of a swim goggle with the goggle lens removed, may raise IOP modestly and decrease the TLPG, thus preventing disc edema in space in susceptible subjects.

11. VIIP Drug Countermeasures

Acetazolamide is a carbonic anhydrase inhibitor and is used as treatment in cases of infantile hydrocephalus, glaucoma, IIH and for prophylaxis of high-altitude illness. Multiple studies have demonstrated that acetazolamide is effective in decreasing CSF pressure in animals and humans. McCarthy and Reed (1974) found that CSF production decreased 50%–60% in rabbits following administration of 20 mg/kg of acetazolamide, while Melby *et al.* (1982) found a 90% reduction in CSF formation in cats using the same dosing regimen. The transport of Na across the apical membrane of the choroid plexus establishes an osmotic gradient that facilitates water diffusion and hence the production of CSF. Acetazolamide decreases CSF production by inhibition of carbonic anhydrase, resulting in decreased sodium ion transport across the choroidal epithelium and a decline in water diffusion and therefore CSF production (Tomsak *et al.*, 1988). Several studies have documented the resolution of papilledema and or improvement in visual field grade in IIH patients following daily oral acetazolamide with doses ranging from 1 to 4 g (Tomsak *et al.*, 1988; Celebisoy *et al.*, 2007). A reduction in ICP secondary to decreased CSF production is believed to be responsible. In long-term ICP monitoring of IIH patients, Gücer and Viernstein (1978) found that 4 g of acetazolamide reduced ICP by nearly 50%, 12 h after administration. In the recent IIH treatment trial (Wall *et al.*, 2014), 86 subjects in the acetazolamide group received an average oral daily dose of 2.5 g for 6 months. The mean CSF pressure decreased from 35.3 cm H_2O prior to treatment to 23.6 cm H_2O after 6 months of therapy, a decline of 11.7 cm H_2O. In addition, peripheral visual field mean defect improved 0.75 dB in the study eye. Given the effectiveness of acetazolamide at ameliorating elevated ICP and papilledema, it may be an effective treatment for VIIP-related disc edema both in-flight and postflight. However, acetazolamide induces a metabolic acidosis due to renal excretion of HCO_3^-. A major concern regarding acidosis in normal subjects is a rise in serum ultrafilterable calcium concentration, and decreased renal tubular calcium reabsorption (Lehmann *et al.*, 1967) causing hypercalciuria and hypocitraturia, both risk factors for kidney stone formation (Paisley and Tomson, 1999). In space, calcium concentration is already elevated above terrestrial levels due to the loss of gravity acting on the skeletal system and a resulting increase in bone resorption. An induced metabolic acidosis may further raise calcium concentrations in the kidney. Ordinarily, urinary citrate forms a soluble complex with calcium, reducing the available ionized calcium, which would otherwise precipitate. However, this risk may be mitigated if it became necessary to treat a crew member in-flight by administering oral potassium citrate. Whitson *et al.* (2009) in a randomized double-blind study administered daily oral potassium citrate (20 mEq) or placebo to 30 long-duration space crew and collected 24-h urine samples before, during, and after drug ingestion. Potassium citrate-treated crew members had decreased urinary calcium excretion and maintained the calcium oxalate supersaturation risk at preflight levels compared to that in controls. Increased urinary pH in the treatment group decreased the risk of uric acid stones. Therefore, it may be prudent to pair administration of in-flight acetazolamide with potassium citrate to decrease the risk of kidney stone formation.

12. Summary

The VIIP syndrome is currently one of NASA's top human spaceflight risks. The syndrome, which is related to microgravity exposure, manifests with changes in visual acuity (hyperopic shifts) and in eye structure (optic disc edema, choroidal folds, globe flattening, and distended optic nerve sheaths). In some cases, elevated CSF pressure has been documented postflight, reflecting ICP. While the eye appears to be the main affected organ of this syndrome, the ocular manifestations are thought to be caused by the combined interaction of the ocular, cardiovascular, and the central nervous system.

Current U.S. astronaut data indicate that after approximately 6 months of spaceflight, 22 of 33 crew members show a range of severity in these signs and symptoms of the VIIP syndrome.

The Medical Operations Group has implemented a clinical monitoring program to observe and record changes in ocular health measures. The spectrum of VIIP signs and symptoms spans a range from mild (choroidal folds, globe flattening, and change in refraction) to more clinically significant findings (optic disc edema, scotomas, and visual field changes such as an enlarged blind spot). Successful countermeasure development will be dependent on a thorough understanding of the cause and progression of this syndrome, including the identification of the most prevalent environmental and individual risk factors that contribute to its onset. The primary research goal is to understand the cause and progression of the VIIP syndrome and the risk factors that most significantly influence the development of VIIP. NASA's Human Research Program, which established the VIIP Research Project, has developed an integrated research plan covering four identified gaps (etiology, technology, analogs, and countermeasures), encompassing more than 70 studies. Understanding the mechanisms and contributing risk factors for the ocular structural and functional changes seen in–flight and postflight in astronauts is currently considered the highest research and clinical priority.

References

Alexander, DJ, CR Gibson, DR Hamilton, SMC Lee, TH Mader, C Otto, CM Oubre, AF Pass, SH Platts, JM Scott, SM Smith, MB Stenger, CM Westby and SB Zanello (2012). NASA Human Research Program Evidence Report: Risk of Spaceflight-Induced Intracranial Hypertension and Vision Alterations. https://human researchroadmap.nasa.gov/evidence/reports/viip.pdf.

Alperin, NJ, SH Lee, F Loth, PB Raksin and T Lichtor (2000). MR–intracranial pressure (ICP): A method to measure intracranial elastance and pressure noninvasively by means of MR imaging: Baboon and human study 1. *Radiology*, 217(3), 877–885.

American College of Surgeons Committee on Trauma (2012). *Advanced trauma life support student course manual*, Chicago: American College of Surgeons.

Anderson, AP, JG Swan, SD Phillips, DA Knaus, NT Kattamis, CM Toutain-Kidd, ME Zegans, AM Fellows and JC Buckey (2016). Acute effects of changes to the gravitational vector on the eye. *Journal of Applied Physiology*, 120(8), 939–946.

Baryshnik, DB and RI Farb (2004). Changes in the appearance of venous sinuses after treatment of disordered intracranial pressure. *Neurology*, 62, 1445–1446.

Bateman, GA and SH Siddique (2014). Cerebrospinal fluid absorption block at the vertex in chronic hydrocephalus: Obstructed arachnoid granulations or elevated venous pressure?. *Fluids and Barriers of the CNS*, 11(1), 1.

Baumann, UA, C Marquis, C Stoupis, TA Willenberg, J Takala and SM Jakob (2005). Estimation of central venous pressure by ultrasound. *Resuscitation*, 64, 193–199.

Bellezza, AJ, RT Hart and CF Burgoyne (2000). The optic nerve head as a biomechanical structure: Initial finite element modeling. *Investigative Ophthalmology and Visual Science*, 41(10), 2991–3000.

Bellner, J, B Romner, P Reinstrup, *et al.* (2004). Transcranial Doppler sonography pulsatility index (PI) reflects intracranial pressure (ICP). *Surgical Neurology*, 62, 45–51. discussion 51.

Bershad, EM, A Anand, SM DeSantis, M Yang, RA Tang, E Calvillo and P Gupta (2015). Clinical validation of a transcranial Doppler based non-invasive ICP meter: A prospective cross-sectional study. *World neurosurgery*, 89, 647s–653.

Blaber, AP, N Goswami, RL Bondar and MS Kassam (2011). Impairment of cerebral blood flow regulation in astronauts with orthostatic intolerance after flight. *Stroke*, 42(7), 1844–1850.

Bringmann, A, T Pannicke, J Grosche, M Francke, P Wiedemann, SN Skatchkov, *et al.* (2006). Muller cells in the healthy and diseased retina. *Progress in Retinal and Eye Research*, 25(4), 397–424.

Celebisoy, N, F Gökçay, H Sirin and Ö Akyürekli (2007). Treatment of idiopathic intracranial hypertension: Topiramate vs acetazolamide, an open-label study. *Acta Neurologica Scandinavica*, 116(5), 322–327.

CSF Production and Outflow: Cranial Lymphatic Drainage and Study of aquaporins, cellular junction proteins, and cellular permeability in the archnoid granulations and choroid plexus of an appropriate animal model. https://humanresearchroadmap.nasa.gov/Tasks/task.aspx?i=1742 [21 May 2016].

Davet, J, B Clavel, L Datas, L Mani-Ponset, D Maurel, S Herbuté and J Gabrion (1998). Choroidal readaptation to gravity in rats after spaceflight and head-down tilt. *Journal of Applied Physiology*, 84(1), 19–29.

Dentinger, AM and K Patwardhan (2014). Multimodality registration and visualization of MR and ultrasound volumes for longitudinal tracking of ocular structures. In *Paper presented at the NASA Human Research Program Investigators' Workshop*, Galveston, TX.

Dentinger, M, DM Mills and A Obi (2014). Integration of a volumetric ophthalmic imaging probe with the ultrasound 2 platform. In *Paper presented at the NASA Human Research Program Investigators' Workshop*, Galveston, TX.

Eklund, A, *et al.* (2016). The pressure difference between eye and brain changes with posture. *Annals of Neurology*, 80(2), 269–276.

Ethier, CR, A Feola, L Mulugeta, JG Myers, E Nelson, J Raykin and B Samuels (2015). Finite Element Modeling of VIIP Syndrome. NASA Human Research Program Investigator's Workshop, Galveston Texas.

Farb, RI, I Vanek, JN Scott, *et al.* (2003). Idiopathic intracranial hypertension: The prevalence and morphology of sinovenous stenosis. *Neurology*, 60, 1418–1424.

Fuller, CA, TM Hoban-Higgins, EL Robinson and CJ Murphy (2014). *Head-Down Tilt as a Model for Intracranial Pressure and Ocular Changes During Spaceflight*. NASA Human Research Program Investigator's Workshop, Galveston, Texas.

Gabrion, J, D Maurel, B Clavel, J Davet, J Fareh, S Herbuté and A Guell (1996). Changes in apical organization of choroidal cells in rats adapted to spaceflight or head-down tilt. *Brain Research*, 734(1), 301–315.

Geeraerts, T, S Merceron, D Benhamou, B Vigue and J Duranteau (2008). Non-invasive assessment of intracranial pressure using ocular sonography in neurocritical care patients. *Intensive Care Medicine*, 34, 2062–2067.

Griffith, JQ, WA Jeffers, *et al.* (1938). Papilledema associated with subarachnoid hemorrhage. *Archives Internal Medicine*, 61, 880–888.

Gücer, G and L Viernstein (1978). Long-term intracranial pressure recording in the management of pseudotumor cerebri. *Journal of Neurosurgery*, 49(2), 256–263.

Hamilton, DR, AE Sargsyan, K Garcia, DJ Ebert, PA Whitson, AH Feiveson and JM Duncan (2012). Cardiac and vascular responses to thigh cuffs and respiratory maneuvers on crewmembers of the International Space Station. *Journal of Applied Physiology*, 112(3), 454–462.

Hannerz, J, JP Antovic, M Blombäck, G Edman, M Khademi and F Piehl (2011). Inflammatory and haemostatic markers in idiopathic intracranial hypertension. *Journal of Internal Medicine*, 270(5), 496–499.

Haykowsky, MJ, ND Eves, DE, RW, *et al.* (2003). Resistance exercise, the Valsalva maneuver, and cerebrovascular transmural pressure. *Medical Science Sports Exercise*, 35, 65–68.

Herault, S, G Fomina, I Alferova, A Kotovskaya, V Poliakov and P Arbeille (2000). Cardiac, arterial and venous adaptation to weightlessness during 6-month MIR spaceflights with and without thigh cuffs (bracelets). *European Journal of Applied Physiology*, 81, 384–390.

Herbuté, S, J Oliver, J Davet, M Viso, RW Ballard, C Gharib and J Gabrion (1994). ANP binding sites are increased in choroid plexus of SLS-1 rats after 9 days of spaceflight. *Aviation Space and Environmental Medicine*, 65(2), 134–138.

Higgins, JNP and JD Pickard (2004). Lateral sinus stenoses in idiopathic intracranial hypertension resolving after CSF diversion. *Neurology*, 62, 1907–1908.

Higgins, JNP, C Cousins, BK Owler, *et al.* (2003). Idiopathic intracranial hypertension: 12 cases treated by venous sinus stenting. *Journal of Neurology, Neurosurgery and Psychiatry*, 74, 1662–1666.

Holman, DW, V Kurtcuoglu and DM Grzybowski (2010). Cerebrospinal fluid dynamics in the human cranial subarachnoid space: An overlooked mediator of cerebral disease. II.

In vitro arachnoid outflow model. *Journal of the Royal Society Interface*, 7(49):1205–1218.

Integrative physiology of VIIP: Cardiopulmonary, sleep and cognitive function assessment during hypercapneic bed rest. Retrieved from https://humanresearchroadmap.nasa.gov/Tasks/task.aspx?i=1424 [22 May 2016].

James, J, V Meyers, W Sipes, R Scully and C Matty (2011). Crew health and performance improvements with reduced carbon dioxide levels and the resource impact to accomplish those reductions. In *Proc. of the 41st International Conference on Environmental Systems*, pp. 2011–5047. Portland: AIAA.

Jennings, T (1990). Space adaptation syndrome is caused by elevated intracranial pressure. *Medical Hypotheses*, 32(4), 289–291.

Karahalios, DG, HL Rekate, MH Khayata, *et al.* (1996). Elevated intracranial pressure as a universal mechanism in pseudotumor cerebri of varying etiologies. *Neurology*, 46, 198–202.

Kharkar, S, S Batra, P Metellus, A Hillis, MA Williams and D Rigamonti (2011). Cognitive impairment in patients with pseudotumor cerebri syndrome. *Behavioural Neurology*, 24(2), 143–148.

King, JO, PJ Mitchell, KR Thomson, *et al.* (2002). Manometry combined with cervical puncture in idiopathic intracranial hypertension. *Neurology*, 58, 26–30.

Kramer, LA, KM Hasan, AE Sargsyan, JS Wolinsky, DR Hamilton, RF Riascos and C Otto (2015). Mr-derived cerebral spinal fluid hydrodynamics as a marker and a risk factor for intracranial hypertension in astronauts exposed to microgravity. *Journal of Magnetic Resonance Imaging*. 42(6), 1560–1571.

Kubota, S, T Kurihara, H Mochimaru, S Satofuka, K Noda, Y Ozawa, *et al.* (2009). Prevention of ocular inflammation in endotoxin-induced uveitis with resveratrol by inhibiting oxidative damage and nuclear factor-kappa B activation. *Investigative Ophthalmology and Visual Science*, 50(7), 3512–3519.

Kutscher, CL (1971). Hematocrit, plasma osmolality, and plasma protein concentration as estimators of plasma volume in hooded rats during food and water deprivation. *Physiology and Behaviour*, 7(2), 283–285.

Lakin, WD, SA Stevens and PL Penar (2007). Modeling intracranial pressures in microgravity: the influence of the blood–brain barrier. *Aviation, Space, and Environmental Medicine*, 78(10), 932–936.

Law, J, M Van Baalen, M Foy, SS Mason, C Mendez, ML Wear and D Alexander (2014). Relationship between carbon dioxide levels and reported headaches on the International Space Station. *Journal of Occupational and Environmental Medicine*, 56(5), 477–483.

Lawley, JS, *et al.* (2017). Effect of gravity and microgravity on intracranial pressure. *The Journal of Physiology*, 595(6), 2115–2127.

Lemann, Jr J, JR Litzow and EJ Lennon (1967). Studies of the mechanism by which chronic metabolic acidosis augments urinary calcium excretion in man. *Journal of Clinical Investigation*, 46(8), 1318.

Lieth, E, AJ Barber, B Xu, C Dice, MJ Ratz, D Tanase, *et al.* (1998). Glial reactivity and impaired glutamate metabolism in short-term experimental diabetic retinopathy. Penn State Retina Research Group. *Diabetes*, 47(5), 815–820.

Marini, JJ and AP Wheeler (2005). Critical Care Medicine: The Essentials. Lippincott Williams & Wilkins, Philadelphia, PA, USA.

Martin, DS, SMC Lee, SP Stein, MB Stenger, AH Feiveson, TP Matz, TL Caine, JM Scott, CM Westby and SH Platts (2015). Pilot study to evaluate a novel non-invasive technology to measure peripheral venous pressure. In *NASA Johnson Space Center*, Houston, TX, Report No. NASA/TM-2015-218572.

Martins AN, JK Wiley and PW Myers (1972). Dynamics of the cerebrospinal fluid and spinal dura mater. *Journal of Neurology, Neurosurgery, and Psychiatry*, 35, 468–473.

Masseguin, C, M Corcoran, C Carcenac, NG Daunton, A Güell, AS Verkman and J Gabrion (2000). Altered gravity downregulates aquaporin-1 protein expression in choroid plexus. *Journal of Applied Physiology*, 88(3), 843–850.

McCarthy, KD and DJ Reed (1974). The effect of acetazolamide and furosemide on cerebrospinal fluid production and choroid plexus carbonic anhydrase activity. *Journal of Pharmacology and Experimental Therapeutics*, 189(1), 194–201.

Melby, JM, LC Miner and DJ Reed (1982). Effect of acetazolamide and furosemide on the production and composition of cerebrospinal fluid from the cat choroid plexus. *Canadian Journal of Physiology and Pharmacology*, 60(3), 405–409.

Moreno, JA, E Mesalles, J Gener, *et al.* (2000). Evaluating the outcome of severe head injury with transcranial Doppler ultrasonography. *Neurosurgical Focus*, 8, e8.

Morey-Holton, ER and RK Globus (1998). Hindlimb unloading of growing rats: A model for predicting skeletal changes during space flight. *Bone*, 22(5), 83S–88S.

Morgan, WH, TS Cunneen, C Balaratnasingam and DY Yu (2008). Wearing swimming goggles can elevate intraocular pressure. *British Journal of Ophthalmology*, 92(9), 1218–1221.

Otto, C (2013). *Risk of microgravity-induced impairment and elevated intracranial pressure (VIIP)*. Washington, DC: BiblioGov.

Otto, C, R Ploutz-Snyder, S Mason, W Taiym, J Garcia and M Van Baalen (2015). Astronaut preflight cardiovascular health is highly correlated with postflight eye outcome measures. In *The Visual Impairment Intracranial Pressure (Viip), Risk*. 86th Annual Scientific Meeting of the Aerospace Medical Association at the Walt Disney Swan and Dolphin Resort, Lake Buena Vista, FL.

Paisley, K and C Tomson (1999). Calcium phosphate stones during long-term acetazolamide treatment for epilepsy. *Postgraduate Medical Journal*, 75(885), 427.

Parsons-Wingerter, P, K Radhakrishnan, MB Vickerman and PK Kaiser (2010). Oscillation of angiogenesis with vascular dropout in diabetic retinopathy by VESsel GENeration Analysis (VESGEN). *Investigative Ophthalmology & Visual Science*, 51(1), 498–507.

Parsons-Wingerter, P, KE Elliott, AG Farr, K Radhakrishnan, JI Clark and EH Sage (2000a). Generational analysis reveals that TGF-beta1 inhibits the rate of angiogenesis in vivo by selective decrease in the number of new vessels. *Microvascular Research*, 59, 221–232.

Parsons-Wingerter, P, KE Elliott, JI Clark and AG Farr (2000b). Fibroblast growth factor-2 selectively stimulates angiogenesis of small vessels in arterial tree. *Arteriosclerosis Thrombosis and Vascular Biology*, 20, 1250–1256.

Parsons-Wingerter, P, TL McKay, D Leontiev, MB Vickerman, TK Condrich and PE Dicorleto (2006). Lymphangiogenesis by blind-ended vessel sprouting is concurrent with hemangiogenesis by vascular splitting. *Anatomical Record. Part A Discoveries in Molecular, Cellular, and Evolutionary Biology*, 288, 233–247.

Patel, NB, AF Pass, CR Gibson and C Otto (2014). SD-OCT analysis of the optic nerve head and surrounding structures in U.S. long duration ISS astronauts compared to terrestrial bound normals. In *Paper presented at the NASA Human Research Program Investigators' Workshop*, Galveston, TX.

Phillips, SD, NT Kattamis, DA Knaus, JG Swan, M Zegans and JC Buckey (2014). Predicting microgravity induced vision changes using a cranial venouscirculatory model. In *NASA Human Research Program Investigator's Workshop*, Galveston, Texas.

Probst, RJ, JM Lim, DN Bird, GL Pole, AK Sato and JR Claybaugh (2006). Gender differences in the blood volume of conscious Sprague-Dawley rats. *Journal of American Association for Laboratory Animal Science*, 45(2), 49–52.

Ragauskas, A, V Matijosaitis, R Zakelis, K Petrikonis, D Rastenyte, 1 Piper and G Daubaris (2012). Clinical assessment of noninvasive intracranial pressure absolute value measurement method. *Neurology*, 78(21), 1684–1691.

Rohr, A, L Dorner, R Stingele, R Buhl, K Alfke and O Jansen (2007). Reversibility of venous sinus obstruction in idiopathic intracranial hypertension. *American Journal of Neuroradiology*, pp. 656–659.

Rohr, AC, C Riedel, M-C Fruehauf, A van Baalen, T Bartsch, J Hedderich, K Alfke, L Doerner and O Jansen (2011). MR imaging findings in patients with secondary intracranial hypertension. *American Journal of Neuroradiology*, 32, 6, 1021–1029.

Schwartz, KM, PH Luetmer, CH Hunt, AL Kotsenas, FE Diehn, LJ Eckel, and EP Lindell (2013). Position-related variability of CSF opening pressure measurements. *American Journal of Neuroradiology*, 34(4), 904–907.

Scott J, D Martin, B Crowell, E Goetchius, C Seponski, R Gonzales, T Matz, R Ploutz-Snyder, M Stenger and L Ploutz-Snyder (2016). Influence of exercise modality on cerebral–ocular hemodynamics and pressures. Poster presented at the NASA Human Research Program Investigators' Workshop, Galveston, TX, United States.

Sigal, IA, JG Flanagan and CR Ethier (2005). Factors influencing optic nerve head biomechanics. *Investigative Ophthalmology and Visual Science*, 46(11), 4189–4199.

Silverberg, GD, E Levinthal, EV Sullivan, DA Bloch, SD Chang, J Leverenz and D McGuire (2002). Assessment of low-flow CSF drainage as a treatment for AD Results of a randomized pilot study. *Neurology*, 59(8), 1139–1145.

Singh, M, SI Savitz, R Hoque, G Gupta, S Roth, PS Rosenbaum, *et al.* (2001). Cell-specific caspase expression by different neuronal phenotypes in transient retinal ischemia. *Journal of Neurochemistry*, 77(2), 466–475.

Skau, M, JP Goetze, JF Rehfeld and R Jensen (2010). Natriuretic pro-peptides in idiopathic intracranial hypertension. *Regulatory Peptides*, 164(2), 71–77.

Sørensen, PS, AM Thomsen and F Gjerris (1986). Persistent disturbances of cognitive functions in patients with pseudotumor cerebri. *Acta Neurologica Scandinavica*, 73(3), 264–268.

Sørensen, PS, F Gjerris and M Hammer (1984). Cerebrospinal fluid vasopressin and increased intracranial pressure. *Annals of Neurology*, 15(5), 435–440.

Sugerman, HJ, *et al.* (2001). Continuous negative abdominal pressure device to treat pseudotumor cerebri. *International Journal of Obesity and Related Metabolic Disorders*, 486–490.

Taylor, CR, M Hanna, BJ Behnke, JN Stabley, DJ McCullough, RT Davis and MD Delp (2013). Spaceflight-induced alterations in cerebral artery vasoconstrictor, mechanical, and structural properties: implications for elevated cerebral perfusion and intracranial pressure. *The FASEB Journal*, 27(6), 2282–2292.

Thalhammer, C, M Aschwanden, A Odermatt, UA Baumann, S Imfeld, D Bilecen, SC Marsch and KA Jaeger (2007). Noninvasive central venous pressure measurement by controlled compression sonography at the forearm. *Journal of American College of Cardiology*, 50, 1584–1589.

Thalhammer, C, M Siegemund, M Aschwanden, M Gassmann, UA Baumann, KA Jaeger and S Imfeld (2009). Non-invasive central venous pressure measurement by compression ultrasound — a step into real life. *Resuscitation,* 80, 1130–1136.

Theriot CA, P Wingerter-Parsons, G Vizzeri and SB Zanello (2014). Hindlimb suspension as a model to study ophthalmic complications in microgravity status report: optimization of rat retina flat mounts staining to study vascular remodeling. In *NASA Human Research Program Investigator's Workshop.*, Galveston, Texas.

Theriot, CA, CM Westby, JLL Morgan, SR Zwart and SB Zanello (2015). High dietary iron increases oxidative stress and radiosensitivity in the rat retina and vasculature after exposure to fractionated gamma radiation. Manuscript in preparation.

Tomsak, RL, AS Niffenegger and BF Remler (1988). Treatment of pseudotumor cerebri with Diamox (acetazolamide). *Journal of Neuro-Ophthalmology*, 8(2), 93–98.

Valenza, F, N Bottino, K Canavesi, A Lissoni, S Alongi, S Losappio, E Carlesso, and L Gattinoni (2003). Intra-abdominal pressure may be decreased non-invasively by continuous negative extra-abdominal pressure (NEXAP). *Intensive Care Medicine*, 29(11), 2063–2067.

Wall, M, MP McDermott, KD Kieburtz, JJ Corbett, SE Feldon, DI Friedman and MJ Kupersmith (2014). Effect of acetazolamide on visual function in patients with idiopathic intracranial hypertension and mild visual loss: The idiopathic intracranial hypertension treatment trial. *Journal of the American Medical Association*, 311(16), 1641–1651.

Waters, WW, MG Ziegler and JV Meck (2002). Postspaceflight orthostatic hypotension occurs mostly in women and is predicted by low vascular resistance. *Journal of Applied Physiology*, 92(2), 586–594.

Whitson, PA, RA Pietrzyk, JA Jones, M Nelman-Gonzalez, EK Hudson and CF Sams (2009). Effect of potassium citrate therapy on the risk of renal stone formation during spaceflight. *The Journal of Urology*, 182(5), 2490–2496.

Wostyn, P (2004). Can chronic increased intracranial pressure or exposure to repetitive intermittent intracranial pressure elevations raise your risk for Alzheimer's disease?. *Medical Hypotheses*, 62(6), 925–930.

Yoffey, JM and CK Drinker (1939). Some observations on the lymphatics of the nasal mucous membrane in the cat and monkey. *Journal of Anatomy*, 74, 45–52.

Yri, HM, B Fagerlund, HB Forchhammer and RH Jensen (2014). Cognitive function in idiopathic intracranial hypertension: A prospective case–control study. *BMJ Open*, 4(4), e004376.

Zanello SB, CA Theriot, CM Prospero-Ponce, P Chevez_Barrios (2013). Spaceflight effects and molecular responses in the mouse eye: Observations after Shuttle Mission STS-133. *Gravitational and Space Research*, 1(1), 29–46.

Zwart, SR, *et al.* (2012). Vision changes after spaceflight are related to alterations in folate- and vitamin B-12-dependent one-carbon metabolism. *The Journal of Nutrition*, 142(3), 427–431.

Zwart, SR, *et al.* (2016). Genotype, B-vitamin status, and androgens affect spaceflight-induced ophthalmic changes. *The FASEB Journal*, 30(1), 141–148.

Advanced Imaging of the Intracranial Physiology of Spaceflight

9

Donna R. Roberts, MD, Thomas McLaren, MD and Michael U. Antonucci, MD

Department of Radiology and Radiological Sciences,
Medical University of South Carolina, 171 Ashley Avenue, Charleston,
South Carolina 29425, USA

1. Introduction

Several unique features of the spaceflight environment may have an impact on brain health and function. In microgravity, there is a loss of gravitational hydrostatic pressure gradients which results in large fluid shifts toward the head (Hargens *et al.*, 2013). Elevated carbon dioxide (CO_2) levels, a potent cerebral arterial vasodilator, have been reported aboard the International Space Station (ISS). While in orbit, astronauts are exposed to higher levels of radiation than on Earth which is of concern (National Research Council, 2008). The physiological consequences of prolonged exposure to the unique environmental parameters of spaceflight on the human central nervous system have not yet been fully investigated and are poorly understood. Despite NASA's extensive history of biomedical investigations characterizing the human body's adaptation to spaceflight, there is surprisingly little data concerning brain structure and function in space and upon readaption to Earth. This knowledge gap has profound implications for astronaut health, influencing performance in essentially every functional domain including cognition, vision, vestibular function, sensorimotor capabilities, and behavioral health.

Initial studies of intracranial adaptation to spaceflight focused on cardiovascular physiology and its role in the development of orthostatic intolerance, a presyncopal/syncopal condition commonly experienced by astronauts upon return to Earth, and on the role of the vestibular system in the development of the space-flight adaptation syndrome. More recently, the identification of the visual impairment intracranial pressure (VIIP) syndrome among the astronaut popula-tion has generated interest in investigating intrinsic intracranial adaptation to microgravity. However, to date, few studies have utilized advanced imaging meth-ods to examine the human brain's physiologic response to long-term spaceflight.

This chapter will review the available literature and postulate mechanisms that could contribute to the development of VIIP syndrome. This will include a thor-ough discussion of the established relevant advanced imaging methods that have been used as well as emerging techniques that may be applicable to future studies of intracranial adaptation to spaceflight.

2. Intracranial Physiology Associated with the Supine Posture

A traditional ground-based analog used by NASA and other international space agencies to study the physiological changes associated with spaceflight is the place-ment of healthy subjects in bed rest for varying periods of time (Nicogossian and Dietlein, 1989; Pavy-Le Traon *et al.*, 2007). As an analog for spaceflight, unloading of the vertical body weight during bed rest results in rapid cephalad fluid shifts. As a result, subjects demonstrate facial puffiness, nasal congestion, distention of the jugular veins, and a sensation of "fullness of the head" (Nicogossian and Dietlein, 1989). These findings are also seen in astronauts on orbit. However, there is a pau-city of dedicated neuroimaging research conducted on healthy subjects during bed rest and therefore, data must be extrapolated from studies of intracranial physiol-ogy in response to postural shifts between the upright and supine body positions.

For example, adjusting head position is routinely used in the treatment of brain injury patients with elevated intracranial pressure (ICP). It is known that the supine position can further increase ICP and therefore, the standard posture for patients with severe head injury is 30° of head elevation (Ng *et al.*, 2004). This position reduces ICP and assists in maintaining adequate cerebral perfusion pres-sure (CPP) according to the equation:

$$CPP = MAP - ICP \tag{1}$$

where MAP is the mean arterial pressure. Increased ICP can compromise cerebral blood flow (CBF) by reducing CPP, and studies have shown that a high ICP (>20–25 mmHg) is associated with increased mortality (Czosnyka *et al.*, 2006).

Neutral positioning of the neck is also used clinically to minimize venous obstruction and optimize venous drainage of the brain.

The intracranial contents include noncompressible fluid and tissue in the fixed volume of the skull. This has been conceptualized in the Monro–Kellie doctrine, which states that the contents of the cranial vault must exist in equilibrium such that an increase in volume of one component results in a compensatory decrease in volume of another component. More specifically, the intracranial contents consist of the brain parenchyma, cerebrospinal fluid (CSF) and blood. Therefore, in the absence of pathology, the intracranial volume ($V_{\text{intracranial}}$) is:

$$V_{\text{intracranial}} \text{ (constant)} = V_{\text{brain}} + V_{\text{CSF}} + V_{\text{blood}} \tag{2}$$

The brain tissue, with a total mass of about 1400 g (Gwinnutt and Saha, 2005), is composed of gray matter which is approximately 80% water, and white matter which is approximately 68% water. The relative importance of brain water can be dramatically increased in the presence of cerebral edema (Gean, 1994). There is approximately 150 mL of blood within the cranium: 50 mL of arterial blood and 100 mL in the venous system (Gwinnutt and Saha, 2005). The total volume of CSF is approximately 150 mL. About half of the CSF is within the confines of the skull in the ventricular system (right and left lateral, third, and fourth ventricles) and within the subarachnoid spaces surrounding the brain and the optic nerves (Fig. 1). The remainder is in the subarachnoid space of the spinal canal surrounding the spinal cord (Gwinnutt and Saha, 2005). The cranium and spinal canal are in continuity with each other through the large opening at the base of the skull called the foramen magnum. The CSF around the spinal cord is contained within a dura-lined space called the thecal sac. CSF is produced at a rate of approximately 20 mL per hour by the choroid plexuses, which are highly vascularized structures located within the ventricles of the brain (Gwinnutt and Saha, 2005). With each heartbeat, as arterial blood enters the cranium, a small net change in blood volume causes CSF to move out of the cranium through the foramen magnum and into the spinal canal in order to maintain a constant $V_{\text{intracranial}}$. This creates an oscillatory flow of a small volume of CSF into and out of the intracranial cavity synchronized to the cardiac and respiratory cycles (Marmarou, 1996).

In a closed system such as the cranium, the relationship between pressure and volume can be studied by injecting a known volume of fluid into the CSF space and measuring the resultant change in pressure, first demonstrated by Marmarou *et al.* (1975). The intracranial pressure–volume curve can be expressed as:

$$\text{ICP} = P_1 e^{EV} \tag{3}$$

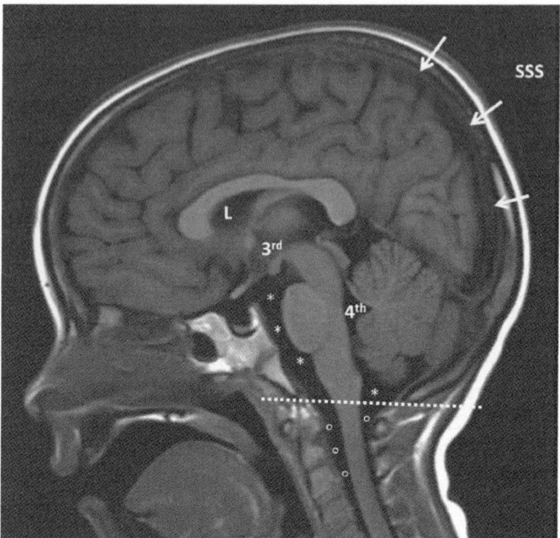

Figure 1. A sagittal view of the brain along the midline (T1-weighted MR image). L = lateral ventricles; 3rd = 3rd ventricle; 4th = 4th ventricle; * = CSF contained with the subarachnoid spaces surrounding the brain; ° = the subarachnoid space of the spinal canal surrounding the spinal cord contained within the thecal sac; dashed line = basion-opisthion line indicating the location of the foramen magnum; superior sagittal sinus (SSS).

where E is an elastance coefficient (units of volume^{-1}; the inverse of compliance), P_1 is a pressure coefficient related to the exponential shape of the curve, and V is the intracranial volume (brain tissue + CSF + blood) (Alperin *et al.*, 2006). The pressure–volume curve is shown in Fig. 2. With each heartbeat, as arterial blood enters the cranium, a small change in volume results in a change in pressure (pulse pressure) that is determined by the compliance of the system. The small net change in blood volume (arterial inflow–venous outflow) during the cardiac cycle is thought to be the driving force behind the cranial-to-spinal flow of CSF (Alperin *et al.*, 1996, 2006).

A concept important to the understanding of CSF flow dynamics is compliance, defined as the ratio of change in volume to the corresponding change in pressure ($\Delta V/\Delta P$), and equivalent to the slope of the pressure volume curve. Intracranial compliance describes the distensibility of the CSF compartment, which in turn, is a significant determinant of the degree that the ICP changes in response to a change in volume of brain tissue, CSF, or blood (Marmarou *et al.*, 1975). For an ideal container, compliance is a constant and therefore, the pressure within the container varies linearly with volume. However, pressure and volume in

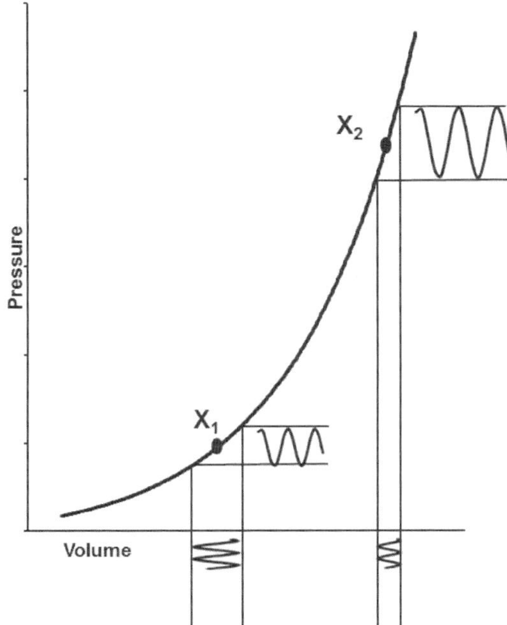

Figure 2. Intracranial pressure volume curve — The initial pressure of the system is represented as X_1. The magnitude of the pulsatile pressure for small changes in volume will be determined by the slope of the pressure volume curve at X_1. A permanent shift to a new operating point at a higher steady-state pressure is represented by X_2. The pulsatile pressure at X_2 will be larger in magnitude due to reduced compliance (Modified from Marmarou *et al.*, 1975).

the CSF compartment are not linearly related. Instead, intracranial compliance decreases at higher pressures. As a result, for equivalent volume increments, a larger change in pressure will occur in a system that is initially in a state of higher pressure than one at a lower pressure. For example, in Fig. 2, point X_1 represents the initial state of a system in which a small change in intracranial volume (such as that which occurs during the cardiac cycle) results in a small change in ICP. The slope at point X_1, reflects the intracranial compliance and determines the magnitude of the pulse pressure. If the system is moved to a higher baseline pressure indicated by point X_2, for example (such as what might occur in a patient with a large brain tumor), the same small change in volume would lead to a much larger change in pulse pressure. This is due to the nonlinearity of the intracranial pressure–volume relationship.

2.1. *Magnetic resonance intracranial pressure (MR-ICP)*

Alperin *et al.* (2006) developed a noninvasive magnetic resonance imaging (MRI)-based method for measuring intracranial compliance and pressure known as MR-ICP. Similar to the principles used by Marmarou *et al.* (1975), MR-ICP estimates intracranial compliance and pressure based on the system's response to a small increase in intracranial volume. However, in place of measuring the response to the administration of a known volume of extrinsic fluid injected into the CSF, MR-ICP measurements are based on the magnitude of the intrinsic, physiologic pulse pressure which occurs naturally during each systolic increase in intracranial volume. This increase in volume is calculated from MR measurements of the momentary difference between volumes of blood and CSF that enter and leave the cranium during the cardiac cycle. The amplitude of the resulting pulse pressure is calculated from the measured craniospinal CSF velocities based on first principles of fluid dynamics (Tain *et al.*, 2011). The mean absolute ICP is then derived from the inverse relationship between compliance and pressure given by the intracranial pressure–volume curve, Eq. 3 (Alperin *et al.*, 2006).

The velocity measurements of blood and CSF flows are obtained using an MRI technique known as velocity-encoded phase contrast (PC) MRI which provides a series of velocity maps with pixel values that are proportional to the velocity of moving blood or CSF at each location (Fig. 3). Total arterial inflow, or CBF, is calculated from the sum of the volumetric flow through both internal carotid and vertebral arteries, which are the main sources of arterial blood to the brain. Venous outflow is obtained from measurement of the venous drainage through the jugular veins and through secondary venous channels such as the epidural, vertebral, and deep cervical veins of the vertebral plexus. CSF flow velocity is evaluated at the level of the foramen magnum. Applying MR-ICP in a group of 23 healthy adults, Alperin *et al.* found CBF values ranged from 514 to 956 mL/min and ICP values ranged from 3.5 to 17.1 mmHg (Alperin *et al.*, 2006).

Alperin *et al.* (2005a,b) further applied the MR-ICP technique to characterize cerebral hemodynamics and CSF flow changes related to posture. Using a vertical gap open MRI scanner, which allows for image acquisition of subjects in the sitting position, 10 healthy subjects were imaged in both the supine and upright, sitting positions. In the supine position: CBF was 12% higher (825±166 mL/min compared with 724±127 mL/min), venous outflow was 57% more pulsatile, a 58% larger volume of CSF flowed between the intracranial compartment and the spinal canal during the cardiac cycle (0.55 ± 0.12 mL compared with 0.23 ± 0.11 mL), intracranial pressure was increased (10.6 ± 3.6 compared with 4.5 ± 1.8 mmHg),

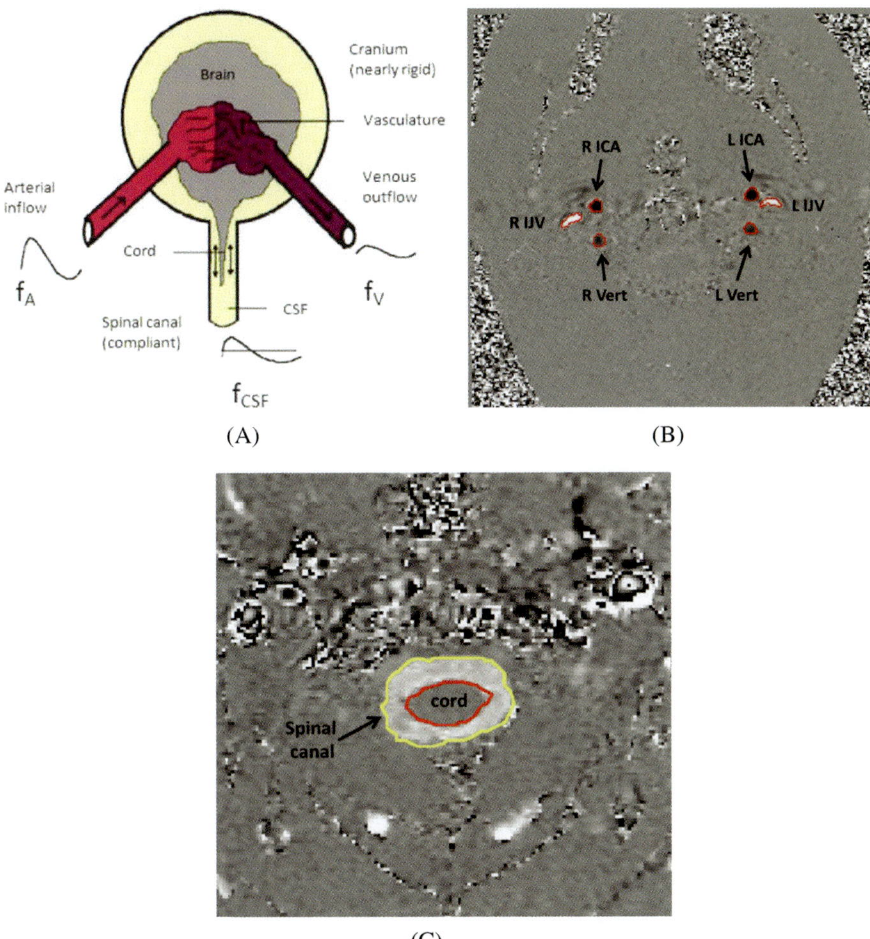

Figure 3. (A) A model of the craniospinal system illustrating arterial inflow, venous out-flow, and the to and fro flow of CSF through the foramen magnum during the cardiac cycle. (B) Velocity-encoded phase contrast MR image through the upper neck at the level of the carotid and vertebral arteries which demonstrates the flow of arterial blood into the head (upward moving fluid is dark) and the internal jugular veins demonstrating the flow of venous blood out of the head (downward moving fluid is white). ICA = internal carotid artery; IJV = internal jugular vein; vert = vertebral artery. (C) Outflow of CSF exiting the cranium during systole and flowing into the upper spinal canal (downward moving fluid is white) around the spinal cord (Courtesy of Dr. Noam Alperin, University of Miami).

and intracranial compliance was decreased by 2.8 fold, compared with the upright position. The arterial waveform was largely unchanged between supine and upright positions. The decrease in intracranial compliance and higher ICP in the supine position were interpreted to be the result of a higher mean intracranial fluid volume when supine (Alperin *et al.*, 2005a,b). Transitioning from the upright to a neutral gravity position results in a shift of blood and CSF into the cranium (Alperin *et al.*, 2005a,b).

Similar to the supine position on Earth, there is a reduction in caudally directed gravitational stimuli during spaceflight. As such, the work of Alperin *et al.* would suggest that during spaceflight (or at least during the initial adaptation phase), compared with the upright posture on Earth, astronauts would experience greater CBF, a larger volume of CSF flow between the intracranial compartment and the spinal canal during each cardiac cycle, and a resultant increase in ICP. In spaceflight, as in the supine position, the brain would be less compliant and there would be a mean increase in intracranial fluid volume with shift of blood and CSF into the cranium. The time course and ultimate consequences of any potential alteration in cranial fluid dynamics during spaceflight compared with daily activity on Earth are unknown; however, such data could provide further insight into the physiology of the VIIP syndrome.

3. The Dural Venous System and ICP

Intracranial pressure can also be calculated according to Davson's Equation as:

$$\text{ICP} = (I_f \times R) + P_d \tag{4}$$

where I_f is the rate of CSF formation, R is the resistance to CSF outflow, and P_d is the pressure in the dural venous sinuses (Marmarou, 1996). According to this equation, ICP depends on pressure within the dural venous sinuses, which in turn is influence by the state of the venous outflow channels.

3.1. *Dural venous sinus anatomy*

Human intracranial venous drainage pathways are complex and involve the deep and superficial cerebral veins, meningeal veins, the dural venous sinuses, diploic and emissary veins, scalp veins, the internal jugular venous system, and the deep cervical venous plexuses (Patel, 2009). Superficial cortical veins and deep cerebral veins drain toward the dural venous sinuses. The walls of the dural venous sinuses

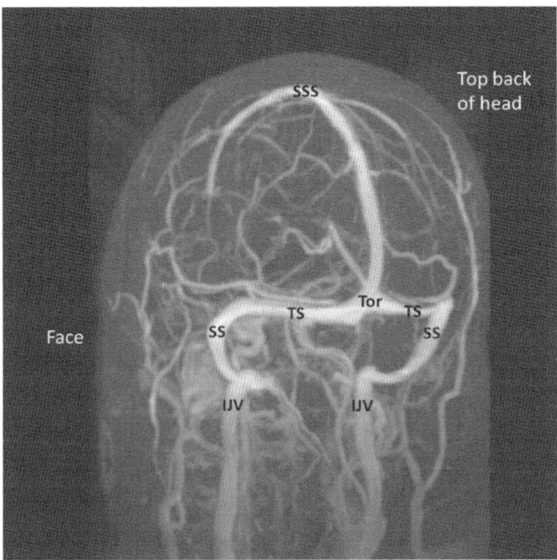

Figure 4. MR image from a venogram study demonstrating the major vessels of the intracranial venous system. SSS = superior sagittal sinus; Tor = torcular herophili; TS = right and left transverse sinuses; SS = right and left sigmoid sinuses; IJV = right and left internal jugular veins.

are rigid and formed from the endosteal and meningeal layers of the dura. In addition to their role in cerebral venous drainage, the dural venous sinuses also contain arachnoid granulations, projections into the venous sinuses which facilitate CSF resorption into the venous system. The superior venous sinuses include the superior sagittal sinus which is joined by the straight sinus to form the torcular Herophili. This, in turn, gives rise to the transverse sinuses which drain into the sigmoid sinuses and ultimately into the internal jugular veins bilaterally (Fig. 4). An anteroinferior group of venous sinuses are also present draining the inferior surface of the brain and orbits which include the cavernous sinuses, the sphenoparietal sinuses, the inferior and superior petrosal sinuses, and the basilar venous plexus. There are numerous anastomoses between both the superior and inferior venous sinuses.

The internal jugular veins represent the main pathway for cerebral venous outflow in the supine position. However, the pathway of intracranial venous drainage is dependent on posture with the vertebral venous plexuses playing a larger role in the upright position (Alperin *et al.*, 2005b; Valdueza *et al.*, 2000). The vertebral venous plexuses include the vertebral artery venous plexuses, the epidural venous plexuses (which lies within the epidural space of the spinal canal), and the deep cervical veins (San Millan Ruiz *et al.*, 2002). In addition to the internal jugular veins, emissary veins also assist in extracranial venous drainage of the dural venous sinuses. The emissary veins are small, valveless veins which pass through foramina in the skull forming connections between the intracranial and extracranial circulation. While typically small, emissary veins can become important alternative routes for venous drainage in pathological states such as seen in chronic increased ICP. Diploic veins, which are small veins within the bones of the skull, are also present and communicate with the dural sinuses and the extracranial venous system via emissary veins.

3.2. *Venous insufficiency due to dural venous sinus obstruction and idiopathic intracranial hypertension*

Various pathologies are associated with abnormalities in intracranial venous outflow including the development of vascular malformations, venous thrombosis, and venous infarction. In particular, some have hypothesized that the syndrome of idiopathic intracranial hypertension (IIH), which has been likened to the VIIP syndrome experienced by astronauts (Mader *et al.*, 2011), may be the result of venous outflow obstruction. IIH, also known as pseudotumor cerebri, is a condition of unknown etiology in which typically occurs in obese, female patients, who present with a constellation of symptoms related to increased ICP. Both patients with IIH and astronauts with VIIP syndrome present with increased intracranial pressure, papilledema, flattening of the posterior contour of the eye, dilated optic nerve sheaths, and visual disturbances (Ball and Clarke, 2006; Degnan and Levy, 2011; Mader *et al.*, 2011). Clinical differences between classic IIH and VIIP include: gender predilection with IIH being more common in women and VIIP more common in men, and an association with obesity in IIH but not in VIIP. However, interestingly, there is a form of IIH that occurs in prepubertal pediatric patients which is more similar to VIIP in that the affected children are typically not obese and there is no gender predilection (Ball and Clarke, 2006). Although the etiologies of both conditions are unknown, there is evidence that IIH may be the result of venous outflow obstruction. For instance, focal areas of tight stenosis are commonly found in one or both of the transverse sinuses in IIH patients (Farb *et al.*, 2003). The resulting increased resistance to venous outflow would result in elevated cerebral venous pressures, and by Davson's equation (Eq. 4), lead to increased ICP. The potential role of venous hypertension in IIH has led researchers to speculate that venous insufficiency or hypertension caused by cephalad fluid shifts during spaceflight may relate to the development of VIIP syndrome in astronauts (Mader *et al.*, 2011).

While the treatment of IIH remains controversial, dilating and placing stents across the narrowed dural venous sinuses has been shown to be an effective treatment in select patients (Higgins *et al.*, 2002). As such, assessment of the dural venous sinuses for areas of flow limiting stenosesis critical in triaging patients for more invasive evaluations/treatments.

3.3. *Imaging of intracranial venous outflow*

Various imaging techniques are available for evaluating the venous sinuses. MRI-based techniques, known as MR venography (MRV), can be used to demonstrate dural venous sinus anatomy and to assess for areas of narrowing. MRV can be performed using either noncontrast MRI sequences that are sensitive to venous blood flow (although these techniques intrinsically underestimate the caliber of the vessels) or using sequences that are obtained after the administration of intravenous contrast agents (which provide superior image quality and allow better depiction of small-sized intracranial venous structures even in the setting of low venous blood flow as in Fig. 4) (Tomasian *et al.*, 2009).

While the noninvasive nature of MRI makes it an appealing screening test, the gold-standard for determining areas of hemodynamically significant stenosis in the venous system is intravascular, catheter-based venography with direct venous pressure measurements. During catheter venography, intravenous access is gained via the femoral vein in the groin and a guidewire is advanced through the inferior vena cava into the internal jugular vein or the desired location in the venous system (Harrigan and Deveikis, 2009). A catheter is then fed over the guidewire and the guidewire is removed. Intravenous contrast material is injected by hand through the catheter and x-rays are taken to visualize the contrast-opacified venous system. Once the anatomy of the sinuses has been established, intravenous pressure measurements are obtained in the superior sagittal sinus, bilateral transverse and sigmoid sinuses, and bilateral internal jugular veins (Harrigan and Deveikis, 2009). Hemodynamically significant stenosis is defined by a pressure gradient of at least 10 mmHg and can be treated with placement of a stent across the area of narrowing (Harrigan and Deveikis, 2009) (Fig. 5).

MRV findings have been shown to correlate with venous pressure measurements obtained at catheter venography and can therefore serve as a noninvasive predictor of clinically relevant pressure drops across the transverse sinuses (Roberts *et al.*, 2015a). Interpretation of noninvasive imaging, however, can be challenging and complicated by the frequent finding of variant venous sinus anatomy. For example, the transverse sinuses are often of unequal size, most commonly with a dominant right transverse sinus and a hypoplastic left transverse sinus (Fig. 6). In about 20% of cases of normal subjects, there is partial or total agenesis of the transverse sinus (Cure *et al.*, 1994). However, while variant sinus anatomy is commonly seen and

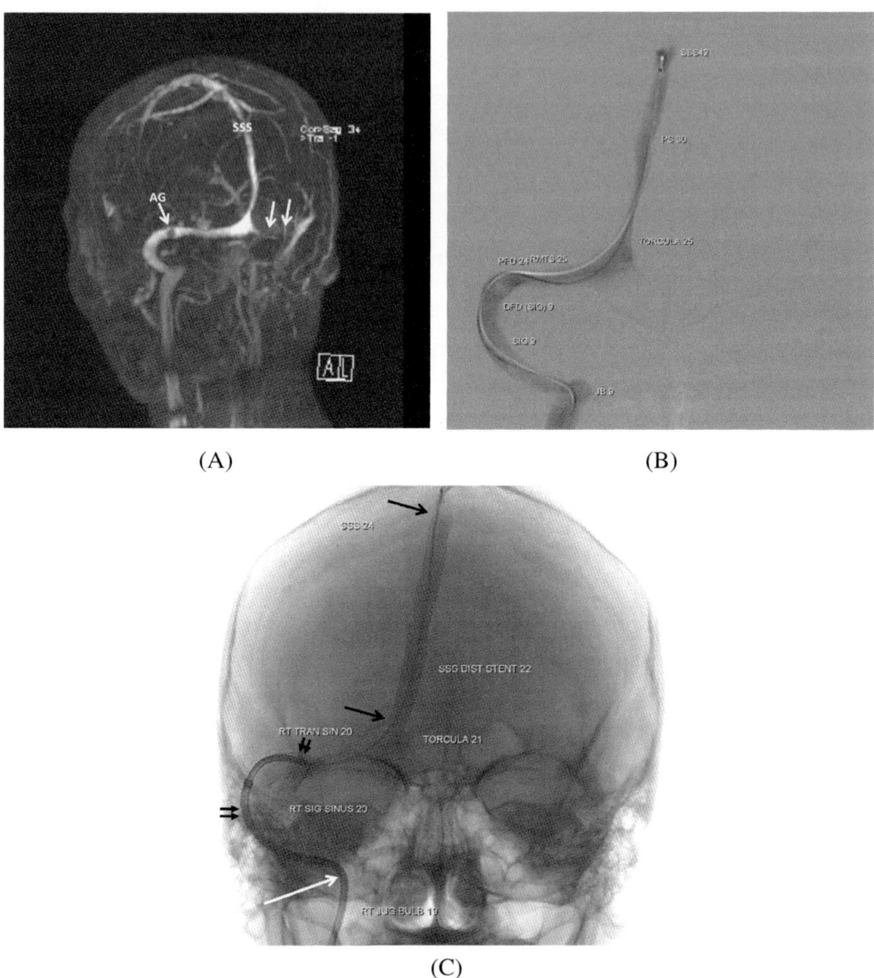

(A)

(B)

(C)

Figure 5. A patient presented with symptoms of increased intracranial pressure with papilledema and headaches. (A) The patient underwent MR venography which demonstrated narrowing of the distal superior sagittal sinus, severe narrowing of the left transverse sinus (two white arrows), and a dominant right transverse sinus which was narrowed by the presence of a prominent arachnoid granulation (AG) at the junction of the right transverse and right sigmoid sinuses. (B) The patient subsequently underwent catheter-based venogram and direct venous pressure measurements. The pressure within the superior sagittal sinus (SSS) was 42 mmHg. At the torcula and medial portion of the right transverse sinus (RMTS), the pressure was 25 mmHg. Within the sigmoid sinus (SIG) and the jugular bulb (JB), the pressure was 9 mmHg. (C) Because the patient was symptomatic with large pressure drops across the superior sagittal sinus and across the right transverse–sigmoid

←——

Figure 5. (*Continued*) junction, the patient underwent stent placement to open up the areas of narrowing with resultant improvement of symptoms and resolution of increased ICP. Long black arrows = stent placed across the superior sagittal sinus; double short black arrows = stent placed across the right transverse–sigmoid sinus junction; white arrow = catheter and guidewire within the venous sinuses.

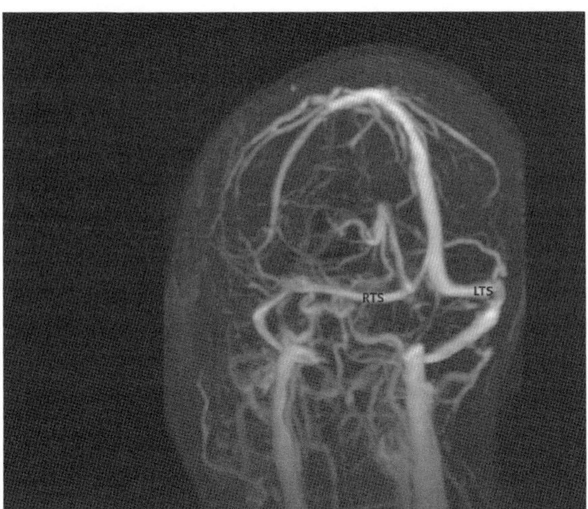

Figure 6. MR venogram showing variant anatomy with a dominant left transverse sinus (LTS) and a smaller diameter right transverse sinus (RTS). The patient underwent catheter-based venogram and direct venous pressure measurements for suspected IIH; however, no significant pressure drops were noted across the dural venous sinuses.

often considered "normal", some anatomical findings can have clinical relevance. For instance, narrowing of one or both of the transverse sinuses near the transverse/ sigmoid sinus junction by the presence of prominent arachnoid granulations can lead to venous outflow obstruction, particularly in symptomatic IIH patients. As such, similar variant anatomy could represent a predisposing factor for the development of VIIP syndrome in the astronaut population, however this remains untested.

A limitation in the radiological evaluation of the intracranial venous system is that both MRV and catheter venography are performed with patients in the supine position. Few studies evaluating the venous system in the upright position are available. However, there is partial collapse of the internal jugular veins in most normal subjects in the upright position with redirection of venous outflow through collateral pathways (Zhou *et al.*, 2014; Valdueza *et al.*, 2000). As humans spend much of their daily life in the upright position, the state of these collateral pathways could be an important determinant of P_d and therefore ICP. Unfortunately, the ability to measure this effect directly is limited by the lack of equipment capable of obtaining imaging in positions other than supine. The spatial limitations of the bore of most MR units preclude patient repositioning. Further, there are limits to the movement of angiographic tables used for catheter-based procedures.

There is no reported data concerning direct venous sinus pressure measurements in the upright position. Head elevation is limited to 15° on most angiographic tables. Venography performed in this position shows no change in pressure measurements in the superior sagittal or bilateral transverse sinuses (personnel communication, Aquilla Turk, MD, January, 2015). However, this small amount of tilt may not be sufficient to result in the physiologic changes seen in the fully upright position, including collapse of the internal jugular venous system and resultant redirection of venous outflow through collateral pathways. Therefore, further research is needed to understand the potential consequences of chronic exposure to the microgravity environment and the resultant lack of daily gravity-dependent variations in venous return on ICP.

4. Imaging of CSF Flow

In the past, it was widely accepted that CSF flow is unidirectional from the ventricular system (where it is produced by the choroid plexus) into the subarachnoid space at the base of the brain, and then coursing superiorly along the surface of the brain, to ultimately be absorbed by the arachnoid granulations into the dural venous sinuses (Dichiro, 1964; Weed, 1914a,b). More recently, however, the nature of CSF flow has generated controversy as advanced imaging techniques have now suggested the presence of alternative pathways of CSF production and resorption (Bradley, 2015).

4.1. *Nuclear medicine CSF flow study*

Nuclear medicine CSF flow studies were introduced in the 1960s to assess CSF flow patterns and are still in clinical use today (Ponto, 2008). Radionuclide cisternography involves a lumbar puncture along the lower back to inject a radiotracer into the thecal sac, within the CSF space surrounding the distal spinal cord and nerve roots. Over time, in all subjects without a blockage to CSF flow, the radiotracer migrates with the flow of CSF superiorly along the spinal canal through the foramen magnum and up to the base of the brain (Ziessman *et al.*, 2006). Patients then undergo serial imaging with a gamma camera, which detects movement of the radiotracer around the brain. Typically, radiotracer injected into the intrathecal space at the lumbar level reaches the base of the brain by 1 h, moves along the cerebral convexities by 12 h, and is absorbed into the superior sagittal sinus by 24 h (Ziessman *et al.*, 2006) (Fig. 7). The movement of the radiotracer, which follows

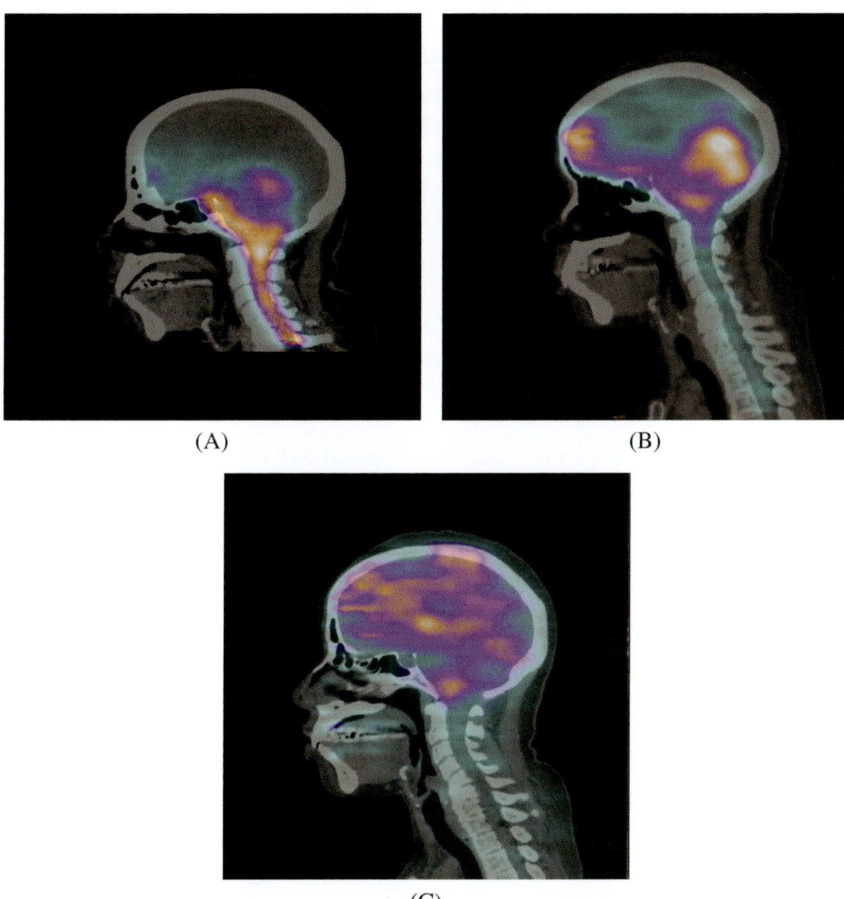

(A)

(B)

(C)

Figure 7. Sagittal images of the brain from a nuclear medicine cisternogram study which have been coregistered to a computer tomography (CT) scan. Radiotracer was injected into the spinal canal at the lumbar level and delayed images were obtained as the radiotracer entered the cranium. The patient had a history of intracranial metastatic disease from breast cancer and therefore, delayed migration of radiotracer along the cerebral convexities was noted (>24 h in this patient versus typically 12–24 h). (A) Image acquired 5 h following radiotracer injection. Radiotracer has reached the base of the brain. (B) Image acquired 24 h following radiotracer injection. Radiotracer has started to move along the cerebral convexities but has not yet reached the superior sagittal sinus at the vertex. (C) Image acquired 48 h following radiotracer injection. Radiotracer now reached the superior sagittal sinus at the vertex.

the bulk flow of CSF from the lumbar level upward to the brain, is not dependent on gravity and will occur even with the patient in the upright position (Alker and Leslie, 1969). In normal subjects, injected radiotracer is not typically seen within the ventricular system, a finding suggesting one-way flow of CSF out of the ventricles toward the dural venous sinuses and thus supportive of the theory of bulk, unidirectional CSF flow (Ziessman *et al.*, 2006). Radionuclide cisternography, however, is limited by temporal resolution (requiring imaging over a period of hours to days) and also by the lack of spatial resolution.

4.2. *MRI-based CSF flow studies: phase contrast and MR time-spatial labeling inversion pulse*

An MRI-based technique known as phase contrast MRI (Fig. 8) has been used to depict CSF flow. However, it also lacks adequate temporal resolution to discern transient turbulence or complex CSF flow patterns as the technique requires an image acquisition time of 2–3 min and time averaging over several cardiac cycles (Yamada, 2014; Yamada *et al.*, 2014). Fortunately, a more recently introduced technique known as time-spatial labeling inversion pulse (time–SLIP) MRI allows visualization of CSF movement over a shorter time interval (up to 5 s) and in any

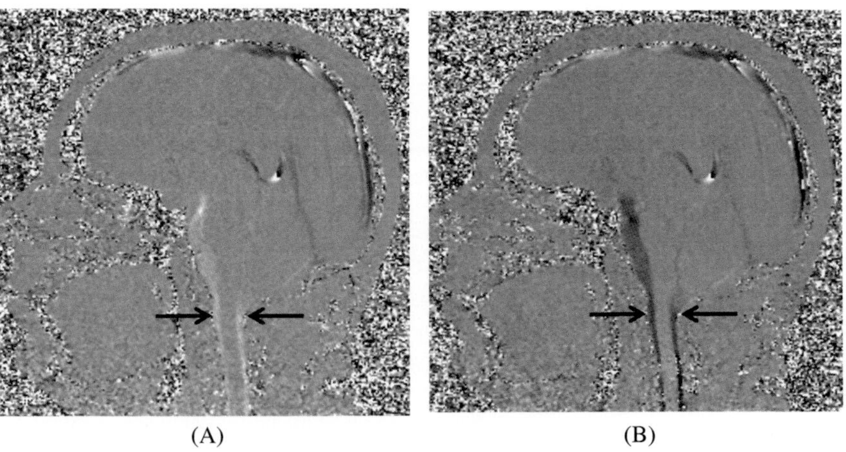

(A)   (B)

Figure 8. MRI CSF flow study using phase contrast technique. (A) A sagittal view of the brain during systole demonstrating CSF flow out of the cranium into the upper cervical canal. Downward movement of fluid is indicated as white. Black arrows = the level of the foramen magnum. (B) A sagittal view of the brain during diastole demonstrating CSF flow into the cranium out of the upper cervical canal. Upward movement of fluid is indicated as dark. Black arrows = the level of the foramen magnum.

selected localized region of the brain or spinal canal (Yamada *et al.*, 2014). Using the excellent temporal resolution afforded by this technique, Yamada and colleagues have identified complex CSF flow patterns within the ventricular system and subarachnoid space (Yamada *et al.*, 2014). Rather than the classically described unidirectional CSF flow out of the ventricles, they identified both anterograde and retrograde motion of CSF between the lateral and third ventricles. In addition, time-SLIP MRI revealed that head motion can create turbulent CSF flow in the body of the lateral ventricles (Yamada, 2014).

Yamada *et al.* further studied the positional dependence of intraspinal CSF flow within the thecal sac of seven patients in both the supine and prone positions (Yamada *et al.*, 2008). In the supine position, there were alterations in the CSF flow with pulsatile flow anterior to the spinal cord but little CSF flow posterior to the spinal cord. When the subjects moved to the prone position, CSF flow anterior to the cord decreased and there was pulsatile flow of CSF posterior to the spinal cord instead (Fig. 9).

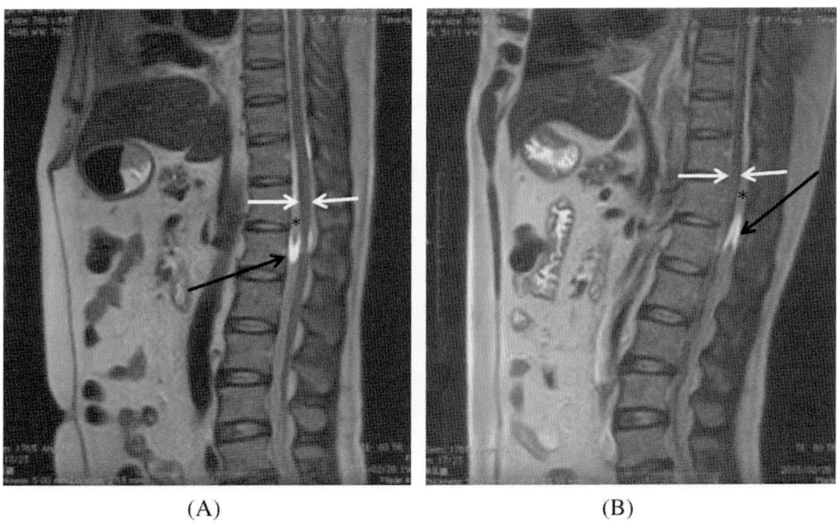

(A)   (B)

Figure 9. MRI CSF flow study using time-SLIP (time-spatial labeling inversion pulse) technique. (A) Subject in supine position: a sagittal view of the spine at the lower thoracic/upper lumbar levels showing the flow of CSF (black arrow) within the spinal arachnoid space (*) anterior to the spinal cord (white arrows). (B) Subject in prone position: a sagittal view of the spine at the lower thoracic/upper lumbar levels showing the flow of CSF (black arrow) within the posterior aspect of the spinal arachnoid space (*). With the subject in the prone position, the spinal cord (white arrows) has moved anteriorly within the spinal canal (Courtesy of Shinya Yamada, MD, PhD, Toshiba Rinkan Hospital, Kanagawa, Japan).

Further published studies of the positional dependence of CSF flow are not available. In particular, intracranial CSF flow patterns have not yet been studied in various body positions. Nevertheless, Yamada *et al.*'s work has important implications. Given that radionuclide cisternography indicates bulk, global flow of CSF within the subarachnoid space independent of gravity, but more complex CSF flow patterns are locally altered based on patient positioning, there is existing evidence to suggest the potential for altered CSF flow dynamics and homeostasis in a microgravity environment.

5. Imaging of Microscopic Tissue Water

The microarchitecture of the brain is complex and formed by a network of different compartments (vascular, intra- and extracellular) and cell types (neurons, glial cells). This microstructural complexity (at the micron level) supports the complex information processing and cognitive functions of the human brain but is beyond the resolution of standard anatomical MRI sequences to visualize (~ 1 mm 3 voxels).

MRI techniques, known in general as diffusion weighted imaging (DWI), measure the diffusion of water molecules within brain tissue. Water, which is the main constituent of brain tissue, is constantly in motion driven by random thermal energy fluctuations (Hagmann *et al.*, 2006; Hess and Mukherjee, 2007). The random motion of free water, or Brownian motion, occurs with equal probability in all directions characterized by a Gaussian probability distribution. However, the diffusion of water in brain tissue is not unrestricted but instead is altered as water molecules encounter barriers such as cell membranes and axons (Jensen and Helpern, 2010). Using DWI, the alteration in water diffusion, in the presence of microstructural barriers, can be measured. In this way, water serves as a "reporter molecule" in that the diffusion properties of water are reflective of the complexity of the microarchitecture. Thus, knowledge of brain water diffusion may be used to study complex function and thus help us understand neurological diseases.

Within the white matter of the brain, white matter tracts are composed of axons tightly packed together surrounded by glial cells and arranged in parallel bundles. As such, movement of water is hindered to a greater extent in a direction perpendicular to white matter tracts and diffuses more easily along a direction parallel to them. The larger degree of water diffusion parallel to white matter bundles can be detected by DWI and is the basis for white matter tractography (Hagmann *et al.*, 2006) (Fig. 10).

Several diffusion weighted MRI techniques are available and have been used in clinical and research applications. The most basic and widely used technique is

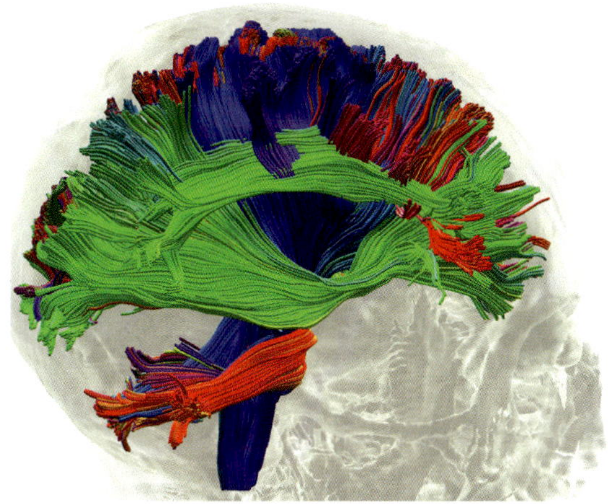

Figure 10.   Three dimensional reconstruction of the white matter tracts in a normal subject based on diffusion kurtosis imaging (DKI). The white matter fiber tracts are color coded such that fiber tracts coursing anterior–posterior are in green, transversely are in red, and superior-inferior are in blue (Courtesy of Jens Jensen, PhD and Russell Glenn, Medical University of South Carolina).

diffusion tensor imaging (DTI), which is based on a Gaussian model of water diffusion (Hagmann *et al.*, 2006). However, as discussed above, the Gaussian model does not accurately depict the true complexity of the microarchitecture of the brain. Also, for tractography applications, while the diffusion tensor model may be sufficient to describe diffusion along parallel white matter bundles, due to its Gaussian probability assumption, DTI cannot accurately measure more complex white matter architectures. This becomes a problem in regions of the brain where multiple white matter tracts intersect (Hagmann *et al.*, 2006).

Therefore, mapping more complex microarchitecture and delineating crossing white matter tracts requires imaging techniques that provide higher angular resolution. Several techniques are available, based on non-Gaussian assumptions, which better model microstructural complexity but require trade-offs of longer imaging times and limited hardware availability. These techniques include diffusion kurtosis imaging, q-ball imaging, spherical deconvolution, and diffusion spectrum imaging. Acquisition times of these sequences ranging from 6 to 60 min (Hagmann *et al.*, 2006; Hess and Mukherjee, 2007; Fieremans *et al.*, 2011; Tabesh *et al.*, 2011).

Although no gross brain edema has been observed following spaceflight, little is known of the microscopic water content of the brain in microgravity. Due to the combined effects of cephalad fluid shifts, venous hypertension, chronic hypercapnia, altered CSF flow dynamics, and potentially altered cerebral autoregulation, one could hypothesize that an increase in brain tissue water (brain edema) could occur on a microscopic level. Alterations in brain tissue water could also be the result of a shift in relative water fractions between the intra- and extra-axonal compartments. The use of advanced diffusion imaging techniques, along with the application of white matter and gray matter modelling, would be valuable in further elucidating the intracranial physiological changes associated with spaceflight and the VIIP syndrome.

6. Structural Brain Changes Following Long-Term Bed Rest

Little is known of any potential structural brain changes that may occur as a result of long-term microgravity exposure. During spaceflight, the removal of the gravitational gradient would be expected to result in unloading of the cranial contents. Similarly, in the long-term bed rest model used as an analog for spaceflight, subjects' heads are maintained in the head-down tilt position, which could lead to a global shift in brain tissue within the cranial vault toward the vertex along the G_z direction. Recently, in a study of eight healthy subjects undergoing approximately 60 days of 6° head-down tilt bed rest, the brain as a whole showed significant displacement superiorly (0.36 ± 0.15 mm, $t = 7.0$, $p < 0.01$) and rotation posteriorly ($0.28 \pm 0.34°$, $t = 2.3$, $p = 0.051$) within the skull (Roberts *et al.*, 2015b). In other words, the brain's center of mass was shifted upward and the brain demonstrated posterior rotation relative to the skull. There was associated contraction of the adjacent extra-axial CSF at the vertex.

No significant differences were seen in the overall volume of gray matter, white matter, CSF, or the ventricles between pre- and postbed rest on the group level. However, there were significant individual changes in the volume of the ventricular system which varied among the subjects and correlated with the degree of posterior brain rotation (Spearman correlation: $r = 0.893$, $p = 0.007$). The largest increase in ventricular size occurred in subjects with the greatest shift in brain structure. Following bed rest, the change in ventricular size ranged from a 10.4% increase to a 22.4% decrease compared with baseline values, an unexpected finding over the course of only two months in young subjects (Fig. 11). For comparison, in elderly, healthy subjects, expansion of the ventricles has been reported to be 1.5%–3.0% per year and 5%–16% per year in patients with Alzheimer's disease (Winkelman, 2000). Of note, ventricular volume can also be influenced by fluid balance, and the bed rest subjects did undergo an initial diuresis. However, this stabilized within three days, and any ventricular volume change attributable to

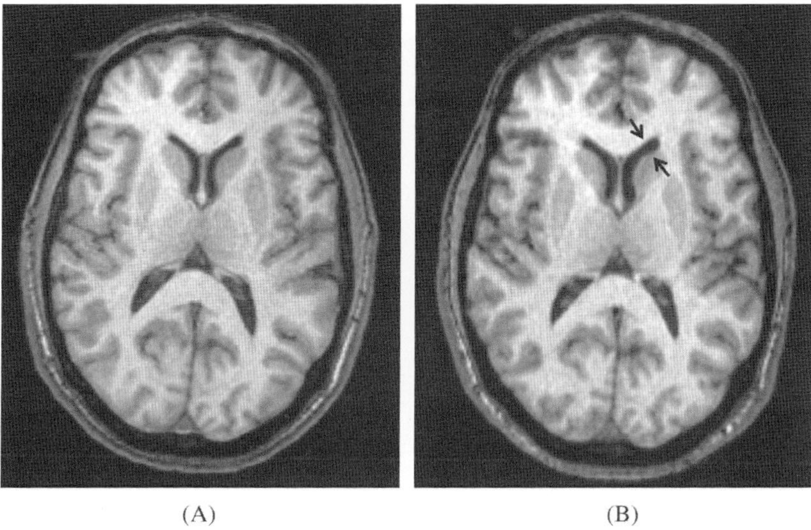

(A)   (B)

Figure 11. Axial T1-weighted MRI images through the brain showing an increase in ventricular size following 60 days of 6° head-down tilt bed rest. (A) Prebed rest baseline. (B) Postbed rest. Notice the increase in the size of the lateral ventricles, particularly the frontal horns (arrows).

such dehydration would be approximately 1%–3% (Bono *et al.*, 2003) — markedly less than the observed ventricular enlargement following bed rest.

The reason for individual changes in ventricular volume during bed rest is unknown. However, the observed upward shift in brain structure and resultant effacement of the subarachnoid spaces at the top of the brain could have two effects: (1) effacement of the subarachnoid spaces altering local CSF flow dynamics and possibly disrupting function of arachnoid granulations located at the vertex, and (2) upward shift of the brain resulting in compression of the adjacent superior sagittal sinus which runs along the vertex of the skull. This, in turn, would contribute to venous outflow obstruction and the spectrum of intraorbital and intracranial findings seen in astronauts presenting with VIIP syndrome, analogous to the role of venous hypertension in IIH as described previously. The hypothesis that an alteration in CSF homeostasis occurs during long-term bed rest is further supported by the observation that the degree of ventricular change and posterior brain rotation are correlated.

Roberts *et al.* (2015b) reported widespread morphological changes in brain tissue following bed rest affecting functionally important areas of the brain (Fig. 12). Compared with baseline, the postbed rest brains showed significant tissue

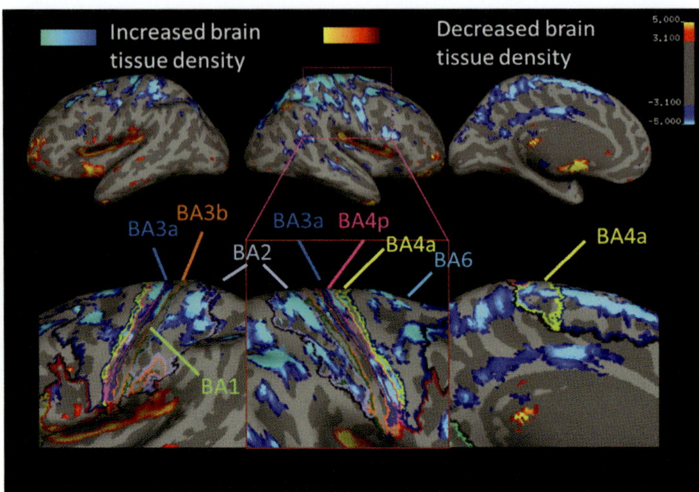

Figure 12. Morphological changes affecting widespread areas of the brain after 60 days of bed rest. Images were threshold at $p = 0.001$ ($t = 3.1$, uncorrected). Most affected areas including premotor cortex, primary motor cortex, sensory cortex, orbitofrontal cortex, cingulate, cuneus, thalami, and cerebellum. The lower part of figure outlines the detailed changes of the central frontoparietal (BA = Brodmann area 1, 2, 3, 4, 6, with subsections a, b, and p) which are involved in sensorimotor function (Courtesy of Xun Zhu PhD, Medical University of South Carolina).

density (both gray and white matter) increase involving the central frontoparietal lobes, posterior cingulate, cuneus, thalami, and superior aspect of the cerebellum. Conversely, tissue density decrease was found in the orbitofrontal cortex, brainstem, corpus callosum, striatum, anterior cingulate, and parietal operculum. There was an associated expansion of the basal extra–axial CSF spaces.

The consequences of these structural changes are unknown but may be crucial given the involvement of these areas in adaptation to microgravity. For example, optimal performance in the microgravity environment requires reinterpretation of sensory input from peripheral receptors (Porcelli *et al.*, 2010). As the role of the lower extremities in locomotion is decreased during spaceflight, new sensorimotor strategies must emerge for the coordination of movement. This requires plasticity at higher cortical levels, including the sensorimotor cortices (Porcelli *et al.*, 2010). Disturbances in perceptual–motor task performance have been found during spaceflight, particularly while simultaneously engaging in a secondary cognitive task (Porcelli *et al.*, 2010). These findings warrant further investigation, including planned and ongoing functional brain imaging studies of astronauts following long-term spaceflight (See Chapter 10).

7. Cerebral Perfusion and Spaceflight

Given that microgravity results in cephalad fluid shifts, one might expect alterations in cerebrovascular structure and function associated with long-duration spaceflight. Under normal circumstances, cerebral perfusion is highly regulated as CBF must be maintained at a constant level to ensure proper neurological function. Normal CBF is approximately 50 mL/100 g/min. Patients become presyncopal when CBF is reduced by 50%–60%, with loss of consciousness occurring with an interruption of CBF for 8–10 s (Franco Folino, 2007). As CBF falls below 16–18 mL/100 g/min, electrical activity ceases and when CBF further declines to 10–12 mL/100 g/min, irreversible tissue damage occurs (Franco Folino, 2007).

The main arterial supply to the human brain is the internal carotid artery system (anterior circulation) and the vertebral-basilar system (posterior circulation). At the base of the brain, these vessels are interconnected via anterior and posterior communicating arteries to form the circle of Willis, an anastomotic system which functions to provide collateral flow should one or more of the main supply arteries become occluded. Six major vessels arise from the circle of Willis: bilateral anterior, middle, and posterior cerebral arteries. These large intracranial vessels supply the brain via pial arteries which penetrate the brain parenchyma, ultimately dividing to form the arterioles and capillaries that provide regional CBF (Fig. 13).

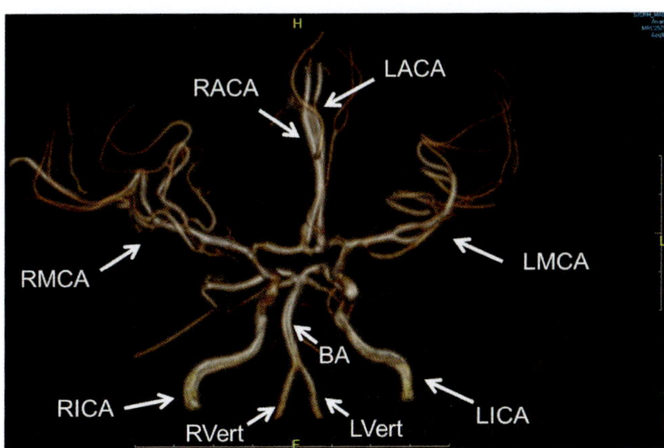

Figure 13. A three dimensional image from a magnetic resonance angiography study demonstrating the main arterial supply to the human brain. The main vascular supply to the anterior circulation is the bilateral internal carotid arteries (RICA and LICA). The main vascular supply to the posterior circulation is the bilateral vertebral arteries (Rvert and Lvert) which give rise to the basilar artery (BA). The six major vessels which arise from the circle of Willis are the bilateral anterior (RACA and LACA), middle (RMCA and LMCA), and posterior cerebral (RPCA and LPCA) arteries.

7.1. *The regulation of cerebral blood flow*

The control of CBF is complex and involves several homeostatic mechanisms. These include cerebrovascular autoregulation, functional hyperemia, partial pressure of CO_2 $\left(Pa_{CO_2}\right)$, partial pressure of oxygen $\left(Pa_{O_2}\right)$, and neurovascular innervation (Attwell *et al.*, 2010; Franco Folino, 2007; Iadecola, 2004; Vavilala *et al.*, 2002).

7.1.1. *Cerebrovascular autoregulation*

While arterial blood pressure is a major determinant of CBF, it can vary widely during the course of normal activity and in pathologic states. Cerebrovascular autoregulation refers to the process through which cerebral perfusion is maintained at a constant rate despite a wide variation in blood pressures. Cerebral perfusion pressure (CPP) is the difference between the mean arterial blood pressure (MAP) and the ICP (Gwinnutt and Saha, 2005). CBF, then, is determined by the mean arterial blood pressure, intracranial pressure, and cerebral vascular resistance according to the following equation:

$$CBF = (MAP - ICP)/(\text{cerebral vascular resistance})$$
$$= CPP/(\text{cerebral vascular resistance}) \tag{5}$$

To maintain CBF over a range of blood pressures and variable ICP, cerebral vascular resistance is altered through adjustments in the diameter of cerebral arterioles and capillaries (Attwell *et al.*, 2010). Under normal conditions, cerebrovascular autoregulation is effective over a range of arterial blood pressures — typically from a lower limit of 60 mmHg to an upper limit of 150 mmHg (Fig. 14A) (Paulson *et al.*, 1990). If autoregulation should fail, at arterial blood pressures beyond the upper or lower limits, CBF becomes pressure passive such that an elevation in blood pressure leads to increased CBF, and in turn, to increased ICP.

7.1.2. *Partial pressure of CO_2*

Importantly, the pressure limits of cerebrovascular autoregulation are not fixed, and the autoregulatory curve may shift depending on global and local physiological conditions. For example, CO_2, which is a potent vasodilator (Kety and Schmidt, 1946), can modify the limits of arterial blood pressures within which cerebrovascular autoregulation is effective. CO_2 rapidly increases CBF by 2%–6% per 1 mmHg increase in Pa_{CO_2} (Ito *et al.*, 2003; Noth *et al.*, 2008; Vavilala *et al.*, 2002). CO_2 indirectly affects cerebral vasomotor tone by reducing extracellular pH. In

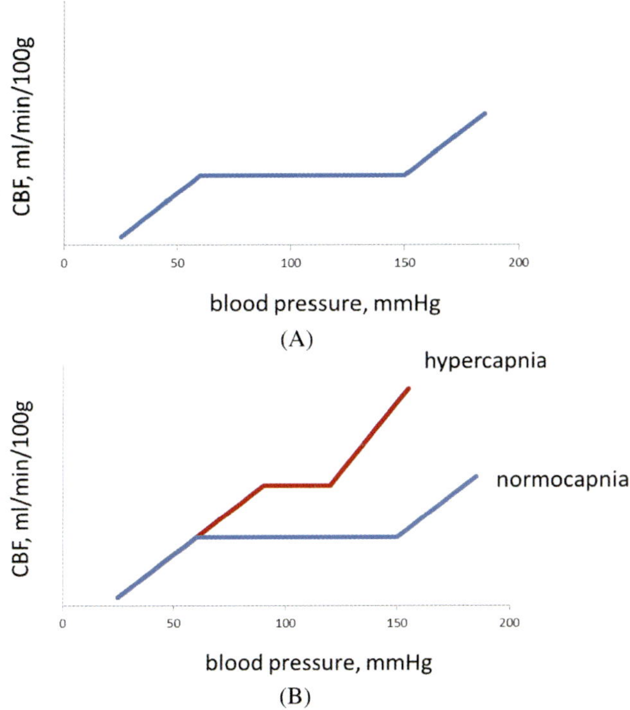

Figure 14. (A) Graph of the cerebrovascular autoregulatory curve. Under normal conditions, cerebrovascular autoregulation is effective over a range of arterial blood pressures — typically from a lower limit of 60 mmHg to an upper limit of 150 mmHg. This is illustrated graphically by the flat portion of the curve known as the plateau. If autoregulation should fail, at arterial blood pressures beyond the upper or lower limits, cerebral blood flow (CBF) becomes pressure passive such that an elevation in blood pressure leads to increased CBF. (B) Compared with normocapnia, under hypercapnic conditions, the plateau of the cerebrovascular autoregulatory curve is elevated and as Pa_{CO_2} rises, the plateau becomes progressively shorter as CBF becomes more dependent on cerebral perfusion pressure (CPP) (Modified from Meng and Gelb, 2015).

response to a lower pH, a complex interaction of secondary mediators including nitrous oxide (NO), cyclic guanosine monophosphate (cGMP), and potassium channels leads to hyperpolarization of vascular smooth muscle cells (Brian, 1998). Membrane hyperpolarization inhibits voltage-gated calcium channels, reducing intracellular calcium and inducing the relaxation of vascular smooth muscle cells with resultant vasodilation (Brian, 1998).

It should be noted that there is a complex interplay between several physiologic responses to chronic CO_2 exposure. As noted above, acute exposure to hypercapnia (elevated Pa_{CO_2}) rapidly and dramatically increases CBF. However, during chronic hypercapnia in anesthetized dogs, CBF returns to baseline levels within 6 h of exposure. This is likely due to the observed increase in CSF bicarbonate which partially neutralizes the initial acidic pH response to the elevated CO_2 (Warner *et al.*, 1987). However, in awake and conscious animals, severe or chronic exposure to CO_2 can increase baseline cerebral metabolism and can result in the release of brain catecholamines. These factors can serve to increase CBF in unanesthetized animals, attenuating the effects of elevated CSF bicarbonate metabolism (Brian, 1998).

Meng and Gelb proposed a model for describing the effect of CO_2 on cerebral autoregulation (Meng and Gelb, 2015) and its effect on the shape of the cerebrovascular autoregulatory curve (Fig. 14B). Hypercapnia increases the baseline level of vasodilation compared with normocapnia (Pa_{CO_2} of $\sim$ 30–50 mmHg) thereby increasing CBF and elevating the plateau of the autoregulatory curve (Meng and Gelb, 2015). This physiologic adaptation to a state of increased Pa_{CO_2} has important ramifications, particularly to the lower and upper limits of the autoregulatory curve.

In a *normocapnic hypotensive* patient, as systemic blood pressure and CPP decrease cerebral vessels dilate to maintain CBF until maximal dilatation occurs and the lower limit of the cerebrovascular autoregulatory curve is reached. However, under *hypercapnic* conditions, as a result of preexisting vasodilatation induced by elevated Pa_{CO_2}, that limit is reached at a higher pressure level. In other words, the lower limit is shifted to the right and physiologic adaptations can no longer maintain CBF over the same lower pressure range. Additional changes affect the upper pressure range. In a *normocapnic, hypertensive* patient, systemic blood pressure and CPP increase, and cerebral vessels constrict to protect against the increasing pressure — until maximal constriction is reached and CBF becomes pressure passive. In a *hypercapnic* patient, however, preexisting vasodilatation induced by elevated Pa_{CO_2} attenuates the degree of vasoconstriction. Therefore, the upper limit of the cerebrovascular autoregulatory curve is reached at a lower pressure level than during normocapnia. In short, under hypercapnic conditions, the plateau of the cerebrovascular autoregulatory curve becomes progressively shorter and CBF becomes more dependent on CPP (Meng and Gelb, 2015).

7.1.3. *Functional hyperemia*

Another mechanism involved in the control of CBF is termed functional hyperemia or neurovascular coupling. Metabolic changes in the microenvironment of the brain due to regional neuronal activity lead to localized increases in CBF (Attwell *et al.*, 2010). The increased CBF supports the greater energy demands of activated neurons and removes byproducts of neuronal metabolism. This process, which results in the objective blood oxygenation changes measured in functional neuro-imaging studies, ensures that CBF is directed to areas of the brain that are most active.

7.1.4. *Neurovascular innervation*

Cerebrovascular tone is regulated through vascular innervation. All segments of the cerebral vasculature are innervated, including both the large intracranial vessels and the smaller intraparenchymal vessels (Gulbenkian *et al.*, 2001; Hamel, 2006; Paulson *et al.*, 1990). Neurovascular innervation of the large vessels at the base of the brain (e.g., the middle cerebral artery in the circle of Willis) is derived from cranial ganglia. These include sympathetic fibers from the superior cervical ganglion and parasympathetic fibers from the sphenopalatine ganglion (Gulbenkian *et al.*, 2001; Hamel, 2006, Paulson *et al.*, 1990). However, when cerebral arteries enter the brain parenchyma, this peripheral innervation is largely absent. Instead, the intraparen-chymal microvasculature receives innervation via central neurons located in the locus coeruleus, raphe nucleus, basal forebrain, as well as from the cortex 2 itself via interneurons (Franco Folino, 2007). In response to sympathetic activation, the larger cerebral vessels may constrict resulting in decreased CBF. However, further downstream, the arterioles supplying functional neuronal tissue will respond to a decrease in global CBF by dilating in order to keep CBF constant under the normal range of blood pressures. In addition, during such a situation, the metabolically active brain tissue can directly increase the amount of oxygen extracted from the blood it receives (increased oxygen extraction fraction) to stave off ischemia.

All of these homeostatic mechanisms act in concert to provide very tight con-trol of CBF ensuring local tissue demands for oxygen and glucose are continuously met. However, it should be noted that the energy demands throughout the brain are not homogenous. Instead, the metabolic requirements of specific neuronal tis-sue are quite variable and can rapidly change with the degree of ongoing neuronal activity and systemic factors. Certainly, the role of the large cerebral arteries in regulating CBF is important. However, it is ultimately the response of the localized microvascular (arteriole and capillaries) that allows for global and regional differ-ences in cerebral perfusion. The relative contribution of the large arteries and microvasculature on CBF can be assessed through the degree of their respective potential vasomotor changes in response to alterations in blood pressure and CO_2

levels. For instance, Giller *et al.* (1993) reported a mean change in diameter of approximately 4% in the large cerebral arteries including the carotid arteries, middle cerebral arteries (MCAs), and the vertebral arteries. In contrast, the smaller arteries (e.g., distal branches of the MCA) showed diameter changes as large as 29%. As such, these smaller vessels have a proportionally larger net effect on CBF. Specifically, while the changes in cerebrovascular resistance of the large intracerebral and pial arteries account for approximately 20%–30% of CBF changes, the balance arises from the arterioles and capillaries at a regional level (Faraci and Heistad, 1990). The role of these small vessels in control of regional CBF and localized neuronal metabolic activity is underscored by the finding that capillary density correlates linearly with local cerebral glucose utilization and varies considerably throughout the brain (Iadecola and Nedergaard, 2007; Klein *et al.*, 1986). Therefore, it is the response of both the large cerebral arteries and the microvasculature that must be investigated in order to characterize fully any adaptation in cerebral autoregulation that might occur in the spaceflight environment.

7.2. *Cerebral autoregulatory adaptation to microgravity*

Several investigators have examined cerebral perfusion in astronauts before, during, and after spaceflight using a technique known as transcranial Doppler (TCD). TCD uses ultrasound technology to measure cerebral blood flow velocity as an indirect marker of cerebral perfusion. The use of TCD to measure relative changes in cerebral blood flow velocity was reported in 1982 by Aaslid *et al.* It is made possible by the fact that at low frequencies, ultrasound can penetrate the human skull (Aaslid *et al.*, 1982; Petty *et al.*, 1990). By directing sound waves toward the base of the brain, frequency shifts can be measured to obtain blood flow velocities in the MCA, one of the large vessels at the base of brain. Cerebral blood flow velocity (CBFV) can then be used to determine CBF according to the following equation (Levine *et al.*, 1994):

$$\text{CBF (mL/min)} = \text{CBFV (cm/min)} \times \text{vessel area (cm}^2) \tag{6}$$

With TCD, CBF can only be inferred from velocity changes, and is based on the assumption that the area of the interrogated vessel, the MCA, remains constant throughout the experimental paradigm (Aaslid *et al.*, 1982; Levine *et al.*, 1994). The results of several studies have suggested that this assumption is fairly accurate. As stated above, Giller *et al.* (1993) reported that the mean change in diameter of the large cerebral arteries, including the MCA, was less than 4% during moderate changes in end tidal CO_2 and blood pressure changes. This finding was based on direct visualization of the cerebral vessels in patients during open brain surgery in which measurements of the external diameter of the vessels were taken through the operative microscope. Likewise, by measuring the loss of signal on MRI created by flow within the MCA, Serrador, *et al.* (2000) found no change in MCA dimensions during −40 mmHg LBNP or during hypo- and hypercapnic challenges.

One of the main advantages of using TCD to assess the response of the cerebrovascular system in spaceflight is the ability to obtain real-time, beat-to-beat determination of CBFV. Therefore, TCD can be used to dynamically assess cerebrovascular autoregulatory mechanisms in response to various experimental protocols, including, for example, shifting of body position from supine to standing, the application of lower body negative pressure, or CO_2 administration. A second major advantage of TCD is that inflight data can be obtained throughout a mission given the presence of an ultrasound device aboard the ISS. This is important, as the time course of cerebrovascular adaptation over the duration of spaceflight is unknown. Additionally, interpretation of postflight data is potentially compounded by physiological changes related to reentry and early readaptation to Earth before postflight measurements can be made.

Using TCD, studies of CBF in astronauts have shown only modest changes in CBFV following spaceflight. The results of these studies have been mixed (Table 1) with various investigators reporting increased CBFV, no change in CBFV, or decreased CBFV compared with preflight values. Meaningful interpretation of the results of these studies is limited by the small number of tested subjects and the paucity of inflight data. In addition, as different missions (Mir, Space Shuttle, and ISS) were studied, important parameters, such as flight duration and level of CO_2 exposure, are nonuniform across the available data. Perhaps most importantly, many of the studies examining cerebrovascular changes of spaceflight were performed to assess orthostatic intolerance. At present, no published reports have specifically investigated the unique and complex adaptation in subjects who present with VIIP syndrome.

Nonetheless, several studies describing dynamic cerebral autoregulation in the astronaut population provide important insight into the effects of spaceflight on cerebral perfusion (Blaber *et al.*, 2011; Iwasaki *et al.*, 2007; Zuj *et al.*, 2012). In a group of 27 (20 male, 7 female) astronauts, Blaber *et al.* (2011) used TCD to assess MCA CBFV before spaceflight, on landing day, and 3 days postflight. They characterized the astronauts as finishers ($n = 19$; 17 male, 2 female) or nonfinishers ($n = 8$; 5 female, 3 male) based on the astronauts' ability to remain standing for 10 min without becoming presyncopal as an indicator of orthostatic intolerance. The nonfinishers had higher preflight CBFV than finishers, suggesting that the former had a higher baseline level of cerebral vasodilatation than the latter. On landing

Table 1. Studies of cerebral perfusion in astronauts using transcranial Doppler.

Investigators	No. of subjects	Mission	Spaceflight duration	Inflight data acquired	Cerebral blood flow velocity (CBFV) of the middle cerebral artery compared with preflight values*	Additional measures*
Fritsch–Yelle et al. (1996)	29	Space shuttle	8–16 days	—	—	CBFV was higher preflight in the orthostatic intolerant astronauts (8/29) compared with astronauts without orthostatic intolerance. Cerebral vascular resistance (mean arterial pressure at the level of the MCA/CBFV) of the MCA was lower while standing in the orthostatic intolerant astronauts (8/29) on landing day compared with astronauts without orthostatic intolerance.
Arbeille et al. (1996)	3	—	—	Yes	One astronaut ↑ CBFV One astronaut slight ↑ CBFV One astronaut ∅ CBFV	—
Arbeille et al. (2001)	12	—	7 days up to 6 months	Yes	↑ CBFV early in flight; ↓ CBFV later in flight	Changes in CBFV during spaceflight were only modest; decreased later in flight, with an associated increase in MCA vascular resistance
Tobal et al. (2001)	10	Mir	6 months	Yes	∅ CBFV during spaceflight or postflight at rest	∅ CBFV in flight or postflight at LBNP A lack of lower limb arterial vasoconstriction and a reduced increase in the cerebral-femoral flow ratio was observed during LBNP inflight and postflight, particularly in orthostatic intolerant cosmonauts

Iwasaki *et al.* (2007)	6	Space shuttle	1–2 weeks	Yes	∅ CBFV during spaceflight or postflight at rest	A large cumulative loss of cerebral perfusion during LBNP was observed preflight in orthostatic intolerant cosmonauts (three subjects) ↓ CBFV during LBNP preflight, but not inflight or postflight ↓↓ CBFV during upright tilt preflight, smaller ↓ CBFV during upright tilt postflight Improved indexes of dynamic cerebrovascular autoregulatory during flight and postflight
Blaber *et al.* (2011)	27	Space shuttle	8–16 days	—	∅ CBFV postflight in astronauts without orthostatic intolerance ($n = 19$; 17 males) ↓ CBFV postflight upon standing in astronauts with orthostatic intolerance ($n = 8$; five females)	Reduced indexes of dynamic cerebrovascular autoregulatory postflight
Zuj *et al.* (2012)	7	ISS	147 ± 49 days	—	∅ CBFV postflight	Reduced indexes of dynamic cerebrovascular autoregulatory postflight ↓CO_2 reactivity

*Key:

↑ indicates increased CBFV

↓ indicates decreased CBFV

∅ indicates no change CBFV

day, only the nonfinishers had CBFV reduced below preflight values upon standing, though on postflight day 3, CBFV was significantly elevated in the nonfinishers. Their data suggested that nonfinishers had a higher baseline level of cerebral vasodilatation than finishers for a given mean arterial pressure. Despite the severe impairments in CBFV in the nonfinishers, blood pressures were not significantly different from preflight values. This would indicate a postflight failure of cerebral autoregulation with the inability to preserve CBF despite normal blood pressures. Within this group, there was also a significant gender effect. Specifically, preflight very low frequency gain (VLFG) in females was double that of males. VLFG is a measure of the correlation between changes in CBF and arterial pressure, with a large gain indicative of ineffective cerebral autoregulation. In addition, females demonstrated higher CBFV than the males on postflight day 3, again suggesting impaired postflight cerebral autoregulation.

Iwasaki *et al.* (2007) studied a group of six astronauts before, during, and after spaceflight, and used head up tilt testing (HUT) and lower body negative pressure (LBNP) as provocative techniques to test cerebral autoregulation. LBNP is a technique in which various levels of negative pressure are applied to the lower body resulting in reduced central blood volume simulating the effects of an upright posture in a 1-gravity environment. LBNP is useful as a means of testing orthostatic intolerance in that it can be performed in space as well as on Earth (Bungo, 1989). Iwasaki *et al.* (2007) found that statistically significant reductions in CBFV were induced by the application of LBNP prior to spaceflight. However, during and after spaceflight, reductions in CBFV were not statistically significant. In addition, the decrease in CBFV observed after 10 min of upright tilt was less after spaceflight. Lastly, VLFG decreased significantly following 1 and 2 weeks in space, and on landing day compared with preflight values. Therefore, Iwasaki *et al.* (2007) concluded that human cerebral autoregulation is preserved and possibly even augmented by exposure to microgravity. While this data are quite compelling, it remains unclear why cerebral autoregulation would be improved during and following spaceflight.

Zuj *et al.* (2012) studied seven astronauts (six males, one female) preflight and postflight within 48 h of landing. CBFV and blood pressure measurements were made during LBNP and following two breaths of 10% CO_2 to assess cerebrovascular CO_2 reactivity. They found no differences pre- to postflight in CBFV during LBNP. There was, however, a blunt vasodilatory response to CO_2 postflight compared with preflight values.

Several studies of orthostatic intolerance included measures of cerebral vascular resistance during spaceflight. Orthostatic intolerance is a common occurrence following long-term spaceflight and numerous studies have evaluated changes in various systemic parameters (such as blood pressure, peripheral vascular resistance, baroreceptor responses, and other changes in cardiovascular physiology) as factors contributing to its occurrence. However, syncope during orthostatic stress ultimately reflects a failure in cerebral autoregulation with a critical reduction in CBF leading to unconsciousness. Therefore, cerebral autoregulation plays the central role in the final step of orthostatic intolerance. In light of this, a few investigators have included measurements of cerebral vascular resistance in their investigation of orthostatic intolerance in astronauts. While this provides useful information, it must be stressed (prior to discussing the specifics of these studies) that no evaluation has assessed physiologic changes/cerebral vascular reactivity at the level of the microvasculature.

In a study of 29 astronauts before and after shuttle missions lasting 8–16 days, Fritsch-Yelle *et al.* (1996) measured several indicators of hemodynamic response to orthostatic stress including cerebral vascular resistance. Their main finding was that susceptibility to orthostatic intolerance immediately after spaceflight was characterized by a decreased adrenergic response to upright posture. They also found a greater compensatory decrease in cerebrovascular resistance to decreased mean arterial pressure postflight compared with preflight values. However, this autoregulatory change was insufficient to maintain CBFV in the face of markedly decreased systemic arterial pressure in subjects who were presyncopal on landing day.

Arbeille *et al.* (2001) studied both astronauts during missions of varying duration and subjects during head down tilt bed rest. They noted a significant increase in cerebral vascular resistance after 4 days of bed rest. Conversely, in spaceflight there was no similar early increase in cerebral vascular resistance, but a more gradual and progressive increase in resistance between weeks 2–3 and months 5–6. Based on TCD velocity measurements, they found no significant decrease in cerebral perfusion in either bed rest or spaceflight subjects as MCA CBFV varied inversely with cerebral vascular resistance.

Animal studies have also been contradictory. For example, in hind-limb suspended rats, a ground-based model for microgravity, enhanced vasoconstriction of cerebral vessels is seen (Lin *et al.*, 2009; Prisby *et al.*, 2006; Wilkerson *et al.*, 1999, 2002, 2005; Zhang *et al.*, 2001). However, in space-flown mice, vasoconstrictor responses were lower, maximal arterial diameter was increased, there was no change in medial vessel wall thickness, and vascular stiffness was decreased (Taylor *et al.*, 2013).

Although cerebrovascular hemodynamics plays a crucial role in intracranial pressure regulation, there is limited knowledge of cerebral autoregulatory mechanisms during and following spaceflight. Published studies were commonly performed using protocols optimized to assess orthostatic intolerance and not VIIP syndrome. Furthermore, all data in both flight and ground-based studies have been acquired using TCD as the method for assessing CBF. Unfortunately, while convenient, TCD provides only an indirect assessment of cerebral perfusion as CBF must be inferred from blood flow velocity measurements. More importantly, the constraints of Doppler imaging limit its utility to the circle of Willis. As such, CBFV can only be determined at the level of the large cerebral arteries, precluding evaluation of the cerebral microvasculature which is implicated in playing a major role in autoregulation.

7.3. *Imaging of cerebral perfusion*

Currently, no data exist concerning cerebral autoregulation in astronauts at the level of the microvasculature, the evaluation of which is not possible with TCD, instead requiring cross-sectional imaging. Numerous imaging techniques are available for evaluating perfusion including: positron emission tomography (PET), single photon emission computed tomography (SPECT), Xenon-enhanced computed tomography (XeCT), dynamic perfusion computed tomography, MRI dynamic susceptibility-weighted contrast, and noncontrast MRI arterial spin labeling. Each technique has unique advantages and disadvantages which determines its utility in specific clinical situations. For a thorough comparative overview of brain perfusion imaging techniques, please see Wintermark *et al.* (2005).

For assessment of cerebral perfusion during spaceflight, important considerations for technique selection include: (1) the lack of exposure to ionizing radiation and (2) the rapid acquisition of as complete a data set as possible during a limited timeframe. MRI meets both of these qualifications and offers a variety of sequences designed to characterize the different physiological responses to changes in cerebral perfusion.

Several methods for performing MR perfusion exist. While the specifics of each technique are based on technical parameters defined during sequence development, they can be broadly characterized into two groups based on whether intravenous contrast is required. Dynamic susceptibility-weighted contrast MRI (DSC-MRI), also known as bolus-tracking MRI, is based on detecting the first passage of an exogenously administered endovascular contrast agent, a chelate of gadolinium, through the blood vessels in the brain (Wintermark *et al.*, 2005; Zaharchuk, 2007). A rapid MR sequence, such as echoplanar imaging, is utilized to tract the contrast bolus through the brain. The gadolinium contrast produces local magnetic field gradients that lead to a decrease in the MR signal which is detected as $T2^*$-weighted signal loss. By applying tracer kinetic models, several parametric maps can be calculated from these signal changes and include: mean transit time (MTT), time to peak (TTP), CBV, and CBF (Fig. 15). An inherent

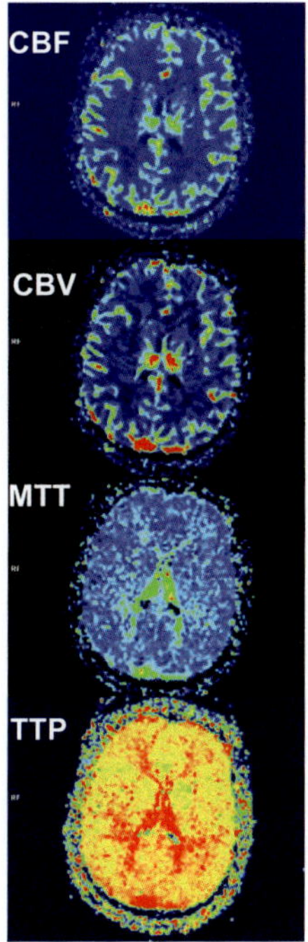

Figure 15. Magnetic resonance (MR) perfusion imaging using dynamic susceptibility-weighted contrast magnetic resonance imaging (DSC-MRI). By applying tracer kinetic models, several parametric maps can be calculated and include: mean transit time (MTT), time to peak (TTP), cerebral blood volume (CBV), and cerebral blood flow (CBF).

limitation of DSC-MRI is that contrast can only serve as an indirect tracer of CBF (in contrast, e.g., to the radioactive tracers used in PET and SPECT). The precise relationship between the DSC-MRI signal and concentration of the paramagnetic tracers is difficult to establish. As such, the relative CBV map acquired using this method is not quantitative. Despite this limitation, DSC-MRI is the most commonly used MRI technique for assessing brain hemodynamics in clinical practice due to its relatively high contrast-to-noise ratio, fast acquisition time, and wealth of available parametric maps (Calamante, 2010).

On the other hand, arterial spin labeling (ASL) is a noncontrast MR perfusion imaging technique in which radio frequency pulses are used to label water protons in blood by inverting their spins along the upper neck before the blood enters the cranium. This labeled water then flows intracranially to the level of capillaries, where a small resulting signal decrease of approximately 1%–2% can be measured using a rapid MR imaging technique based on proton density-weighted images.

A quantitative measurement of CBF is provided by pair-wise subtracting of this signal from a baseline control (nonlabeled) acquisition. The advantages of ASL imaging include its quantitative capabilities and its noncontrast and noninvasive nature. Its limitations include its relatively low signal-to-noise ratio, potential for artifacts, and its inability to measure perfusion parameters other than CBF (Fig. 16).

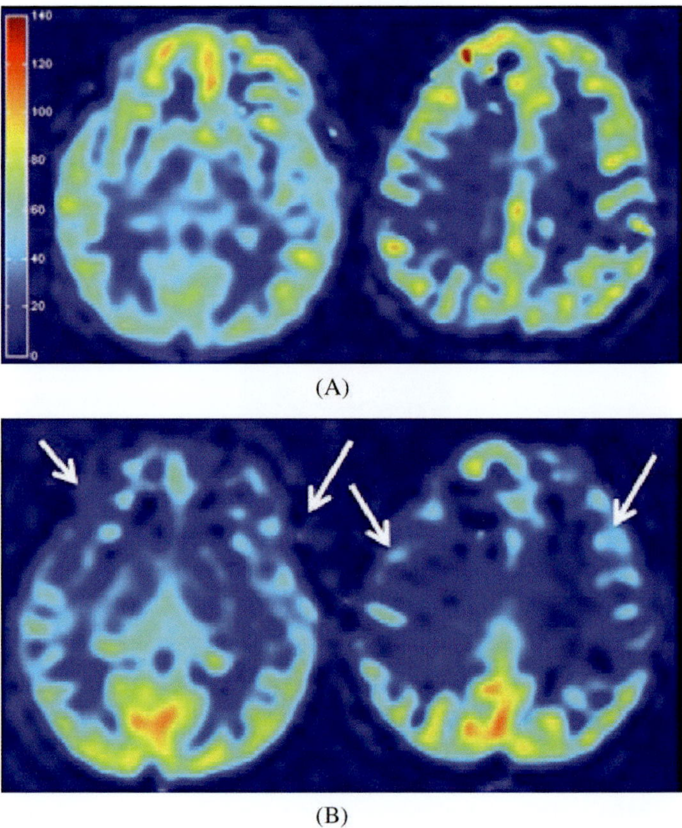

(A)

(B)

Figure 16. Cerebral vascular reactivity (CVR) assessment with arterial spin labeling (ASL). Twenty-nine-year-old female with Moyamoya resulting in severe bilateral internal carotid artery steno-occlusive disease with chronic borderzone ischemic change. (A) ASL demonstrating cerebral blood flow at baseline. (B) The patient was administered a dose of Diamox which results in diffuse vasodilation of the cerebral vasculature. Following the dose of Diamox, ASL was again performed. The post-Diamox ASL reveals a paradoxical decrease in cerebral blood flow to the frontal lobes. This indicates severe CVR impairment with bilateral steal phenomenon (arrows) (Courtesy of Greg Zaharchuk, M.D., Stanford University).

As noted, perfusion-MR provides direct measurement of regional brain perfusion, while transcranial Doppler (TCD) can only indirectly assess it from blood velocity measurements. While TCD studies have implicated cerebral vasoconstriction as a possible precipitating factor in orthostatic intolerance, this is an indirect observation. As Doppler only assesses the large vessels at the base of the brain, waveform increased pulsatility indices measured at the level of the MCA is used as a surrogate marker of elevated vascular resistance in smaller, downstream vessels. The ideal technique to either confirm or refute this finding is MRI, which can directly measure perfusion changes at the regional level for any specific region of brain parenchyma.

This assessment is independent of any priori assumptions concerning alterations in vascular diameter, which are likely to be substantial when considering the extensive network of small vessels which supply neuronal tissue (Giller *et al.*, 1993). MR perfusion techniques can provide measurements of not only CBF, but with DSC-MRI, also provide additional parametric maps as well, allowing a more complete characterization of cerebral autoregulation. However, it is important to note that perfusion MR lacks the real-time continuous monitoring capability offered by TCD. Additionally, unlike TCD, perfusion MR imaging cannot presently be performed in orbit. Therefore, perfusion MR will provide vital, but complementary, information to prior TCD studies.

8. Carbon dioxide Exposure During Spaceflight and Cerebral Perfusion

Symptoms of chronic hypercapnia include headache, papilledema, mental dullness, drowsiness, confusion, stupor, and coma (Ropper *et al.*, 2014). Carbon dioxide is a major by-product of human metabolism and is exhaled by a typical resting adult at a rate of approximately 200 mL per min (Guyton, 1986). Carbon dioxide is also produced aboard the ISS by other sources, for example, specific payloads, accidental combustion of materials, and from the use of CO_2 fire extinguishers (James, 2008). Reduced convection in space can create local alterations in CO_2 with pockets of elevated CO_2 levels particularly in confined spaces with little air flow such as in sleeping quarters (James, 2007). ISS life support systems function to keep CO_2 at acceptable levels. However, because of tradeoffs between power and expendable supplies, it is impossible to maintain ambient CO_2 aboard spacecraft at atmospheric levels (Frey *et al.*, 1998). Therefore, a set of spacecraft maximal allowable concentrations (SMACs) for CO_2 have been set by the National Research Council SMACs Subcommittee along with NASA environmental control engineers and the ISS Program Office (James, 2008). According to the current guidelines, the NASA exposure standards for CO_2 concentration are: 15 mmHg for 1 h, 10 mmHg for 24 h, 5 mmHg for 7–180 days, and 4 mmHg for 1000 days (James, 2008).

Of note, the data that were used to inform NASA concerning safe CO_2 levels for spacecraft personnel (and also the Navy concerning submarine personnel) were often based on studies that included a limited number of subjects without identifying an effect response level (James, 2008, National Research Council, 2007). Therefore, a mathematical correction was often applied to compensate for the "small n factor". Furthermore, the studies mostly predate the availability of TCD and advanced imaging techniques such as MRI which limits conclusions that can be drawn from them in regards to intracranial physiology in conditions of chronic hypercapnia.

For example, Glatte $et\ al.$ (1967) exposed seven subjects to a 21 mmHg CO_2 concentration for 5 days. Physiological measurements, psychomotor performance (such as problem-solving, memory, and tracking tasks), and documentation of subjective complaints were evaluated. No significant changes were seen in psychomotor performance during hypercapnia compared with a normocapnic baseline period. The subjects tolerated hypercapnia well with only complaints of mild to moderate headaches during the first 2 days of CO_2 exposure in four of the seven subjects. The headaches resolved either spontaneously or with analgesic medication and did not recur on days 3–5. Several similar studies have been reported exposing subjects to various chronic CO_2 levels up to approximately 30 mmHg for short periods of time, again with only reports of mild headaches that resolved during the first few days of exposure (Guillerm and Radziszewski, 1979; Radziszewski $et\ al.$, 1988 Sinclair $et\ al.$, 1969, Sinclair $et\ al.$, 1971).

A more recent study, jointly sponsored by NASA, the European Space Agency, and the Deutsche Agentur fur Raumfahrtangelegenheiten (German Space Agency), included four male participants in a dive chamber for two separate month-long campaigns (Frey $et\ al.$, 1998). During the first campaign, subjects were exposed to 5.3 mmHg CO_2 for 23 days, and during the second campaign, the same four subjects were exposed to 9.1 mmHg CO_2 also for 23 days. As in the studies of the effect of spaceflight on CBF described above, the effect of the chronic hypercapnia on CBF was investigated using TCD to measure CBFV within the MCA as a surrogate for CBF (Sliwka $et\ al.$, 1998). In both campaigns, CBFV was found to be significantly elevated by 35% above baseline levels during the first 1–3 days of hypercapnia. However, over the course of the study, CBFV returned to baseline preexposure levels. Interestingly, no significant difference was found in CBFV responses to the 5.3 and 9.1 mmHg CO_2 exposure levels. The authors also performed provocative tests of cerebrovascular reactivity, measuring CBFV in response to rebreathing a CO_2-enriched gas mixture (5% CO_2, 95% Oxygen) in both the supine position and following 19 min of 10° head-down tilt (to simulate microgravity). Cerebrovascular reactivity to acute elevations in CO_2 during rebreathing showed prompted increases in CBFV which were greater in magnitude during the early days of chronic hypercapnia but readjusted to baseline over the course of the study. CBFV in response to CO_2 rebreathing did not significantly change with positional alterations, suggesting maintenance of CO_2 cerebrovascular reactivity during head–down tilt. The authors concluded that cerebrovascular autoregulation is preserved during chronic exposure to 5.3 and 9.1 mmHg CO_2. Interestingly, while elevations in CBFV, and presumably CBF, were similar at the different CO_2 concentrations, subjective complaints of headaches were only made during the early days of exposure to 9.1 mmHg CO_2.

Although the average 7-day CO_2 levels on the ISS has been 3.39 mmHg (data from Expeditions 2–31), anecdotal reports of headaches by ISS crew members prompted NASA to investigate the relationship between headaches and station CO_2 levels (Law *et al.*, 2014). Between March 2001 and May 2012, there were 46 reported headaches among 49 crew members. ISS CO_2 levels were found to be significantly associated with reports of headaches. For each 1 mmHg increase in CO_2, the odds of a crew member reporting a headache doubled. The authors stated that the average CO_2 levels would have to be maintained below 2.5 mmHg to keep the risk of headache below 1%.

The levels of CO_2 on the ISS are below levels the US Environmental Protection Agency has reported to be tolerable by normal subjects on Earth for extended periods of time (U.S. Environmental Protection Agency, 2000) and are in line with the studies of hypercapnia discussed above. For example, the average 7-day CO_2 level on the ISS of 3.39 mmHg is well below the 5.3 mmHg CO_2 which was asymptomatic in the study of Sliwka *et al.* (1998) and the peak CO_2 level of 8.32 mmHg on the ISS (Law *et al.*, 2014) is below the symptomatic CO_2 level of 9.1 mmHg (Sliwka *et al.*'s study).

This discrepancy between ground and flight data suggests that unique factors of the spaceflight environment may exacerbate the sequelae of chronic hypercapnia among ISS crew members. For example, numerous physiological changes occur during spaceflight including loss of red cell mass, loss of plasma volume, and decreased total body water (James, 2007). In addition, as discussed above, cephalad fluid shifts in microgravity may contribute to the development of venous hypertension and ultimately increased ICP, particularly in astronauts susceptible to the development of VIIP syndrome. Exposure to mild hypercapnia on the ISS may further increase ICP by concomitantly increasing CBF. Interestingly, CO_2 responsiveness differed between astronauts postflight compared to a ground–based study of hypercapnia despite the similarities in CO_2 levels on the ISS and those used in the ground-based study of Sliwka *et al.* (1998). Astronauts postflight demonstrated diminished CO_2 cerebral vascular reactivity compared with preflight values, whereas CO_2 cerebral vascular reactivity was maintained in a ground-based study of chronic hypercapnia (Sliwka *et al.*, 1998; Zuj *et al.*, 2012). Altered responsiveness to certain central nervous system–active compounds on orbit may also play a role. For example, one study of promethazine administration reported achieving only a 5% sedation rate on orbit, whereas the sedation rate was 60%–73% in ground-based studies (Bagian and Ward, 1994). Finally, spatial differences in CO_2 concentration within the various components of the ISS may lead to intermittent exposure to higher CO_2 levels than those suggested by average values (James, 2007).

8.1. *Imaging of CO_2 cerebral vascular reactivity*

According to a model proposed by Sobczyk *et al.* (2014), it is regional cerebral vascular reactivity (CVR) that determines the distribution of cerebral blood flow. In patients, altered CVR can result in regions throughout the brain where the cerebral blood flow is paradoxically reduced in response to an acute CO_2 vasodilatory stimulus. This paradoxical decrease in blood flow is termed vascular steal. These areas where vascular steal occurs have apparently normal neurological function, however, closer examination reveals structural changes such as cortical thinning (Fierstra *et al.*, 2010) and associated reductions in fine cognitive function (Balucani *et al.*, 2012). Global measurements used in the studies described above (Sliwka *et al.*, 1998; Zuj *et al.*, 2012) would not detect this regional variability in CVR response or the presence of vascular steal.

The dynamic response of the cerebral vasculature is commonly measured by exposing subjects to a hemodynamically significant stimulus such as an acute elevation in CO_2 levels. Several methods can be used to achieve elevated CO_2 levels. The most common technique that has been used clinically is the administration of a single dose of Diamox, a carbonic anhydrase inhibitor that results in an increase in carbonic acid, H_2CO_3, and subsequent vasodilation of the cerebral vessels (Fig. 16B). Another method that is easy to implement is simply having the subject alternate between periods of normal breathing and holding their breath (Fig. 17). More controlled methods also exist using automated technology to administer CO_2 in a way that is customized to each subject. This ensures equivalent changes in Pa_{CO_2} are achieved regardless of body size or pattern of breathing — in other words, a standardized vasoactive stimulus (Spano *et al.*, 2013; Han *et al.*, 2011;

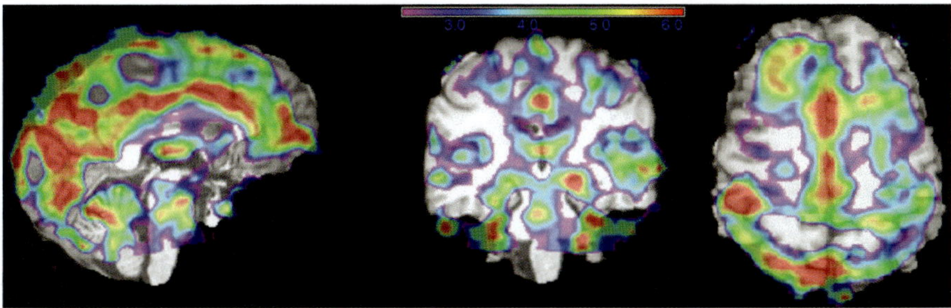

Figure 17. Cerebral vascular reactivity (CVR) imaging using the breath-hold technique. During imaging acquisition using a blood oxygen level dependent (BOLD) sequence, the subject alternates between periods of normal breathing and holding their breath. A subtraction image is then calculated. Regions of the brain which demonstrate a statistically significant increase in signal during breath-hold is color-coded and overlaid upon the anatomical images.

Mandell *et al.*, 2008; Vesely *et al.*, 2001). Vascular responses can then be examined with reference to a standard database of normal responses (Sobczyk *et al.*, 2015; Poublanc *et al.*, 2015). Imaging typically involves the acquisition of a fast MR sequence such as echoplanar imaging based on blood oxygen level dependent (BOLD) contrast. Axial images are acquired allowing determination of regional CVR throughout the brain.

9. Conclusion

Over the past half century of manned spaceflight, humans have adapted remarkably well to the challenges of the spaceflight environment, living and working in space for extended periods of time. Almost certainly, this has been possible due to significant, beneficial adaptive responses of the brain and cerebrovasculature to the microgravity environment. However, there are hints that brain function can be adversely affected by spaceflight, with overt symptoms becoming more evident as the duration of space missions increase. Some astronauts, during the first few days on orbit, describe difficulties initially adapting to the spaceflight with reports of sleep disturbance, decreased ability to perform high precision tasks, and impairments in mental performance, particularly during multitasking, known as space adaptation syndrome (Clement and Reschke, 2008). Astronauts commonly demonstrate symptoms of orthostatic hypotension upon return to Earth indicating impairment of the cerebrovascular autoregulatory response. More recently, astronauts have experienced headaches and visual problems onboard the ISS, some with documented structural changes of the eyes and increased intracranial pressure upon return to Earth referred to as VIIP syndrome. This chapter summarizes the research to date of the physiological mechanisms involved in intracranial adaptation to spaceflight emphasizing the use of advanced imaging techniques to address potential etiologies of VIIP syndrome.

The control of CBF is complex and involves several homeostatic mechanisms to ensure the metabolic needs of the brain for glucose and oxygen are continually met including cerebrovascular autoregulation, functional hyperemia, Pa_{CO_2} levels, Pa_{O_2} levels, and neurovascular innervation. These mechanisms act in concert to maintain a constant blood supply to the brain in spite of fluctuating systemic factors. For example, moving from the upright to supine position acutely normalizes the hydrostatic pressure gradient. Homeostatic mechanisms respond by increasing CBF and venous outflow. There is redirection of venous outflow from the vertebral venous plexuses to the less resistant internal jugular veins. With a shift of blood and CSF into the cranium, the brain becomes less compliant and the ICP is increased within physiological limits (as experienced on Earth on a nightly basis).

However, obstruction to intracranial venous outflow can result in to a pathological increase in ICP. In patients with IIH, areas of anatomical narrowing of the intracranial venous outflow tracts can result in intracranial venous hypertension and increased ICP. Dilating and placing stents within the venous sinuses across these areas of narrowing has been shown to be an effective treatment for IIH. Similarly, if increased ICP is a defining feature of VIIP syndrome in astronauts, it can be hypothesized that venous hypertension may contribute to the development of increased ICP. Factors that may lead to intracranial venous hypertension during spaceflight include the loss of hydrostatic pressure gradients with resultant cephalad fluid shifts, variant venous anatomy with varying degrees of susceptibility to VIIP syndrome among the astronaut population, and potentially, gravity-depended structural changes within the cranial vault.

Although an untested hypothesis, the removal of gravitational gradients during spaceflight could result in unloading of the cranial contents. During long-term head-down tilt bed rest, which is considered an analog for spaceflight, the brain's center of mass has been shown to shift upward and rotate posteriorly relative to the skull. This results in compression of brain tissue at the top of the brain and contraction of the adjacent extra-axial CSF spaces. With shift of the brain upward, there is the potential for anatomical distortion and partial effacement of the superior sagittal sinus, a major intracranial venous outflow pathway which runs along the top of the brain beneath the skull. Investigations for any potential alteration in venous anatomy following spaceflight are currently underway.

A change in the size of the ventricular system is also seen during long-term bed rest (comparable to annual ventricular volume changes seen in patients with Alzheimer's disease), which correlates with the degree of posterior brain rotation. The change in ventricular volume suggests an alteration in CSF homeostasis during long-term bed rest. The upward shift of the brain, with resultant contraction of the adjacent extra-axial CSF spaces, may alter local CSF flow dynamics and possibly disrupt the function of arachnoid granulations located at the vertex impairing resorption of CSF. Unlike the traditional concept of bulk, unidirectional CSF flow, advanced imaging methods have depicted CSF flow patterns that are complex and can be gravity dependent. CSF homeostasis is critical for the maintenance of normal ICP.

At the same time, astronauts onboard the ISS are exposed to mild levels of hypercapnia. During acute exposure to hypercapnic conditions, as Pa_{CO_2} rises, CBF dramatically increases and becomes more dependent on CPP. Much less is known about the response of hemodynamic mechanisms to chronic hypercapnia, although one study found that CBFV was significantly elevated by 35% above preexposure levels during the first one to three days of hypercapnia, but, over the course of the study, CBFV returned to baseline preexposure levels. While ground-based studies suggest an adaptive response to mildly elevated levels of CO_2 such as those that astronauts experience onboard the ISS, symptoms suggestive of chronic hypercapnia (headache, papilledema, mental dullness, drowsiness, and confusion) have been reported by astronauts. The levels of CO_2 on the ISS are below levels the US Environmental Protection Agency has reported to be tolerable by normal subjects on Earth for extended periods of time (US Environmental Protection Agency, 2000) and are in line with previous human studies of chronic hypercapnia. Therefore, it is unclear why astronauts would exhibit symptoms of mild hypercapnia. This discrepancy between ground and flight data suggests that unique factors of the spaceflight environment, or a combination of factors, may exacerbate the sequelae of chronic hypercapnia among ISS crew members. For example, cephalad fluid shifts in microgravity may play a role in the development of increased ICP seen in some astronauts who present with VIIP syndrome. Exposure to mild hypercapnia on the ISS may then further exacerbate symptoms of elevated ICP by concomitantly increasing CBF.

However, despite the attributes of the space environment expected to impact brain and cerebrovasculature function (cephalad fluid shifts, chronic hypercapnia) and clinical evidence for neurological compromise (VIIP syndrome), investigations of CBF in astronauts have consistently shown only modest changes in CBFV following spaceflight. Furthermore, results have been mixed with various investigators reporting increased CBFV, no change in CBFV, or decreased CBFV compared with preflight values. It is difficult to interpret the results of these studies given the small number of subjects, various protocols used, limited inflight data, and the various missions involved (Mir, Space Shuttle, and ISS) suggesting the need for systematic investigations by NASA and other space agencies. In addition, all studies to date have used ultrasound-based TCD technology to assess cerebral perfusion changes. However, as detailed above, it is the response of the smaller vessels, which cannot be interrogated by TCD technology that must be investigated in order to fully characterize the cerebral autoregulatory response that occurs in the spaceflight environment. In contrast, perfusion MR lacks the real-time continuous monitoring capability offered by TCD. Also, unlike TCD, perfusion MR imaging cannot be performed in orbit. Therefore, perfusion MR will provide vital, but complementary, information to prior and ongoing TCD studies.

The time course and ultimate consequences of any adaptive response of the brain and the cerebrovasculature during spaceflight are unknown; however, such data could provide further insight into the physiology of the VIIP syndrome. With astronauts demonstrating sequelae of altered intracranial pressure even months following return from spaceflight, it is now imperative to fully characterize intracranial adaptation to microgravity and its consequences upon return to Earth. This knowledge gap has profound implications for astronaut health, influencing performance in essentially every functional domain including cognition, vision, vestibular function, sensorimotor capabilities, and behavioral health.

Acknowledgment

The authors wish to thank Ms. Judy Yost for editorial assistance.

References

Aaslid, R, TM Markwalder and H Nornes (1982). Noninvasive transcranial Doppler ultrasound recording of flow velocity in basal cerebral arteries. *Journal of Neurosurgery*, 57, 769–774.

Alker, GJ, Jr and EV Leslie (1969). Isotope cisternography and ventriculography. *Acta Radiologica Diagnosis (Stockh)*, 9, 589–596.

Alperin, N, SG Hushek, SH Lee, A Sivaramakrishnan and T Lichtor (2005a). MRI study of cerebral blood flow and CSF flow dynamics in an upright posture: the effect of posture on the intracranial compliance and pressure. *Acta Neurochirurgica Supplement*, 95, 177–181.

Alperin, N, SH Lee, A Sivaramakrishnan and SG Hushek (2005b). Quantifying the effect of posture on intracranial physiology in humans by MRI flow studies. *Journal of Magnetic Resonance Imaging*, 22, 591–596.

Alperin, N, M Mazda, T Lichtor and SH Lee (2006). From cerebrospinal fluid pulsation to noninvasive intracranial compliance and pressure measured by MRI flow studies. *Current Medical Imaging Reviews*, 2, 117–129.

Alperin, N, EM Vikingstad, B Gomez-Anson and DN Levin (1996). Hemodynamically independent analysis of cerebrospinal fluid and brain motion observed with dynamic phase contrast MRI. *Magnetic Resonance Medicine*, 35, 741–754.

Arbeille, P, F Achaibou, G Fomina, JM Pottier and M Porcher (1996). Regional blood flow in microgravity: adaptation and deconditioning. *Medicine and Science in Sports and Exercise*, 28, S70–79.

Arbeille, P, G Fomina, J Roumy, I Alferova, N Tobal and S Herault (2001). Adaptation of the left heart, cerebral and femoral arteries, and jugular and femoral veins during short- and long-term head-down tilt and spaceflights. *European Journal of Applied Physiology*, 86, 157–168.

Attwell, D, AM Buchan, S Charpak, M Lauritzen, BA Macvicar and EA Newman (2010). Glial and neuronal control of brain blood flow. *Nature*, 468, 232–243.

Bagian, JP and DF Ward (1994). A retrospective study of promethazine and its failure to produce the expected incidence of sedation during space flight. *Journal of Clinical Pharmacology*, 34, 649–651.

Ball, AK and CE Clarke (2006). Idiopathic intracranial hypertension. *Lancet Neurology*, 5, 433–442.

Balucani, C, G Viticchi, L Falsetti and M Silvestrini (2012). Cerebral hemodynamics and cognitive performance in bilateral asymptomatic carotid stenosis. *Neurology*, 79, 1788–1795.

Blaber, AP, N Goswami, RL Bondar and MS Kassam (2011). Impairment of cerebral blood flow regulation in astronauts with orthostatic intolerance after flight. *Stroke*, 42, 1844–1850.

Bono, F, MR Lupo, A Lavano, L Mangone, F Fera, K Pardatscher and A Quattrone (2003). Cerebral MR venography of transverse sinuses in subjects with normal CSF pressure. *Neurology*, 61, 1267–1270.

Bradley, WG, Jr (2015). CSF flow in the brain in the context of normal pressure hydrocephalus. *AJNR American Journal of Neuroradiology*, 36, 831–838.

Brian, JE, Jr (1998). Carbon dioxide and the cerebral circulation. *Anesthesiology*, 88, 1365–1386.

Bungo, MW (1989). The cardiopulmonary system. In *Space Physiology and Medicine*, Nicogossian, AE, EL Huntoon and SL Pool (eds.), 2nd Ed. Philadelphia: Lea and Febiger.

Calamante, F (2010). Perfusion MRI using dynamic-susceptibility contrast MRI: Quantification issues in patient studies. *Topics in Magnetic Resonance Imaging*, 21, 75–85.

Cure, JK, P Van Tassel and MT Smith (1994). Normal and variant anatomy of the dural venous sinuses. *Seminars in Ultrasound CT, and MR*, 15, 499–519.

Clement, G and MF Rescheke (2008). *Neuroscience in Space*. New York, New York, Springer.

Czosnyka, M, PJ Hutchinson, M Balestreri, M Hiler, P Smielewski and JD Pickard (2006). Monitoring and interpretation of intracranial pressure after head injury. *Acta Neurochirurgica Supplement*, 96, 114–118.

Degnan, AJ and LM Levy (2011). Pseudotumor cerebri: Brief review of clinical syndrome and imaging findings. *AJNR American Journal of Neuroradiology*, 32, 1986–1993.

Dichiro, G (1964). Movement of the cerebrospinal fluid in human beings. *Nature*, 204, 290–291.

Faraci, FM and DD Heistad (1990). Regulation of large cerebral arteries and cerebral microvascular pressure. *Circulation Research*, 66, 8–17.

Farb, RI, I Vanek, JN Scott, DJ Mikulis, RA Willinsky, G Tomlinson and KG Terbrugge (2003). Idiopathic intracranial hypertension: the prevalence and morphology of sino-venous stenosis. *Neurology*, 60, 1418–1424.

Fieremans, E, JH Jensen and JA Helpern (2011). White matter characterization with diffusional kurtosis imaging. *Neuroimage*, 58, 177–188.

Fierstra, J, J Poublanc, JS Han, F Silver, M Tymianski, AP Crawley, JA Fisher and DJ Mikulis (2010). Steal physiology is spatially associated with cortical thinning. *Journal of Neurology Neurosurgery, and Psychiatry*, 81, 290–293.

Franco Folino, A (2007). Cerebral autoregulation and syncope. *Progress in Cardiovascular Diseases*, 50, 49–80.

Frey, MA, FM Sulzman, H Oser and G Ruyters (1998). The effects of moderately elevated ambient carbon dioxide levels on human physiology and performance: A joint NASA-ESA-DARA study — Overview. *Aviation, Space, and Environmental Medicine*, 69, 282–284.

Fritsch-Yelle, JM, PA Whitson, RL Bondar and TE Brown (1996). Subnormal norepinephrine release relates to presyncope in astronauts after spaceflight. *Journal of Applied Physiology*, 81, 2134–2141.

Gean, A (1994). *Imaging of Head Trauma*. New York: Raven Press, Ltd.

Giller, CA, G Bowman, H Dyer, L Mootz and W Krippner (1993). Cerebral arterial diameters during changes in blood pressure and carbon dioxide during craniotomy. *Neurosurgery*, 32, 737–741, discussion 741–742.

Glatte, HA, Jr, GJ Motsay and BE Welch (1967). Carbon dioxide tolerance studies. SAM-TR-67-77. *Technical Report SAM-TR*, 1–22.

Guillerm, R and E Radziszewski (1979). Effects on man of 30-day exposure to a $PICO_2$ of 14 torr (2%): Application to exposure limits. *Undersea Biomedical Research*, 6 (Suppl), S91–114.

Gulbenkian, S, R Uddman and L Edvinsson (2001). Neuronal messengers in the human cerebral circulation. *Peptides*, 22, 995–1007.

Guyton, AC (1986). Physical principles of gaseous exchange; diffusion of oxygen and carbon dioxide through the respiratory membrane. *Textbook of Medical Phsiology*, 7th Ed. Philadelphia: W. B. Saunders Company.

Gwinnutt, C and B Saha (2005). Cerebral blood flow and intracranial pressure. *Anaesthesia and Intensive Care Medicine*, 6, 153–156.

Hagmann, P, L Jonasson, P Maeder, JP Thiran, VJ Wedeen and R Meuli (2006). Understanding diffusion MR imaging techniques: from scalar diffusion-weighted imaging to diffusion tensor imaging and beyond. *Radiographics*, 26 (Suppl 1), S205–223.

Hamel, E (2006). Perivascular nerves and the regulation of cerebrovascular tone. *Journal of Applied Physiology*, 100, 1059–1064.

Han, JS, DJ Mikulis, A Mardimae, A Kassner, J Poublanc, AP Crawley, GA Deveber, JA Fisher and WJ Logan (2011). Measurement of cerebrovascular reactivity in pediatric patients with cerebral vasculopathy using blood oxygen level-dependent MRI. *Stroke*, 42, 1261–1269.

Hargens, AR, R Bhattacharya and SM Schneider (2013). Space physiology VI: Exercise, artificial gravity, and countermeasure development for prolonged space flight. *European Journal of Applied Physiology*, 113, 2183–2192.

Harrigan, MR and JP Deveikis (2009). *Handbook of Cerebrovascular Disease and Neurointerventional Technique*. New York: Humana Press.

Hess, CP and P Mukherjee (2007). Visualizing white matter pathways in the living human brain: Diffusion tensor imaging and beyond. *Neuroimaging Clinics of North America*, 17, 407–426, vii.

Higgins, JN, BK Owler, C Cousins and JD Pickard (2002). Venous sinus stenting for refractory benign intracranial hypertension. *Lancet*, 359, 228–230.

Iadecola, C (2004). Neurovascular regulation in the normal brain and in Alzheimer's disease. *Nature Reviews Neuroscience*, 5, 347–360.

Iadecola, C and M Nedergaard (2007). Glial regulation of the cerebral microvasculature. *Nature Neuroscience*, 10, 1369–1376.

Ito, H, I Kanno, M Ibaraki, J Hatazawa and S Miura (2003). Changes in human cerebral blood flow and cerebral blood volume during hypercapnia and hypocapnia measured by positron emission tomography. *Journal of Cerebral Blood Flow and Metabolism*, 23, 665–670.

Iwasaki, K, BD Levine, R Zhang, JH Zuckerman, JA Pawelczyk, A Diedrich, AC Ertl, JF Cox, WH Cooke, CA Giller, CA Ray, LD Lane, JC Buckey, Jr, FJ Baisch, DL Eckberg, D Robertson, I Biaggioni and CG Blomqvist (2007). Human cerebral autoregulation before, during and after spaceflight. *Journal of Physiology*, 579, 799–810.

James, JT (2007). The headache of carbon dioxide exposures. *37th International Conference on Environmental Systems*, July 9–12 Chicago, IL: SAE International.

James, JT (2008). Carbon dioxide. *In Spacecraft Maximum Allowable Concentrations for Selected Airborne Contaminants, National Research Council* (ed.), Vol. 5, Washington, DC: The National Academies Press.

Jensen, JH and JA Helpern (2010). Progress in diffusion-weighted imaging: Concepts, techniques and applications to the central nervous system. *NMR in Biomedicine*, 23, 659–660.

Kety, SS and CF Schmidt (1946). The effects of active and passive hyperventilation on cerebral blood flow, cerebral oxygen consumption, cardiac output, and blood pressure of normal young men. *Journal of Clinical Investigation*, 25, 107–119.

Klein, B, W Kuschinsky, H Schrock and F Vetterlein (1986). Interdependency of local capillary density, blood flow, and metabolism in rat brains. *American Journal of Physiology*, 251, H1333–1340.

Law, J, M Van Baalen, M Foy, SS Mason, C Mendez, ML Wear, VE Meyers and D Alexander (2014). Relationship between carbon dioxide levels and reported headaches on the international space station. *Journal of Occupational and Environmental and Medicine*, 56, 477–483.

Levine, BD, CA Giller, LD Lane, JC Buckey and CG Blomqvist (1994). Cerebral versus systemic hemodynamics during graded orthostatic stress in humans. *Circulation*, 90, 298–306.

Lin, LJ, F Gao, YG Bai, JX Bao, XF Huang, J Ma and LF Zhang (2009). Contrasting effects of simulated microgravity with and without daily — Gx gravitation on structure and function of cerebral and mesenteric small arteries in rats. *Journal of Applied Physiology*, 107, 1710–1721.

Mader, TH, CR Gibson, AF Pass, LA Kramer, AG Lee, J Fogarty, WJ Tarver, JP Dervay, DR Hamilton, A Sargsyan, JL Phillips, D Tran, W Lipsky, J Choi, C Stern, R Kuyumjian and JD Polk (2011). Optic disc edema, globe flattening, choroidal folds, and hyperopic shifts observed in astronauts after long-duration space flight. *Ophthalmology*, 118, 2058–2069.

Mandell, DM, JS Han, J Poublanc, AP Crawley, JA Stainsby, JA Fisher and DJ Mikulis (2008). Mapping cerebrovascular reactivity using blood oxygen level-dependent MRI in patients with arterial steno-occlusive disease: Comparison with arterial spin labeling MRI. *Stroke*, 39, 2021–2028.

Marmarou, A (1996). Pathophysiology of intracranial pressure. In *Neurotrauma*, RJ Narayan, JE Wilberger and JT Povlishock (eds.), New York: McGraw-Hill.

Marmarou, A, K Shulman and J Lamorgese (1975). Compartmental analysis of compliance and outflow resistance of the cerebrospinal fluid system. *Journal of Neurosurgery*, 43, 523–534.

Meng, L and AW Gelb (2015). Regulation of cerebral autoregulation by carbon dioxide. *Anesthesiology*, 122, 196–205.

National Research Council (2007). *Emergency and Continuous Exposure Guidance Levels for Selected Submarine Contaminants*, Vol.1, Washington, DC: National Academies Press.

National Research Council (2008). *Managing Space Radiation Risk in the New Era of Space Exploration*, Washington, DC: The National Academies Press.

Ng, I, J Lim and HB Wong (2004). Effects of head posture on cerebral hemodynamics: its influences on intracranial pressure, cerebral perfusion pressure, and cerebral oxygenation. *Neurosurgery*, 54, 593–597, discussion 598.

Nicogossian, AE and LF Dietlein (1989). Microgravity: simulations and analogs. In *Space Physiology and Medicine*, Nicogossian, AE, EL Huntoon and SL Pool (eds.), 2nd Ed. Philadelphia: Lea and Febiger.

Noth, U, F Kotajima, R Deichmann, R Turner and DR Corfield (2008). Mapping of the cerebral vascular response to hypoxia and hypercapnia using quantitative perfusion MRI at 3 T. *NMR in Biomedicine*, 21, 464–472.

Patel, N (2009). Venous anatomy and imaging of the first centimeter. *Seminars in Ultrasound CT and MR*, 30, 513–524.

Paulson, OB, S Strandgaard and L Edvinsson (1990). Cerebral autoregulation. *Cerebrovascular Brain Metabolism Reviews*, 2, 161–192.

Pavy-Le Traon, A, M Heer, MV Narici, J Rittweger and J Vernikos (2007). From space to Earth: Advances in human physiology from 20 years of bed rest studies (1986–2006). *European Journal of Applied Physiology*, 101, 143–194.

Petty, GW, DO Wiebers and I Meissner (1990). Transcranial Doppler ultrasonography: Clinical applications in cerebrovascular disease. *Mayo Clinic Proceeding*, 65, 1350–1364.

Ponto, JA (2008). Special safety considerations in preparation of technetium Tc-99m DTPA for cerebrospinal fluid-related imaging procedures. *Journal of American Pharmacists Association (2003)*, 48, 413–416.

Porcelli, S, M Marzorati, F Lanfranconi, P Vago, R Pisot and B Grassi (2010). Role of skeletal muscles impairment and brain oxygenation in limiting oxidative metabolism during exercise after bed rest. *Journal of Applied Physiology*, 109, 101–111.

Poublanc, J, AP Crawley, O Sobczyk, G Montandon, K Sam, DM Mandell, P Dufort, L Venkatraghavan, J Duffin, DJ Mikulis and JA Fisher (2015). Measuring cerebrovascular reactivity: the dynamic response to a step hypercapnic stimulus. *Journal of Cerebral Blood Flow and Metabolism*, 35(11),1746–1756.

Prisby, RD, MK Wilkerson, EM Sokoya, RM Bryan, Jr, E Wilson and MD Delp (2006). Endothelium-dependent vasodilation of cerebral arteries is altered with simulated microgravity through nitric oxide synthase and EDHF mechanisms. *Journal of Applied Physiology*, 101, 348–353.

Radziszewski, E, L Giacomoni and R Guillerm (1988). Physiological effects in man as a result of long duration confinement in an atmosphere enriched with carbon dioxide. In *Proceedings of the Colloquium on Space and Sea*, TD Guyenne (ed.), Marseille, France: European Space Agency November 24–27, 1987 (as cited in James, 2008).

Roberts, DR, R Arjal, R Kellogg, T Mclaren, H Collins, S Stalcup and R Turner (2015a). The correlation of MR venograms, catheter venograms, and catheter based venous pressure measurements. *American Society of North American 53rd Annual Meeting & Symposium*, 25–30 April, Oral Presentation, Chicago, IL.

Roberts, DR, X Zhu, A Tabesh, EW Duffy, DA Ramsey and TR Brown (2015b). Structural brain changes following long-term 6 degrees head-down tilt bed rest as an analog for spaceflight. *AJNR American Journal of Neuroradiology*, 36(11): 2048–2054..

Ropper, AH, MA Samuels and JP Klein (2014). The acquired metabolic disorders of the nervous system. In *Adam and Victor's Principles of Neurology*, 10th Ed. AM Sydor and KJ Davis (Eds). China: McGraw-Hill Education.

San Millan Ruiz, D, P Gailloud, DA Rufenacht, J Delavelle, F Henry and JH Fasel (2002). The craniocervical venous system in relation to cerebral venous drainage. *AJNR American Journal of Neuroradiology*, 23, 1500–1508.

Serrador, JM, PA Picot, BK Rutt, JK Shoemaker and RL Bondar (2000). MRI measures of middle cerebral artery diameter in conscious humans during simulated orthostasis. *Stroke*, 31, 1672–1678.

Sinclair, RD, JM Clark and BE Welch (1969). Carbon dioxide tolerance levels for space cabins. *Proc. of the 5th Annual Conference on Atmospheric Contamination in Confined Spaces*, September 16–18. Dayton, OH: Wright-Patterson Air Force Base.

Sinclair, RD, JM Clark and BE Welch (1971). Comparison of physiological responses of normal man to exercise in air and in acute and chronic hypercapnia. In *Underwater Physiology*, CJ Lambertsen (ed.), New York: Academic Press.

Sliwka, U, JA Krasney, SG Simon, P Schmidt and J Noth (1998). Effects of sustained low-level elevations of carbon dioxide on cerebral blood flow and autoregulation of the intracerebral arteries in humans. *Aviation, Space, and Environmental Medicine*, 69, 299–306.

Sobczyk, O, A Battisti-Charbonney, J Fierstra, DM Mandell, J Poublanc, AP Crawley, DJ Mikulis, J Duffin and JA Fisher (2014). A conceptual model for CO-induced redistribution of cerebral blood flow with experimental confirmation using BOLD MRI. *Neuroimage*, 92, 56–68.

Sobczyk, O, A Battisti-Charbonney, Poublanc, J, AP Crawley, K Sam, J Fierstra, DM Mandell, DJ Mikulis, J Duffin and JA Fisher (2015). Assessing cerebrovascular reactivity abnormality by comparison to a reference atlas. *Journal of Cerebral Blood Flow and Metabolism*, 35, 213–220.

Spano, VR, DM Mandell, J Poublanc, K Sam, A Battisti-Charbonney, O Pucci, JS Han, AP Crawley, JA Fisher and DJ Mikulis (2013). CO_2 blood oxygen level-dependent MR mapping of cerebrovascular reserve in a clinical population: safety, tolerability, and technical feasibility. *Radiology*, 266, 592–598.

Tabesh, A, JH Jensen, BA Ardekani and JA Helpern (2011). Estimation of tensors and tensor-derived measures in diffusional kurtosis imaging. *Magnetic Resonance in Medicine*, 65, 823–836.

Tain, RW, AM Bagci, BL Lam, EM Sklar, B Ertl-Wagner and N Alperin (2011). Determination of cranio-spinal canal compliance distribution by MRI: Methodology and early application in idiopathic intracranial hypertension. *Journal of Magnetic Resonance Imaging*, 34, 1397–1404.

Taylor, CR, M Hanna, BJ Behnke, JN Stabley, DJ Mccullough, RT Davis, 3rd, P Ghosh, A Papadopoulos, JM Muller-Delp and MD Delp (2013). Spaceflight-induced alterations in cerebral artery vasoconstrictor, mechanical, and structural properties: Implications for elevated cerebral perfusion and intracranial pressure. *FASEB Journal*, 27, 2282–2292.

Tobal, N, J Roumy, S Herault, G Fomina and P Arbeille (2001). Doppler measurement of cerebral and lower limb flow during a lower body negative pressure test for predicting orthostatic intolerance. *Journal of Ultrasound Medicine*, 20, 1207–1217.

Tomasian, A, N Salamon, MS Krishnam, JP Finn and JP Villablanca (2009). 3D high-spatial-resolution cerebral MR venography at 3T: a contrast-dose-reduction study. *AJNR American Journal of Neuroradiology*, 30, 349–355.

U.S. Environmental Protection Agency (2000). *Carbon Dioxide as a Fire Suppressant: Examining the Risks*. Washington, DC.

Valdueza, JM, T Von Munster, O Hoffman, S Schreiber and KM Einhaupl (2000). Postural dependency of the cerebral venous outflow. *Lancet*, 355, 200–201.

Vavilala, MS, LA Lee and AM Lam (2002). Cerebral blood flow and vascular physiology. *Anesthesiology Clinics of North America*, 20, 247–264.

Vesely, A, H Sasano, G Volgyesi, R Somogyi, J Tesler, L Fedorko, J Grynspan, A Crawley, JA Fisher and D Mikulis. (2001). MRI mapping of cerebrovascular reactivity using square wave changes in end-tidal PCO_2. *Magnetic Resonance in Medicine*, 45, 1011–1013.

Warner, DS, DM Turner and NF Kassell (1987). Time-dependent effects of prolonged hypercapnia on cerebrovascular parameters in dogs: acid-base chemistry. *Stroke*, 18, 142–149.

Weed, LH (1914a). Studies on cerebro-spinal fluid. No. II: The theories of drainage of cerebro-spinal fluid with an analysis of the methods of investigation. *Journal of Medicine Research*, 31, 21–49.

Weed, LH (1914b). Studies on cerebro-spinal fluid. No. III: The pathways of escape from the subarachnoid spaces with particular reference to the Arachnoid Villi. *Journal of Medicine Research*, 31, 51–91.

Wilkerson, MK, PN Colleran and MD Delp (2002). Acute and chronic head-down tail suspension diminishes cerebral perfusion in rats. *American Journal of Physiology Heart and Circulatory Physiology*, 282, H328–334.

Wilkerson, MK, LA Lesniewski, EM Golding, RM Bryan, Jr, A Amin, E Wilson and MD Delp (2005). Simulated microgravity enhances cerebral artery vasoconstriction and vascular resistance through endothelial nitric oxide mechanism. *American Journal of Physiology Heart and Circulatory Physiology*, 288, H1652–1661.

Wilkerson, MK, J Muller-Delp, PN Colleran and MD Delp (1999). Effects of hindlimb unloading on rat cerebral, splenic, and mesenteric resistance artery morphology. *Journal of Applied Physiology*, 87, 2115–2121.

Winkelman, C (2000). Effect of backrest position on intracranial and cerebral perfusion pressures in traumatically brain-injured adults. *American Journal of Critical Care*, 9, 373–380. quiz 381–382.

Wintermark, M, M Sesay, E Barbier, K Borbely, WP Dillon, JD Eastwood, TC Glenn, CB Grandin, S Pedraza, JF Soustiel, T Nariai, G Zaharchuk, JM Caille, V Dousset and H Yonas (2005). Comparative overview of brain perfusion imaging techniques. *Journal of Neuroradiology*, 32, 294–314.

Yamada, S (2014). Cerebrospinal fluid physiology: Visualization of cerebrospinal fluid dynamics using the magnetic resonance imaging Time-Spatial Inversion Pulse method. *Croation Medical Journal*, 55, 337–346.

Yamada, S, M Miyazaki, H Kanazawa, M Higashi, Y Morohoshi, S Bluml and JG Mccomb (2008). Visualization of cerebrospinal fluid movement with spin labeling at MR imaging: Preliminary results in normal and pathophysiologic conditions. *Radiology*, 249, 644–652.

Yamada, S, K Tsuchiya, WG Bradley, M Law, ML Winkler, MT Borzage, M Miyazaki, EJ Kelly and JG Mccomb (2014). Current and emerging MR imaging techniques for the diagnosis and management of CSF flow disorders: A review of phase-contrast and time-spatial labeling inversion pulse. *AJNR American Journal of Neuroradiology*, 36(4):623–630.

Zaharchuk, G (2007). Theoretical basis of hemodynamic MR imaging techniques to measure cerebral blood volume, cerebral blood flow, and permeability. *AJNR American Journal of Neuroradiology*, 28, 1850–1858.

Zhang, LN, LF Zhang and J MA (2001). Simulated microgravity enhances vasoconstrictor responsiveness of rat basilar artery. *Journal of Applied Physiology*, 90, 2296–2305.

Zhou, Y, Y Wang, LL Rao, ZY Liang, XP Chen, D Zheng, C Tan, ZQ Tian, CH Wang, YQ Bai, SG Chen and S Li (2014). Disrutpted resting-state functional architecture of the brain after 45-day simulated microgravity. *Front Behavioural Neuroscience*, 8, 200.

Ziessman, HA, JP O'malley and JH Thrall (2006). *Nuclear Medicine: The Requisites in Radiology*, Philadelphia, PA: Elsevier Mosby.

Zuj, KA, P Arbeille, JK Shoemaker, AP Blaber, DK Greaves, D Xu and RL Hughson (2012). Impaired cerebrovascular autoregulation and reduced CO_2 reactivity after long duration spaceflight. *Amrican Journal of Physiology. Heart and Circulatory Physiology*, 302, H2592–H2598.

10

Sensory and Sensorimotor Changes with Spaceflight: Implications for Functional Performance

Rachael D. Seidler, PhD, Vincent Koppelmans, PhD*, Jacob Bloomberg, PhD[†] and Ajitkumar P. Mulavara, PhD[‡]*

**School of Kinesiology, University of Michigan, 1402 Washington Heights, Ann Arbor, Michigan 48109-2013, USA*
[†]Johnson Space Center, 2101 E NASA Pkwy, Houston, Texas 77058, USA
[‡]KBRwyle, 1960 East Grand Ave, Suite 900, El Segundo, California, USA

1. Introduction

Recent studies have documented optic changes with spaceflight, including flattening of the back of the globe, optic disc edema, and choroidal folding (Mader *et al.*, 2011). A retrospective analysis of magnetic resonance imaging (MRI) scans of 27 astronauts showed optic nerve sheath distention, globe flattening, optic disc protrusion, and an increase of the optic nerve diameter in some but not all astronauts (Kramer *et al.*, 2012). Mice flown in space exhibit increased cerebral artery diameter, suggestive of increased intracranial pressure (Taylor *et al.*, 2013) which may contribute to the optic changes that have been reported. These effects have been termed the visual impairment intracranial pressure (VIIP) syndrome.

Numerous factors have been suggested to play a role in creating the VIIP syndrome, many of which are reviewed elsewhere in this book. The expertise of our group is on documenting and identifying the etiology of the untoward effects of spaceflight on multisensory integration and sensorimotor control, particularly in terms of altered vestibular-visual interactions and their impact on functional motor control. In this chapter, we review our work and that of others on this topic. We will outline what is known about the effects of spaceflight on neurocognitive function, with a particular emphasis on multisensory integration and sensory weighting in relation to motor control, balance, and sensorimotor adaptation. For example, it is known that exposure to microgravity induces adaptive central reinterpretation of visual, vestibular, and proprioceptive information (Paloski *et al.*, 1992, 1993, 1994; Reschke *et al.*, 1998). This microgravity adaptive state, however, is inappropriate for a gravitational environment so that astronauts must spend time readapting to Earth's gravity following their return. During this readaptation period they experience disturbances in perception, spatial orientation, posture, gait, and eye-head coordination (Reschke *et al.*, 1994a, 1994b, 1998). These changes include disruption in spatial orientation during over ground walking, alterations in muscle activation variability (Layne *et al.*, 1997, 1998, 2001, 2004), modified lower limb kinematics (McDonald *et al.*, 1996; Miller *et al.*, 2010), alterations in head-trunk coordination (Bloomberg and Mulavara, 2003), and reduced visual acuity during walking (Peters *et al.*, 2011, Bloomberg and Mulavara, 2003). These postflight changes contribute to impaired mobility on an obstacle course (Mulavara *et al.*, 2010) and decreased ability to coordinate effective landing strategies during a jump down task (Newman *et al.*, 1997). We have also shown changes in postural stability when subjects were forced to rely primarily on vestibular feedback postflight (Paloski *et al.*, 1993; Black *et al.*, 1995, 1999), that is, the visual and proprioceptive feedback was altered and/or absent.

In this chapter, we emphasize contact points between VIIP and sensorimotor control. In Part I, we discuss the known links between intracranial pressure, brain structure, and neurocognitive function, and highlight important directions for future research. In Part II, we review spaceflight effects on sensorimotor control, and highlight potential impacts that altered visual acuity could have on multisensory integration and sensory weighting. We have established that spaceflight impairs dynamic visual acuity (DVA), which has important mission relevance. We will close by highlighting avenues for investigating the impact of VIIP and potential visual acuity changes on multisensory integration and mission relevant behaviors. Future studies should include retrospective data mining investigations as well as data sharing from ongoing, prospective experiments.

2. Effects of Elevated Intracranial Pressure on Brain Structure and Neurocognitive Function

The exact mechanisms behind spaceflight-induced vision changes are still largely unknown. An experimental study testing rodents after less than 2 weeks of spaceflight in low-Earth orbit revealed that oxidative stress, neuronal damage, and mechanical injury affect various parts of the visual system, including the retina, lens, and optic nerve (Zanello *et al.*, 2013). It has been proposed that one of the main causes of this degeneration is increased intracranial pressure due to cephalad fluid shifts that occur in microgravity because of the absence of hydrostatic pressure (Lathers *et al.*, 1989; for a review, see Kawai *et al.*, 2003). An experimental study showed that indeed simulated microgravity induced by head-down tilt results in increased intracranial pressure measured directly through a catheter chronically implanted into the subarachnoid space (Tatebayashi *et al.*, 2003). In humans, indications for fluid shift increasing intracranial pressure have been observed in the form of plasma fluid shift into the interstitial spaces in the head and neck during 8 h of head-down tilt bed rest (Parazynski *et al.*, 1985), that has in turn been linked to an increase in intracranial pressure (Alperin *et al.*, 2005; Lakin *et al.*, 2007). Moreover, flattening of the globe (Mader *et al.*, 2011; Kramer *et al.*, 2012), together with other symptoms that have been observed in astronauts, such as optic disc edema (Mader *et al.*, 2011), and elevated lumbar puncture opening pressure (Mader *et al.*, 2011; Kramer *et al.*, 2012) have all been associated with increased intracranial pressure. This is in line with the ophthalmologic changes observed in patients with idiopathic intracranial hypertension (IIH). IIH is also known as pseudotumor cerebri and is a condition in which there is increased intracranial hypertension in the absence of a clear identifiable etiology. IIH patients often present with similar symptoms of the visual system as astronauts postflight including posterior globe flattening, optic nerve sheath distention, inward protrusion of the optic nerve head, optic disc edema, and thickening of the nerve fiber layer (Degnan and Levy, 2011; Passi *et al.*, 2013). In addition, both IIH patients and astronauts postflight often complain about headaches (Degnan and Levy, 2011; Law *et al.*, 2014), although headaches in astronauts could also be related to increased CO_2 levels (Law *et al.*, 2014).

A contributing factor for vision impairments after spaceflight is alterations in folate and vitamin metabolism (Zwart *et al.*, 2012). A study in astronauts returning from the international space station (ISS) revealed that astronauts who presented with vision impairments postspaceflight had higher concentrations of serum homocysteine, cysthionine, 2-methylcitric acid, and methylmalonic acid concentrations than astronauts who did not show ophthalmic changes (Zwart *et al.*, 2012). These findings indicate that astronauts with polymorphisms of the enzymes in folate-dependent and vitamin B_{12} dependent 1-carbon metabolism genes are more sensitive to the effects of spaceflight on vision compared to astronauts who do not have these polymorphisms.

In addition to sensorimotor changes with flight, there is some indication that astronauts experience problems with cognitive functioning during and after spaceflight, especially in cognitive and motor dual-tasking and visuo-motor tracking (Eddy *et al.*, 1998; Manzey *et al.*, 1995, 1998a, 1998b). Evidence for impaired performance in other cognitive domains has not yet been reliably validated in a sufficiently large set of astronauts (Eddy *et al.*, 1998; Kane *et al.*, 2005; Strangman and Bevan, 2013). A 45-day head-down tilt bed rest study in 16 healthy young men reported impaired executive functioning as a result of head-down tilt (Liu *et al.*, 2012). Impairments in mental spatial representation of words and geometrical figures and mental image transformations of the whole body or body parts have also been reported in astronauts and subjects during parabolic flight, though these effects were ascribed to the absence of the gravito-inertial force and were not considered to be effects of intracranial hypertension because the effects decayed with accumulating time in microgravity (Grabherr and Mast, 2010).

Whether increased intracranial pressure contributes to cognitive and sensori-motor dysfunction in astronauts is yet to be determined. This could be possible considering that IIH patients have shown cognitive dysfunction in various domains, including reaction time, processing speed, verbal functioning, and memory (Sørensen *et al.*, 1986; Arseni *et al.*, 1992; Kharkar *et al.*, 2011; Yri *et al.*, 2014) that might be reversible with pressure alleviating treatment (Sorenson *et al.*, 1986). These findings suggest that cognitive problems with spaceflight could be related to microgravity-induced intracranial hypertension.

Concerns about the effects of spaceflight on the brain have triggered neuro-imaging studies in astronauts and subjects in spaceflight analog settings (Koppelmans *et al.*, 2013). MRI allows the noninvasive investigation of brain structure and water distribution and can indirectly qualify brain activation with high spatial resolution. Bed rest studies have identified various effects of simulated microgravity on brain function and structure. A study in five subjects in whom intracranial and intraocular water content was measured using T2-weighted MRI in supine position and after 40 min of head-down tilt showed a significant reduction in the water fraction in the eyes and subarachnoid cerebrospinal fluid during head-down tilt compared to the supine position (Caprihan *et al.*, 1999). No increases in water content were observed. It was argued that these outcomes were not indicative for global cerebral edema and that the local decreases in water could be due to an increase in intracranial pressure. To support this hypothesis, Caprihan *et al.*, refer to studies conducted in primates and humans in the early nineties that showed increases in intracranial pressure as a function of head-down tilt (for a review of effects of simulated microgravity on cerebral hemodynamics (Kawai *et al.*, 2003)). In line with these reports is the previously described study by Kramer *et al.* who besides ocular effects of microgravity also reported that microgravity was associated with concavity of the pituitary gland with posterior stalk displacement (Kramer *et al.*, 2012). Concavity of the pituitary or "empty sella" is associated with endocrine dysfunction (Guitelman *et al.*, 2013). Because these symptoms are also associated with IIH it was suggested that the pituitary malformations were related to intracranial hypertension. While there is evidence for increased intracranial pressure in microgravity, no studies have shown an association between intracranial hypertension and cerebral edema in microgravity, though it has been proposed that increased venous pressure across the capillary bed could result in greater filtration into cerebral tissue causing cerebral edema (Kawai *et al.*, 2003; Wilson *et al.*, 2011).

In addition to brain structural changes, long-duration head-down tilt has also been associated with an increase in activation of the motor cortex coding for leg movements following bed rest (Roberts *et al.*, 2010). Leg activation was induced in four subjects with transcranial magnetic stimulation, a noninvasive technique to stimulate the cerebral cortex using time-varying magnetic fields. Cortical excitability and activation were measured respectively with transcranial magnetic stimulation (TMS)-derived recruitment curves and functional magnetic resonance imaging (fMRI). Only the TMS measures significantly increased from pre- to postbed rest. The authors ascribed the increased excitability of the primary motor cortex to relearning of leg control after long-term disuse during head-down tilt. Another study in which resting-state fMRI (i.e., spontaneous brain activation during rest) was recorded from 12 male participants before and after 72 h of head-down tilt revealed a decrease in left thalamus activation after head-down tilt (Liao *et al.*, 2012). This finding was ascribed by the authors to cephalad fluid shifts. The thalamus is a relay station for sensory and motor information that also plays an important role in executive cognitive functioning. Therefore, these results could potentially explain part of the effects of microgravity on cognitive and motor dysfunction. Whether these functional changes are associated with intracranial hypertension, functional cortical reorganization due to adaptation to the head-down environment, or both is not known. It has been suggested that the duration of symptoms is an indication of whether they are caused by intracranial hypertension or adaptation to the microgravity environment (Grabherr and Mast, 2010). Effects of adaptation processes while in microgravity are expected to be of shorter duration where effects of intracranial hypertension are expected to be long lasting with gradual increases. The paucity of structural imaging studies in astronauts prevents us from linking the observed functional brain changes to structural alterations. Similarly, the lack of functional studies in IIH patients prevents us from making direct links to increased intracranial pressure in microgravity. We are currently conducting a study which combines both structural and functional brain imaging as well as cognitive and motor performance tests (Koppelmans *et al.*, 2013). The pattern of normal and abnormal outcomes of such studies will help to unravel the pathophysiological mechanisms of the effects of microgravity on the brain.

3. Effects of Spaceflight on Multisensory Integration and Sensorimotor Function

3.1. *Multisensory integration and sensory weighting for balance and functional mobility*

There are multiple sensory cues which provide information about the body's location and orientation, including visual, vestibular, and proprioceptive inputs. Fusing information from multiple sensory sources has been shown to improve both detection of stimuli (Stein and Wallace, 1996; Lovelace *et al.*, 2003) and localization of stimuli (Nelson *et al.*, 1998; Wilkinson *et al.*, 1996). Early on it was thought that only the thalamus was capable of sensory integration (Penfield, 1938) but more recent work has demonstrated the existence of higher order cortical brain regions which integrate information across multiple sensory domains (Wallace *et al.*, 1992; Calvert *et al.*, 2000) to produce an integrated percept. Single neurons in the primate intraparietal cortex respond to visual, vestibular, tactile, and auditory stimuli (Seilheimer *et al.*, 2014). It has been found that even primary sensory areas of the brain such as primary visual, auditory, and somatosensory cortices can be affected by information from other sensory modalities (Stein, 2005; Ghazanfar *et al.*, 2005). This multisensory integration appears to be a learned process; children tend to rely on one sensory input at a time, with integration increasing across development (Seilheimer *et al.*, 2014).

Sensory weighting refers to the capacity of the nervous system to attribute different weights to redundant sources of sensory information (Nashner and Berthoz, 1978). Intermodal reweighting refers to shifting reliance onto one sensory cue versus another, whereas intramodal reweighting refers to the relative gain of a single input. These mechanisms allow the central nervous system (CNS) to change the prominence of a particular sensory input due to injury, disease, or sensory conflict arising from changes in the environment.

Dynamic sensory reweighting has been studied in the context of human posture control. Vestibular inputs can be modified via galvanic vestibular stimulation, leading to the percept of self-motion. Proprioceptive inputs can be manipulated with tendon vibration at specific frequencies, producing the illusion of changing muscle length. Dynamic visual displays or surround motion provide visual cues of self-motion. These inputs can be flexibly reweighted to adjust for noisy or unreliable signals. Vestibular inputs can be noisy but they are interpreted as a "true" signal when corroborated with proprioceptive and visual information. For example, when one is seated on a train at a busy station awaiting departure, the neighboring train may start moving first. This visual flow input can initially lead to the conclusion that one's own train has started to move, particularly for individuals that are more visually dependent. After a short period, however, vestibular signals resolve the conflict and the passenger realizes that they are not yet in motion.

Using the sensory perturbation techniques described above, Hwang *et al.* (2014) and Asslander and Peterka (2014) have demonstrated that human subjects can rapidly reweight sensory modalities for a given context. These perturbations can be delivered at specific frequencies, and then the frequency and phase lag of the postural responses can be recorded and matched to a given input. These authors have demonstrated that sensory reweighting occurs quickly and in a complementary fashion. For example, when subjects down-weight visual inputs they concomitantly rely more on proprioception or vestibular information.

Sensory reweighting occurs for normal daily behaviors as well, because we move in a complex and noisy environment. Sensory receptors do not operate with perfect fidelity, and internal neural representations are noisy as well. Interestingly, recent work demonstrates that multisensory integration occurs in a probabilistic fashion (Seilheimer *et al.*, 2014). That is, not only are sensory inputs coded in neural systems, but also the reliability of inputs is coded. Moreover, there is evidence that prior information is taken into account for sensory weighting and integration, suggesting that the brain operates in a Bayesian fashion (Seilheimer *et al.*, 2014).

The degree to which sensory inputs are weighted and reorganized under sensory discordant conditions varies by individual (Golomer *et al.*, 2005; Isableu *et al.*, 2010; Streepey *et al.*, 2007). Sensory weighting preferences have been reported for special populations and observed in healthy individuals under certain conditions. For example, higher visual dependence has been documented for stroke patients (Bonan *et al.*, 2004a, 2004b; deHaart *et al.*, 2004), the elderly (van Hedel and Dietz, 2004), and vestibularly-intact individuals with high-trait anxiety scores (Viaud-Delmon *et al.*, 2000). Vestibular weighting has been shown to increase just before initiating a turn while walking (Kennedy *et al.*, 2005). Autistic children (Masterton and Biederman, 1983) and individuals susceptible to motion aftereffects (mal de debarquement syndrome, Nachum *et al.*, 2004) depend more heavily on somatosensory cues. Astronauts' responses of illusory self-motion and the simultaneous compensation for these motions when viewing a rotating display of dots on the inside of a rotating drum, or vertical optokinetic stimulation in microgravity, suggest that reliance on visual cues is increased and dependence on graviceptor signals is reduced (cf. Mueller *et al.*, 1992, 1994). In some astronauts, local tactile cues from bungee cord-induced foot pressure inhibited these visually induced motion illusions (Young *et al.*, 1992). These illusions of self-motion continue to be reported during reentry and immediately after landing in response to voluntary pitch or roll head movements or passive roll stimulation in darkness immediately after landing (Reschke and Parker, 1987). Adaptation to microgravity results in lack of bipedal balance control under postflight test conditions requiring accurate feedback from the vestibular inputs and ankle proprioception on computerized dynamic posturography (Paloski *et al.*, 1992, 1994; Paloski, 1998). Most subjects have increased reliance on feedback from vision during their postflight recovery process as a result of degraded performance of the other two feedback systems during adaptation to microgravity (Reschke *et al.*, 1998). Proprioceptive function also adapts to microgravity (Roll *et al.*, 1993, 1998), causing the reduction in relevance and coding of standing posture and body movements, and enhanced reports of movement illusions in response to tendon vibrations (Reschke *et al.*, 1998, Roll *et al.*, 1993, 1998). Crewmembers have also reported related illusions of floor and object movement when doing pushoffs in 0-G and squats upon return to earth (Parker *et al.*, 1989). Approximately 30% of healthy individuals are "highly" visually dependent (Keshner, 2004; Brady *et al.*, 2009; Warren *et al.*, 1996). We have shown that visual dependency may predict decreased ability to adapt to discordant sensory environments.

3.2. *Strategic and adaptive motor learning mediating recovery as a function of spaceflight*

We showed previously that exposure to visual distortions during treadmill walking induces rapid readjustments over the short-term through strategic modifications (Richards *et al.*, 2004) and longer term after-effects through plastic-adaptive modifications (Mulavara *et al.*, 2005b; Nomura *et al.*, 2005) in locomotor function. We have demonstrated the dynamic interplay between strategic and plastic-adaptive mechanisms by showing that subjects display a gradual reduction in the strategic modification of trunk movements during exposure to varied optic flow during treadmill walking as plastic-adaptive mechanisms begin to predominate. Importantly, the rate at which strategic control is reduced is related to the magnitude of the ensuing plastic-adaptive response (Richards *et al.*, 2007). We previously performed a pre- and postflight functional assessment on 18 ISS crewmembers (Functional Mobility Test, FMT) to determine an astronaut's ability to complete challenging locomotor maneuvers similar to those encountered during an egress from a space vehicle following long-duration spaceflight (Mulavara *et al.*, 2010). Adaptation to spaceflight led to a 48% increase in time to complete the course one day after landing. Recovery to preflight scores took an average of 2 weeks after landing. Rapid strategic and slower adaptive motor learning processes influenced astronauts' ability to re-adapt to

Earth's gravity environment over 2 weeks (Mulavara *et al.*, 2010). Also, measures of plastic-adaptive learning and strategic learning were correlated indicating that the strategic recovery processes can influence astronaut's long-term rate of adaptability to Earth's gravity environment. Early motor learning helps astronauts make rapid modifications in their motor control strategies during the first hours after landing. This early motor learning appears to reinforce the adaptive realignment, facilitating re-adaptation to Earth's 1-g environment on return from spaceflight. The early phase of motor learning engages multiple brain regions, such as the basal ganglia, thalamo-cortical loops, medial cerebellum, the anterior cingulate cortex, the inferior frontal gyrus, and visual and parietal cortical areas (Seidler *et al.*, 2006; Anguera *et al.*, 2010). Thus, early in training these specific brain regions are linked to strategic modifications that employ online adjustments to reduce the erroneous motor outputs. Activation of these areas supports cognitive aspects of the task, such as error detection and correction, working memory, and attention. The later phase of motor learning engages the lateral cerebellum, parietal, and cingulate motor cortical areas and thus contributes to the plastic-adaptive component of the motor learning response. The composition and timing of sensory challenges experienced during sensorimotor adaptability training sessions can be optimized to facilitate the ability to engage rapid strategic mechanisms while adapting to novel sensory discordant environments. Thus, a training regimen that focuses on activating strategic control maximally promotes rapid response gait adaptability. These results have important implications for the development of sensorimotor adaptation training regimens as proficiency in rapid, online strategic modifications may be the most critical for producing immediate adaptive responses like those following the initial landing on a planetary surface.

4. Effects of Spaceflight on Dynamic Visual Acuity (DVA)

In addition to documented changes in static near visual acuity in several astronauts, DVA or the ability to read while the head is in motion is also impacted by spaceflight. Gaze control coordinated by the CNS is critical to DVA. The gaze stabilization system coordinates movement of the eyes and head so that a stable retinal image is maintained during head and body motion. An important component of this control system is the vestibulo–ocular reflex (VOR). VOR response properties are modified during and after spaceflight, but the degree of adaptation varies among subjects and experimental conditions (reviewed in Clement and Reschke, 2008). These data suggest that, initially on orbit and following the return to Earth, the VOR is continually in adaptive flux, searching for a new dynamic equilibrium.

Under these conditions, the VOR maintains plasticity and, given sufficient time, adaptively modifies to reestablish stable vision during head perturbations. It has been previously demonstrated that exposure to the microgravity of spaceflight induces modification in eye–head coordination during visual target acquisition. Deficient gaze control during periods of adaptive change, such as the first days of microgravity exposure or reexposure to a gravitational environment, could cause oscillopsia (illusory movement of the visual world), blurred vision, and decrements in DVA. In such cases, stationary objects may appear to bounce up and down or move back and forth during head movements. Inappropriate or inadequate ocular compensation results in an inability to stabilize the visual image on the retina. It has been shown that for values above 2°/s, increases in retinal slip velocity are accompanied by increasingly worse visual acuity (Demer and Amjadi, 1993). Decreased DVA caused by spaceflight can lead to misperception of sensory information and poses a unique set of problems for crewmembers, especially during entry, approach, and landing on planetary surfaces. Visual disturbances could adversely affect entry and landing task performance, such as reading instruments, locating switches on a control panel, or evacuating a vehicle in suboptimal visual conditions (e.g., smoke in the cabin).

We have documented decrements in DVA while walking immediately after spaceflight. First, in a ground-based study, we demonstrated that a DVA test was effective at identifying differences in visual performance between labyrinthine deficient (LD) patients (patients with vestibular system abnormalities) and a group of normative control subjects (Hillman *et al.*, 1999). The same paradigm was then used to demonstrate decreased DVA performance in astronaut subjects following return from long-duration spaceflight (Bloomberg and Mulavara, 2003). More recently, a second-generation test (using Landolt C characters instead of numbers) was used to document decrements in DVA performance as a function of time after flight in 14 crewmembers returning from long-duration space missions (Peters *et al.* 2011; Peters and Bloomberg, 2005). Treadmill walking was used to induce head motion and visual acuity was determined by sequentially presenting Landolt ring optotypes on a computer display placed 4 m in front of subjects. These data indicate that postflight changes in gaze control produced decreases in DVA during walking. For some subjects the decrement was greater than the mean acuity decrement seen in a population of vestibular impaired patients collected using a similar protocol. The overall mean for the population showed a consistent improvement in DVA performance during the postflight recovery period, although the individual recovery rates varied. Visual disturbances like these could adversely affect the performance of critical mission tasks.

4.1. *Spaceflight effects on head movement control during locomotion: impacts on vision*

Head angular motion with respect to the environment has been shown to be stabilized in the vertical and horizontal plane during the performance of various motor tasks including jumping, walking, running, hopping, and tasks requiring maintaining equilibrium on a beam or a moving platform (Pozzo *et al.*, 1995; Assaiante and Amblard, 1993). The head serves as a stable platform to provide a veridical reference frame for visual-vestibular integration facilitating the organization of postural and locomotor control patterns. Another system that benefits from head stabilization with respect to the environment is the system for maintaining gaze during body movement. Head movements actually contribute to gaze stabilization during locomotion. An example of this is the pitch head rotation (as in nodding the head), which compensates for the vertical translation of the trunk that occurs with each step during the gait cycle (Pozzo *et al.*, 1995; Assaiante and Amblard, 1993). The magnitude of these head rotations was observed to be controlled and also dependent on the distance of the visual target to the eyes. Thus, the goal-directed response of these head movements during concurrent locomotion and visual target fixation suggests that head movements are not completely dependent on passive inertial and viscoelastic properties of the head-neck system but are actively modulated to respond to altered gaze control requirements. Thus, head stabilization mechanisms help both in providing postural adjustments for maintaining balance of the moving body and in maintaining visual acuity for navigational control through a constantly varying environment during locomotion.

In an initial study Bloomberg and colleagues examined whether short-duration exposure (7–16 days) to the microgravity environment of spaceflight during Shuttle missions induces alteration in postflight head-trunk coordination during locomotion (Bloomberg *et al.*, 1997). Twenty-three astronaut subjects were asked to walk (6.4 km/h, 20 s trials] on a motorized treadmill while visually fixating on a centrally located earth-fixed target positioned either 2 m (FAR) or 30 cm (NEAR) from the eyes. Head, trunk and lower limb kinematics were determined with the aid of a video-based motion analyzing system. Data were collected preflight (10 days prior to launch) and postflight (2–4 h, and 2, 4, and 8 days after landing).

One aspect of head movement control that was investigated in this data set was the relationship between vertical translation of the trunk occurring during each step and the corresponding pitch angular head movement during treadmill locomotion at 6.4 km/h. Before spaceflight, pitch head movements act in a compensatory fashion to oppose vertical trunk translation during locomotion. For example, as the trunk translates upward, the head pitched forward/downward, assisting in maintaining target fixation. Following spaceflight, there was a significant alteration in coordination between compensatory pitch angular head movements and vertical trunk translation. This is evidenced by a breakdown in the smooth, sinusoidal nature of pitch head movements into a number of subcomponents.

The degree of association between vertical trunk translation and corresponding compensatory pitch head movement was characterized using a coherence function which describes the relation between head and trunk movements (Bloomberg *et al.*, 1997). The mean coherence between pitch head and vertical trunk movements during gaze fixation of both FAR and NEAR targets was significantly reduced following spaceflight indicating decreased coordination between the head and trunk. This change in head-trunk coordination strategy may account, in part, for the reported oscillopsia that occurs during postflight locomotion and may contribute to disruption in descending control of locomotor function.

One of the interesting features of the short-duration data set concerned individual subject differences (Bloomberg *et al.*, 1997). Compensatory pitch head movement waveforms were subjected to Fourier analysis to determine the amplitude of the predominant frequency. Astronauts showed varying postflight responses in the frequency spectra of pitch head movements. Comparison of responses from multi- and first-time astronauts indicated that multitime astronauts (i.e., those who had experienced more than one spaceflight) demonstrated less postflight alteration in the frequency spectra of pitch head movements than subjects on their first flights. Postflight behavioral differences between astronauts based on their experience level have been previously observed in tests of dynamic postural equilibrium control (Paloski *et al.*, 1994). In these tests, inexperienced astronauts show greater postflight decrements in postural stability than their more experienced counterparts. Such differences may be the result of many factors. However, they could indicate that repeated exposure to spaceflight leads to facilitation in formulating the appropriate adaptive sensorimotor response during the transition from a microgravity to a terrestrial environment. The variability in adaptive responses between subjects may be the result of individual susceptibility to adaptive neural modification. Alternatively, this variability may reflect the response of a control system looking for a new equilibrium point by assessing the veracity of multiple sensory inputs. Indeed, the requirement to maintain gaze stability may not fully account for the variety of head movement strategies observed during locomotion. Head movement strategies adopted during locomotion may reflect specific task constraints and the requirement for reliance on specific sources of sensory information for the effective organization of coordinated movement. Nashner (1985) described two possible head-trunk coordination strategies for maintenance of dynamic postural equilibrium. The first strategy ("strap down") calls for the head to be fixed to the trunk during body movement, so that the head and trunk are considered a single unit. Adopting this strategy means that head-trunk control is simplified; however, the ability to resolve complex movements into their linear and angular components by the otoliths and semi-circular canals becomes complex. Alternatively, the "stable platform strategy" fixes orientation of the head with respect to the gravitational force vector, essentially stabilizing the head in space while the body moves underneath. The advantage of this strategy is that larger sustained rotations of the head are actively nulled, permitting the simplification of the otolithic process responsible for detecting linear acceleration and static orientation of the head. The "cost" incurred by this strategy is that complex head-trunk patterns of coordination are required to successfully execute this control scheme. The significant postflight reduction in predominant frequency amplitude of pitch head movements may be caused by attempts to reduce the amount of angular head movement during locomotion, and reduce potential canal-otolith ambiguities during the critical period of terrestrial readaptation. This in turn, further simplifies the coordinate transformation between the head and trunk, presumably allowing an easier determination of head position relative to space. Yet, this strategy is not optimal for gaze stabilization because it results in a disruption in the regularity of the compensatory nature of pitch head movements during locomotion. This strategy also restricts behavioral options for visual scanning during locomotion. Consequently, there may be trade-offs between head movement strategies depending on the imposed constraints. Once significant readaptation takes place, a decrease in constraints on the degrees-of-freedom of head movement likely occurs, returning performance back to preflight levels. Importantly, patients with vestibular deficits (Mulavara *et al.*, 2012) and children, prior to development of the mature head stabilization response (Assaiante and Amblard, 1993), show head movement restriction during locomotion.

Various compensatory head movement strategies may play a central role in facilitating optimal sensory-motor transformations between the head and trunk required for descending control of locomotion. Zangemeister *et al.* (1991) demonstrated that normal locomotion performed with the head in a retroflexed position induces alterations in lower limb muscle activity patterns. They concluded that a functional linkage exists between otolith signals generated by various head positions and the muscle activity patterns generated in the lower limbs during locomotion. Given this functional linkage, it can be argued that if spaceflight induces adaptive modification in head-trunk coordination, this would cause a disruption in the organization of coordinated body movement during postflight terrestrial locomotion. It follows that active body movement in the unique inertial environment encountered during spaceflight may require subjects to adaptively acquire novel head-trunk control strategies. These strategies, however, may be maladaptive for locomotion in a terrestrial 1-g environment leading to impairment of locomotor function during the readaptation period following the return to Earth.

To quantify the performance to orient during free walking after spaceflight, astronaut subjects were asked to walk preflight and postflight a previously seen triangular path with normal vision and vision occluded (Glasauer *et al.*, 1995). The path, marked on the ground by a cross at each corner, consisted of a right triangle with two legs of 3 m in length. The trajectories of three infrared–reflective markers fixed on a helmet were recorded using a video–based motion analysis system. Subjects showed inter-individual differences especially for directional deviations from the path in the vision occluded condition even preflight; the characteristics of these differences persisted throughout all experimental sessions. However, the absolute directional errors turned out to be larger postflight, which means that subjects had larger directional errors but in different directions. There was, however, a trend to a larger underestimation of the angle turned at each corner in the postflight condition. In contrast to directional errors, the length of the legs walked was similar pre- and postflight. These data suggest that the perception of self-displacement during turning, but not during linear motion was changed due to the stay in microgravity. A possible explanation could be the development of a mismatch between information from otoliths and semicircular canals during whole-body turns in microgravity. This change in canal-otolith interaction may underlie the disturbances in locomotion experienced by returning astronauts.

4.2. *Effects of plastic adaptive modification of the vestibulo-ocular reflex (VOR) on full body gaze control*

In order to test the general hypothesis that the whole body can serve as an *integrated* gaze stabilization system, we investigated how the multiple, interdependent full-body sensorimotor subsystems respond to changes in gaze stabilization task constraints during locomotion (Mulavara and Bloomberg 2003). Nine subjects performed two gaze stabilization tasks while walking at 6.4 km/h on a motorized treadmill: (1) focusing on a central point target; (2) reading numeral characters; both presented at 2 m in front at eye level. While reading numeral characters as compared to the central point target: (1) the compensatory head pitch movement was on average 22% greater, (2) the peak acceleration measured at the head was significantly reduced by an average of 13% in four of the six subjects, and (3) the knee joint total movement was on average 11% greater during the period from the heel strike event to the peak knee flexion event in stance phase of the gait cycle. These results suggest that the full body contributes to gaze stabilization during locomotion, and that its different functional elements respond to changes in visual task constraints.

We further investigated how introducing a plastic adaptive modification of eye-head coordination — by modifying the VOR gain — alters eye-head-trunk coordination and causes reorganization of lower limb joint configurations to help preserve gaze stabilization during locomotion (Mulavara *et al.*, 2005a and b). The adaptive stimulus was a 30 min exposure to 0.5 × minifying lenses worn during self-generated sinusoidal vertical head rotations while the subject was seated. During the adaptation phase, subjects were seated facing a projected complex visual scene. Before and after VOR adaptation fourteen subjects walked (6.4 km/h) on a motorized treadmill while performing a number recognition task. There was a significant increase in the duration of stance and stride times, alteration in the amplitude of head movement with respect to space, and a significant increase in the amount of knee flexion during the initial stance phase of the gait cycle. Thus, preliminary results indicate that visual–vestibular conflict induced by the minifying lenses caused alteration in full-body strategies consistent with the requirement to aid gaze stabilization during locomotion. These strategic changes returned to pre-adaptation levels within the 10 repeated trials completed immediately after the adaptation period. Thus, a limited plastic adaptation to one subsystem of the gaze stabilization mechanism during locomotion causes strategic modifications and reorganization among its different functional elements.

4.3. *Effects of long-duration spaceflight on full body gaze control*

Changes in head-trunk coordination during locomotion were characterized in six crewmembers who lived on the Mir Space Station for periods that ranged from 4 to 6 months (Bloomberg and Mulavara, 2003). These subjects walked (6.4 km/h) on a treadmill before and after spaceflight while visually fixating on an earth-fixed target. At this walking, speed head pitch movements serve to compensate for the vertical trunk movements that occur during each step (Pozzo *et al.*, 1990, 1995; Bloomberg *et al.*, 1997; Hirasaki *et al.*, 1999). Head and trunk pitch movements, along with trunk vertical movement with respect to space were determined using motion analysis data. Head and trunk pitch waveforms were transformed into the frequency domain. The power in these signals was summed in the frequency range of 1.5–2.5 Hz reflecting the contributions of reflexive head stabilization mechanisms (Keshner *et al.*, 1995). Subjects showed a reduction in power in this frequency range during postflight locomotion followed by a recovery trend spanning several days. This reduction in head pitch movement occurred despite no significant change in trunk pitch or vertical movement. Therefore, during postflight locomotion head movement amplitude with respect to space was reduced.

During foot contact with the ground, weight transfers from one foot to the other and the push off with the toe from the ground are critical phases as these interactions result in forces that create vibrations, which if unattenuated, could interfere with the visual–vestibular sensory systems in the head (Ito *et al.*, 1997; Lafortune *et al.*, 1996; McDonald *et al.*, 1997; Mulavara *et al.*, 2002; Mulavara and Bloomberg, 2003; Pozzo *et al.*, 1990; Smeathers, 1989; Valiant, 1990; Voloshin, 1988; Whittle, 1999). The musculoskeletal system controls these vibrations: muscles and joints act as filters to minimize the perturbing effects of impacts with the ground and help to maintain a stable trajectory at the head (Holt *et al.*, 1995; McDonald *et al.*, 1997). After long-duration spaceflight, astronauts showed that during treadmill walking, knee flexion during the stance phase significantly increased and then subsequently returned to normal within 6–10 days (Bloomberg and Mulavara, 2003). This increase in knee flexion during locomotion will result in reduction of the axial stiffness of the lower limb complex during the critical stance phase following heel strike leading to reduced perturbations being transmitted to the head during locomotion. In support of this concept an analysis of accelerations measured along the superior inferior axis at the head and tibia showed a significant reduction of the shock experienced at the tibia (40% average reduction) and the head (20% average reduction) segments during postflight locomotion (Mulavara *et al.*, 2012). However, the mean shock experienced by the head normalized to per unit tibial shock showed a significant increase of 40% during locomotion testing one day postflight (Mulavara *et al.*, 2012).

Therefore, adaptation to long-duration spaceflight led to: modified reflexive head stabilization mechanisms; decreased DVA; modified transmission characteristics of the shock-wave at heel strike; and increased total knee movement during the subsequent stance phase during postflight walking. Hence, appropriate attenuation of energy transmission during locomotion, achieved by the modulation of the lower limbs' joint configuration coupled with appropriate eye-head-trunk coordination strategies, form the fundamental features of an integrated gaze stabilization system. From this point of view, the whole body is an integrated gaze stabilization system, in which several subsystems contribute, leading to accurate visual acuity during body motion.

4.4. *Vestibular-somatosensory convergence in head movement control during locomotion after long-duration spaceflight*

Consistent with previous work in our laboratory and elsewhere (cf. Mulavara *et al.*, 2005a and b), we have observed that tasks requiring sensorimotor integration after an adaptive exposure are associated with a wide range of adaptive behavioral responses. Specifically, after short duration spaceflight astronauts showed diverse responses, with some people showing increases, and other people showing decreases in the magnitude of head pitch movement during walking (Bloomberg *et al.*, 1997; Bloomberg and Mulavara, 2003). Our recent report confirms and extends this observation of response variability one day after return from long-duration spaceflight (Mulavara *et al.*, 2012). For the spaceflight study, each subject's data collected after spaceflight (post) were compared to their corresponding data collected before spaceflight (pre). We have classified subjects based on the pre and post average of the magnitude of head pitch movements with respect to space during the locomotion paradigm. Thus, subjects were classified into two groups: a "decreaser" group wherein subjects' post flight averages decreased with respect to their pre-flight average responses, and an "increaser" group, wherein subjects' post-flight averages exceeded their pre-flight responses. The paired t-tests showed that while magnitude of head pitch movements was significantly changed (increased or decreased in the corresponding increasers or decreaser's groups, respectively, $p < 0.05$), the vertical torso translation was not significantly different ($p > 0.05$) after exposure to spaceflight.

Previous spaceflight data have shown postflight increases in vestibule–spinal reflexes in humans (Reschke *et al.*, 1984) and increased utricular afferent sensitivity to translation shown in toadfish (Boyle *et al.*, 2001). Reschke *et al.* (1984) showed reduction in in-flight responses compared to pre-flight values followed by increased activity post-flight. Boyle *et al.* (2001) reported that the magnitude of response of the vestibular nerve afferents in toadfish supplying the utricularotolith organ to an applied translation was on average three times greater than for controls on the first post-flight day. This may be a general phenomenon of upregulation of the sensitivity of the utricular afferents after adaptation to the microgravity environment of spaceflight. This indeed may be the case in the "increaser" group of astronaut subjects and the outcome seen in the adaptation of body weight support locomotion. However, a similar increase in vestibular sensitivity would tend to generate larger head pitch for the same trunk vertical translation during locomotion (Moore *et al.*, 2006). This is not the case for the subjects in the "decreaser" group of astronaut subjects. Data from our experiments with labyrinthine deficient patients and experiments in which we used galvanic vestibular stimulation (GVS) to induce acute vestibular disturbances indicate that a reduction in head movement response could be a voluntary strategic response to reduce sensory conflict. Pitch head movements as well as vertical eye movements act together to stabilize gaze during vertical trunk translation (Pozzo *et al.*, 1990, 1991). Patients with bilateral vestibular weakness experience increased head oscillations and oscillopsia during walking (Pozzo *et al.*, 1991). Astronauts returning from spaceflight often experience oscillopsia during locomotion associated with vestibular dysfunction as well as postural and gait instabilities. This suggests a breakdown in head–trunk coordination due to conflicting sensorimotor input during transition from microgravity to a 1-g environment. These results suggest that spaceflight may cause a central adaptation of the converging vestibular and body load-sensing somatosensory systems. The significant post-flight changes in the predominant frequency amplitude of pitch head movement in the two groups of astronauts were similar to that demonstrated by our adaptation to body load supported locomotion and labyrinthine deficient (LD) subjects (Mulavara *et al.*, 2012). If the increased vestibular response sensitivity due to spaceflight were to be uniformly applied across subjects, then we may have had only one group with increasers in head movements during locomotion. However, half of the astronaut subjects showed a reduction in head movement responses similar to our LD subjects study (Mulavara *et al.*, 2012) and to that reported for subjects exposed to GVS during locomotion (Moore *et al.*, 2006). These responses may represent attempts to reduce the amount of angular head movement during locomotion dependent on the weightings afforded to sensorimotor integration of available sensory inputs during the adaptation process when exposed to weightlessness. Thus, the "decreaser" group of subjects may show an increased weighting of vestibular signals and hence sensory weighting may be a marker of post flight disturbance. This strategy may also reflect the response of a control system looking for a new equilibrium point. The goal of establishing this new end point would be to reduce potential canal-otolith ambiguities. This strategy, however, is not optimal for gaze stabilization, which may account for the decreased dynamic visual acuity in astronauts and LD subjects. This idea is supported by the finding that compensatory pitch head movement in all LD subjects was reduced while all subjects exposed to acute adaptation to body weight supported locomotion was increased despite no change in vertical trunk translation. The kinematic measurements give additional information regarding compensatory strategies during locomotor testing. The lack of change in vertical trunk translation indicates that the input disturbances to the gaze control system remain unchanged. Taken together these findings indicate that body load-sensing mediated somatosensory input centrally modulates vestibular input and can adaptively modify vestibularly mediated head movement control during locomotion. Thus, spaceflight may cause a central adaptation of the converging vestibular and body load-sensing somatosensory systems leading to alterations in head movement control.

5. Looking Forward: Conclusions and Future Directions

Our work and that of others clearly demonstrates that spaceflight impairs sensory reweighting and therefore sensorimotor control due to central reinterpretation of visual, vestibular, and proprioceptive inputs. We believe that a better understanding of VIIP, its consequences, and its mechanisms should be predicated upon an integrative approach which amalgamates across all systems affected by microgravity. Moreover, as the underlying factors contributing to VIIP are elucidated, spaceflight physiologists will need to consider their broader impact on mission relevant behaviors. Such an endeavor can only be accomplished via data sharing and collaboration across a range of scientists. One productive approach would include retrospective data mining to determine whether ocular structural changes are linked to changes in static visual acuity, DVA, sensory integration and reweighting, gait and balance. Collaborative teams should also be assembled for prospective studies examining relationships between cephalad fluid levels, intracranial pressure, ocular changes, and functional behaviors, such as gait, balance, and DVA tasks. Understanding the relationship between spaceflight, VIIP, and sensorimotor function is a necessary first step for the development of prevention approaches and countermeasures that are necessary for successful return missions to the moon and next generation space missions to mars.

References

Alperin, N, SH Lee, A Sivaramakrishnan and SG Hushek (2005). Quantifying the effect of posture on intracranial physiology in humans by MRI flow studies. *Journal of Magnetic Resonance Imaging*, 22(5), 591–596.

Anguera, JA, PA Reuter-Lorenz, DT Willingham and RD Seidler (2010). Contributions of spatial working memory to visuomotor learning. *Journal of Cognitive Neuroscience*, 22(9), 1917–1930.

Arseni, C, I Simoca, I Jipescu, E Leventi, P Grecu, A Sima, *et al.* (1992). Pseudotumorcerebri: Risk factors, clinical course, prognostic criteria. *Rom Journal of Neurology Psychiatry*, 30(2), 115–132.

Assaiante, C and B Amblard (1993). Ontogenesis of head stabilization in space during locomotion in children: Influence of visual cues. *Experimental Brain Research*, 93, 499–515.

Asslander, L and RJ Peterka (2014). Sensory reweighting dynamics in human postural control. *Journal of Neurophysiology*, 111, 1852–1864.

Black, FO, WH Paloski, MF Reschke, M Igarashi, F Guedry, and DJ Anderson (1999). Disruption of postural readaptation by inertial stimuli following space flight. *Journal of Vestibular Research*, 9(5), 369–378.

Black, FO, WH Paloski, DD Doxey-Gasway and MF Reschke (1995). Vestibular plasticity following orbital spaceflight: Recovery from post-flight postural instability. *Acta Oto-laryngologica*, 520, Pt 2, 450–454.

Bloomberg JJ and AP Mulavara (2003). Changes in walking strategies after spaceflight. *IEEE Engineering in Medicine Biology Magazine*, 22, 58–62.

Bloomberg, JJ, BT Peters, SL Smith, WP Huebner and MF Reschke (1997). Locomotor head-trunk coordination strategies following space flight. *Journal of Vestibular Research*, 7, 161–177.

Boyle, R, AF Mensinger, K Yoshida, S Usui, F Intravaia, T Tricas and SM Highstein (2001). Neural readaptation to earth's gravity following return from space. *Journal of Neurophysiology*, 86, 2118–2122.

Bonan, IV, FM Colle, JP Guichard, E Vicaut, M Eisenfisz, P Tran Ba Huy and AP Yelnik (2004a). Reliance on visual information after stroke. Part I: Balance on dynamic pos-turography. *Archives of Physical Medicine Rehabilitation*, 85, 268–273.

Bonan, IV, AP Yelnik, FM Colle, C Michaud, E Normand, B Panigot, P Roth, JP Guichard and E Vicaut (2004b). Reliance on visual information after stroke. Part II: Effectiveness of a balance rehabilitation program with visual cue deprivation after stroke: A rand-omized controlled trial. *Archives of Physical Medicine Rehabilatation*, 85, 274–278.

Brady, RA, BT Brian and JJ Bloomberg (2009). Strategies of healthy adults walking on a laterally oscillating treadmill. *Gait and Posture*, 29(4), 645–649.

Calvert, GA, R Campbell and MJ Brammer (2000). Evidence from functional magnetic resonance imaging of crossmodal binding in the human hetermodal cortex. *Current Biology*, 10(11), 649–57.

Caprihan, A, JA Sanders, HA Cheng and JA Loeppky (1999). Effect of head-down tilt on brain water distribution. *European Journal of Applied Physiology and Occupational Physiology*, 79(4), 367–373.

Clement, G and MF Reschke (2008). *Neuroscience in Space*. New York: Springer.

deHaart, M, AC Geurts, SC Huidekoper, L Fasotti and J van Limbeek (2004). Recovery of standing balance in post acute stroke patients: A rehabilitation cohort study. *Archives of Physical Medicine Rehabilitation*, 85, 886–895.

Degnan, AJ and LM Levy (2011). Pseudotumorcerebri: Brief review of clinical syndrome and imaging findings. *AJNR American Journal of Neuroradiology*, 32(11), 1986–1993.

Demer, JL and F Amjadi (1993). Dynamic visual acuity of normal subjects during vertical optotype and head motion. *Investigative Ophthalmology & Visual Science*, 34, 1894–1906.

Eddy, DR, SG Schiflett, RE Schlegel and RL Shehab (1998). Cognitive performance aboard the life and microgravity spacelab. *Acta Astronautica*, 43(3-6), 193–210.

Ghazanfar, AA, JX Maier, KL Hoffman and NK Logothetis (2005). Multisensory integra-tion of dynamic faces and voices in rhesus monkey auditory cortex. *Journal of Neuroscience*, 25(20), 5004–5012.

Glasauer, S, MA Amorim, JJ Bloomberg, MF Reschke, BT Peters, SL Smith and A Berthoz (1995). Spatial orientation during locomotion [correction of locomation] following space flight. *Acta Astronautica*, 36(8–12), 423–431.

Golomer, E, E Guillou, M Testa, C Lecoq and T Ohlmann (2005). Contribution of neck proprioception to subjective vertical perception among experts in physical activities and untrained women. *Neuroscience Letters*, 381, 31–35.

Grabherr, L and FW Mast (2010) Effects of microgravity on cognition: The case of mental imagery. *Journal of Vestibular Research*, 20(1), 53–60.

Guitelman, M, N Garcia Basavilbaso, M Vitale, A Chervin, D Katz, K Miragaya, J Herrera, D Cornalo, M Servidio, L Boero, M Manavela, K Danilowicz, A Alfieri, G Stalldecker, M Glerean, P Fainstein Day, C Ballarino, MS Mallea Gil and A Rogozinski (2013). Primary empty sella (PES): A review of 175 cases. *Pituitary*, 16(2), 270–274.

Hillman, EJ, JJ Bloomberg, PV McDonald and HS Cohen (1999). Dynamic visual acuity while walking in normals and labyrinthine-deficient patients. *Journal of Vestibular Research*, 9, 49–57.

Hirasaki, E, ST Moore, T Raphan and B Cohen (1999). Effects of walking velocity on vertical head and body movements during locomotion. *Experimental. Brain Research*, 127, 117–130.

Holt, KG, SF Jeng, R Ratcliffe and J Hamill (1995). Energetic cost and stability during human walking at the preferred stride frequency. *Journal of Motor Behavior*, 27, 164–178.

Hwang, S, P Agada, T Kiemel and J Jeka (2014). Dynamic reweighting of three modalities for sensor fusion. *PLoS One*, 9, e88132.

Isableu, B, T Ohlmann, J Cremieux, N Vuillerme, B Amblard and MA Gresty (2010). Individual differences in the ability to identify, select and use appropriate frames of reference for perceptuo-motor control. *Neuroscience*, 169(3), 1199–1215.

Ito, Y, S Corna, M von Brevern, A Bronstein and M Gresty (1997). The functional effectiveness of neck muscle reflexes for head righting in response to sudden fall. *Experimental Brain Research*, 117, 266–272.

Kane, RL, P short, W Sipes and CF Flynn (2005). Development and validation of the spaceflight cognitive assessment tool for windows (WinSCAT). *Aviation, Space and Environmental Medicine*, 76(6 Suppl), B183–B191.

Kawai, Y, M Doi, A Setogawa, R Shimoyama, K Ueda, Y Asai and K Tatebayashi (2003). Effects of microgravity on cerebral hemodynamics. *Yonago Acta Medica*, 46, 1–8.

Kennedy, PM, EK Cressman, AN Carlsen and R Chua (2005). Assessing vestibular contributions during changes in gait trajectory. *Neuroreport*, 16, 1097–1100.

Keshner, EA (2004). Head-trunk coordination in elderly subjects during linear anteriorposterior translations. *Experimental Brain Research*, 158, 213–222.

Keshner, EA, RL Cromwell and BW Peterson (1995). Mechanisms controlling human head stabilization, II, Head-neck characteristics during random rotations in the vertical plane, *Journal of Neurophysiology*, 73, 2302–2312.

Kharkar, S, *et al.* (2011). Cognitive impairment in patients with Pseudotumor Cerebri Syndrome. *Behavioural Neurology*, 24(2), 143–148.

Koppelmans, V, *et al.* (2013). Study protocol to examine the effects of spaceflight and a spaceflight analog on neurocognitive performance: Extent, longevity, and neural bases. *BMC Neurology*, 13, 205.

Kramer, LA, *et al.* (2012). Orbital and intracranial effects of microgravity: Findings at 3-T MR imaging. *Radiology*, 263(3), 819–827.

Lafortune, MA, MJ Lake and EM Hennig (1996). Differential shock transmission response of the human body to impact severity and lower limb posture. *Journal of Biomechanic*, 29(12), 1531–1537.

Lakin, WD, SA Stevens and PL Penar (2007). Modeling intracranial pressures in microgravity: The influence of the blood-brain barrier. *Aviation Space and Environmental Medicine*, 78(10), 932–936.

Lathers, CM, JB Charles and MW Bungo (1989). Pharmacology in space. Part 1. Influence of adaptive changes on pharmacokinetics. *Trends in Pharmacological Science*, 10(5), 193–200.

Law, J, M Van Baalen, M Foy, SS Mason, C Mendez, ML Wear, VE Meyers and D Alexander (2014). Relationship between carbon dioxide levels and reported headaches on the international space station. *Journal of Occupational and Environmental Medicine*, 56(5), 477–483.

Layne, CS, GW Lange, CJ Pruett, PV McDonald, LA Merkle, AP Mulavara, SL Smith, IB Kozlovskaya and JJ Bloomberg (1998). Adaptation of neuromuscular activation patterns during treadmill walking after long-duration space flight. *Acta Astronautica*, 43, 107–119.

Layne, CS, PV McDonald and JJ Bloomberg (1997). Neuromuscular activation patterns during treadmill walking after space flight. *Experimental Brain Research*, 113, 104–116.

Layne, CS, AP Mulavara, PV McDonald, CJ Pruett, IB Kozlovskaya, and JJ Bloomberg (2001). Effect of long-duration spaceflight on postural control during self-generated perturbations. *Journal of Applied Physiology*, 90, 997–1006.

Layne, CS, AP Mulavara, PV McDonald, CJ Pruett, IB Kozlovskaya and JJ Bloomberg (2004). Alterations in human neuromuscular activation during overground locomotion after long-duration spaceflight. *Journal of Gravitational Physiology*, 11, 1–16.

Liao, Y, J Zhang, Z Huang, Y Xi, Q Zhang, T Zhu and X Liu (2012). Altered baseline brain activity with 72 h of simulated microgravity — Initial evidence from resting-state fMRI. *PLoS One*, 7(12), e52558.

Liu, Q, R Zhou, S Chen and C Tan. (2012) Effects of head-down bed rest on the executive functions and emotional response. *PLoS One*, 7(12), e52160.

Lovelace, CT, BE Stein and MT Wallace (2003). An irrelevant light enhances auditory detection in humans: A psychophysical analysis of multisensory integration in stimulus detection. *Brain Research Cognitive Brain Research*, 17(2), 447–453.

Mader, TH, CR Gibson, AF Pass, LA Kramer, AG Lee, J Fogarty, WJ Tarver, JP Dervay, DR Hamilton, A Sargsyan, JL Phillips, D Tran, W Lipsky, J Choi, C Stern, R Kuyumjian and JD Polk (2011). Optic disc edema, globe flattening, choroidal folds, and hyperopic shifts observed in astronauts after long-duration space flight. *Ophthalmology*, 118(10), 2058–2069.

Manzey, D and B Lorenz (1998a). Mental performance during short-term and long-term spaceflight. Brain research. *Brain Research Reviews*, 28(1-2), 215–221.

Manzey, D, B Lorenz and V Poljakov (1998b). Mental performance in extreme environments: Results from a performance monitoring study during a 438-day spaceflight. *Ergonomics*, 41(4), 537–559.

Manzey, D, B Lorenz, A Schiewe, G Finell and G Thiele (1995). Dual-task performance in space: Results from a single-case study during a short-term space mission. *Human Factors*, 37(4), 667–681.

Masterton, BA and GB Biederman (1983). Proprioceptive versus visual control in autistic children. *Journal of Autism and Developmental Disorders*, 13, 141–152.

McDonald, PV, C Basdogan, JJ Bloomberg and CS Layne (1996). Lower limb kinematics during treadmill walking after space flight: Implications for gaze stabilization. *Experimental Brain Research*, 112, 325–334.

McDonald, PV, JJ Bloomberg and CS Layne (1997). A review of adaptive change in musculoskeletal impedance during space flight and associated implications for postflight head movement control. *Journal of Vestibular Research*, 7, 239–250.

Miller, CA, BT Peters, RR Brady, JR Richards, RJ Ploutz-Snyder, AP Mulavara, JJ Bloomberg (2010). Changes in toe clearance during treadmill walking after long-duration spaceflight. *Aviation, Space and Environmental Medicine*, 81(10), 919–928.

Moore, ST, HG MacDougall, BT Peters, JJ Bloomberg, IS Curthoys and HS Cohen (2006). Modeling locomotor dysfunction following spaceflight with Galvanic vestibular stimulation. *Experimental Brain Research*, 174(4), 647–659.

Mueller, C, L Kornilova, G Wiest and L Deecke (1992). *Optovert Vertical Optokinetic Stimulation Used to Examine Central Orientational Processes*. Health from Space Research. Austrian Accomplishments. The Austrian Society for Aerospace Medicine (ed.), pp. 5–165. New York: Springer-Verlag, Wien.

Mueller, C, L Kornilova, G Wiest, N Steinhoff and L Deecke (1994). Results from vertical vection experiments in short and long term space flights. In *Proc. of the 5th European Symposium on Life Sciences Research in Space, ESA SP-366*, pp. 373–376. Arcachon, France, Sept. 26–Oct. 1, 1993, CNES/ESA 1994.

Mulavara, AP and JJ Bloomberg (2003). Identifying head-trunk and lower limb contributions to gaze stabilization during locomotion. *Journal of Vestibular Research*, 12(5-6), 255–269.

Mulavara, AP, A Feiveson, J Feidler, HS Cohen, BT Peters, CA Miller, R Brady and JJ Bloomberg (2010). Locomotor function after long-duration space flight: Effects and motor learning during recovery. *Experimental Brain Research*, 202(3), 649–659.

Mulavara, AP, J Houser, C Miller and JJ Bloomberg (2005a). Full-body gaze control mechanisms elicited during locomotion: Effects of VOR adaptation. *Journal of Vestibular Research*, 15(5-6), 279–289.

Mulavara, AP, JT Richards, T Ruttley, A Marshburn, Y Nomura and JJ Bloomberg (2005b). Exposure to a rotating virtual environment during treadmill locomotion causes adaptation in heading direction. *Experimental Brain Research*, 166(2), 210–219.

Mulavara, AP, T Ruttley, HS Cohen, BT Peters, C Miller, R Brady, L Merkle and JJ Bloomberg (2012). Vestibular-somatosensory convergence in head movement control during locomotion after long-duration space flight. *Journal of Vestibular Research*, 22(2), 153–166.

Mulavara, AP, MC Verstraete and JJ Bloomberg (2002). Modulation of head movement control in humans during treadmill walking. *Gait Posture*, 16(3), 271–282.

Nachum, Z, A Shupak, V Letichevsky, J Ben-David, D Tal, A Tamir, Y Talmon, CR Gordon and M Luntz (2004). Mal de debarquement and posture: Reduced reliance on vestibular and visual cues. *Laryngoscope*, 114, 581–586.

Nashner, L and A Berthoz (1978). Visual contribution to rapid motor responses during postural control. *Brain Research*, 150(2), 403–407.

Nelson, WT, LJ Hettinger, JA Cunningham, BJ Brickman, MW Haas and RL McKinley (1998). Effects of localized auditory information on visual target detection performance using a helmet-mounted display. *Human Factors*, 40(3), 452–460.

Newman, DJ, DK Jackson, JJ Bloomberg (1997). Altered astronaut lower limb and mass center kinematics in downward jumping following space flight. *Experimental Brain Research*, 117(1), 30–42.

Nomura, Y, AP Mulavara, JT Richards, R Brady and JJ Bloomberg (2005). Optic flow dominates visual scene polarity in causing adaptive modification of locomotor trajectory. *Cognitive Brain Research*, 3, 624–631.

Paloski, WH (1998). Control of posture and movement. In *Neuromusculo-skeletal Interaction and Organizational Principles*, J Winters and P Crago (eds.). Heidelberg: Springer-Verlag.

Paloski, WH, FO Black, MF Reschke, DS Calkins and C Shupert (1993). Vestibular ataxia following shuttle flights: Effects of microgravity on otolith-mediated sensorimotor control of posture. *American Journal of Otolaryngology*, 14, 9–17.

Paloski, WH, JJ Bloomberg, MF Reschke and DL Harm (1994). Spaceflight induced changes in posture and locomotion. *Journal of Biomechanics*, 27, 812.

Paloski, WH, MF Reschke, FO Black, DD Doxey and DL Harm (1992). Recovery of postural equilibrium control following space flight. In *Sensing and Controlling Motion: Vestibular and Sensorimotor Function*, B Cohen, DL Tomko, and F Guedry (eds.), pp. 682, 747–754. New York: Acadamy of Science.

Parazynski, SE, AR Hargens, B Tucker, M Aratow, J Styf and A Crenshaw (1985). Transcapillary fluid shifts in tissues of the head and neck during and after simulated microgravity. *Journal of Applied Physiology*, 71(6), 2469–2475.

Parker, DE, MF Reschke and NG Aldrich (1989). Performance. In *Space Physiology and Medicine*, AW Nicogossian, C Leach-Huntoon, SL Pool (eds.), pp. 167–178. Philadelphia: Lea & Febiger.

Passi, N, AJ Degnan and LM Levy (2013). MR imaging of papilledema and visual pathways: Effects of increased intracranial pressure and pathophysiologic mechanisms. *AJNR American Journal of Neuroradiology*, 34(5), 919–924.

Penfield, WB (1938). The cerebral cortex in man. I. The cerebral cortex and consciousness (Harvey Lecture 1936). *Archive Neurological Psychiatric*, 40, 417.

Peters, BT and JJ Bloomberg (2005). Dynamic visual acuity using FAR and NEAR targets. *Acta Oto-laryngologica*, 125(4), 353–357.

Peters, BT, CA Miller, JT Richards, RA Brady, AP Mulavara and JJ Bloomberg (2011). Dynamic visual acuity during walking after long-duration spaceflight. *Aviation, Space and Environmental Medicine*, 82(4), 463–466.

Paloski, WH, MF Reschke, FO Black, DD Doxey and DL Harm (1992). Recovery of postural equilibrium control following spaceflight. *Annals of the New York Acadamy of Science*, 656, 747–754.

Pozzo, T, A Berthoz and L Lefort (1990). Head stabilization during various locomotor tasks in humans I. Normal Subjects. *Experimental Brain Research*, 82, 97–106.

Pozzo, T, A Berthoz, L Lefort and E Vitte (1991). Head stabilization during various locomotor tasks in humans II. Patients with bilateral peripheral vestibular deficits. *Experimental Brain Research*, 85, 208–217.

Pozzo, T, Y Levik and A Berthoz (1995). Head and trunk movements in the frontal plane during complex dynamic equilibrium tasks in humans. *Experimental Brain Research*, 106(2), 327–338.

Reschke, MF, JJ Bloomberg, DL Harm, WH Paloski, C Layne and V McDonald (1998). Posture, locomotion, spatial orientation, and motion sickness as a function of space flight. *Brain Research Reviews*, 28(1-2), 102–117.

Reschke, MF, DJ Anderson and JL Homick (1984). Vestibulospinal reflexes as a function of microgravity. *Science*, 225(4658), 212–214.

Reschke, MF and DE Parker (1987). Effects of prolonged weightlessness on self-motion perception and eye movements evoked by Roll and Pitch. *Aviation, Space, and Environmental Medicine*, 58, A153–A158.

Reschke, MF, JJ Bloomberg, DL Harm and WH Paloski (1994a). Space flight and neurovestibular adaptation. *Journal of Clinical Pharmacology*, 34, 609–617.

Reschke, MF, JJ Bloomberg, WH Paloski, DL Harm and DE Parker (1994b). Physiological adaptation to space flight; neurophysiological aspects: Sensory and sensory-motor function. In *Space Physiology and Medicine*, AE Nicogossian, C Leach-Huntoon, and SL Pool (eds.), pp. 261–285. Philadelphia: Lea & Febiger.

Reschke, MF, JJ Bloomberg, DL Harm, WH, Paloski C Laynea and V McDonald (1998). Posture, locomotion, spatial orientation, and motion sickness as a function of space flight. *Brain Research Reviews*, 28, 102–117.

Richards, JT, AP Mulavara and JJ Bloomberg (2004). Postural stability during treadmill locomotion as a function of the visual polarity and rotation of a three-dimensional environment. *Presence TeleoperVir Real*, 13, 371–384.

Richards, JT, AP Mulavara and JJ Bloomberg (2007). The interplay between strategic and adaptive control mechanisms in plastic recalibration of locomotor function. *Experimental Brain Research*, 78(3), 326–338.

Roberts, DR, *et al.* (2010). Cerebral cortex plasticity after 90 days of bed rest: Data from TMS and fMRI. *Aviation Space and Environmental Medicine*, 81(1), 30–40.

Roll, JP, K Popov, V Gurfinkel, M Lipshits, AC Deshays, JC Gilhodes and C Quoniam (1993). Sensorimotor and perceptual function of muscle proprioception in microgravity. *Journal of Vestibular Research*, 3, 259–273.

Roll, R, JC Gilhodes, JP Roll, K Popov, O Charade and V Gurfinkel (1998). Proprioceptive information processing in weightlessness. *Experimental Brain Research*, 122(4), 393–402.

Seidler, RD, DC Noll, and P Chintalapati (2006). Bilateral basal ganglia activation associated with sensorimotor adaptation. *Experimental Brain Research*, 175(3), 544–555.

Seilheimer, RL, Rosenberg A and DE Angelaki (2014). Models and process of sensory cue combination. *Current Opinion Neurobiology*, 25, 38–46.

Smeathers, JE (1989). Transient vibrations caused by heel strike. *Engineering Medicine*, 203, 81–186.

Sørensen, PS, AM Thomsen and F Gjerris (1986). Persistent disturbances of cognitive functions in patients with pseudotumor cerebri. *Acta Neurologica Scandinavica*, 73(3), 264–268.

Stein, BE (2005). The development of a dialogue between cortex and midbrain to integrate multisensory information. *Experimental Brain Research*, 166(3–4), 305–315.

Stein BE and MT Wallace (1996). Comparisons of cross-modality integration in midbrain and cortex. *Progress in Brain Research*, 112, 289–299.

Strangman, G and G Bevan (2013). Review of human cognitive performance in spaceflight. In *84th Annual Scientific Meeting of the Aerospace Medical Association*, pp. 12–16. Chicago, IL.

Streepey, JW, RV Kenyon and EA Keshner (2007). Visual motion combined with base of support width reveals variable field dependency in healthy young adults. *Experimental Brain Research*, 176, 182–187.

Tatebayashi, K, *et al.* (2003). Effects of head-down tilt on the intracranial pressure in conscious rabbits. *Brain Research*, 977(1), 55–61.

Taylor, CR, M Hanna, BJ Behnke, JN Stabley, DJ McCullough, RT Davis 3rd, P Ghosh, A Papadopoulos, JM Muller-Delp and MD Delp, (2013). Spaceflight-induced alterations in cerebral artery vasoconstrictor, mechanical, and structural properties: implications for elevated cerebral perfusion and intracranial pressure. *FASEB Journal*, 27(6), 2282–2292.

Valiant, GA (1990). Transmission and attenuation of heel-strike accelerations. In *Biomechanics of Distance Running*, PR Cavanagh (ed.), pp. 225–247. Champaign, IL: Human Kinetics.

Van Hedel, HJ and V Dietz (2004). The influence of age on learning a locomotor task. *Clinical Neurophysiology*, 115, 2134–2143.

Viaud-Delmon II, YP, A Berthoz and R Jouvent (2000). Adaptation as a sensorial profile in trait anxiety: A study with virtual reality. *Journal of Anxiety Disorders*, 14, 583–601.

Voloshin, AS (1988). Shock absorption during running and walking. *Journal of the American Podiatric Medical Association*, 78(6), 295–299.

Wallace, MT, MA Meredith and BE Stein (1992). Integration of multiple sensory modalities in cat cortex. *Experimental Brain Research*, 91(3), 484–488.

Warren, WH, BA Kay and EH Yilmaz (1996). Visual control of posture during walking: functional specificity. *Journal of Experimental Psychology: Human Perception & Performance*, 22, 818–838.

Whittle, MW (1999). Generation and attenuation of transient impulsive forces beneath the foot: A review. *Gait Posture*, 10, 264–275.

Wilson, MH, CH Imray and AR Hargens (2011). The headache of high altitude and microgravity — similarities with clinical syndromes of cerebral venous hypertension. *High Alt Medicine & Biology*, 12(4), 379–386.

Wilkinson, LK, MA Meredith and BE Stein (1996). The role of anterior ectosylvian cortex in cross-modality orientation and approach behavior. *Experimental Brain Research*, 112(1), 1–10.

Young, LR, DK Jackson, N Groleau and S Modestino (1992). Multisensory integration in microgravity. *Annals of the New York Academy of Sciences*, 682, 340–353.

Yri, HM, B Fagerlund, HB Forchhammer and RH Jensen (2014). Cognitive function in idiopathic intracranial hypertension: A prospective case–control study. *BMJ Open*, 4(4), e004376.

Zanello, SB, *et al.* (2013). Spaceflight effects and molecular responses in the mouse eye: Preliminary observations after shuttle mission STS-133. *Gravitational and Space Research*, 1(1), 29–46.

Zangemeister, WH, MV Bulgheroni and A Pedotti (1991). Normal gait is differentially influenced by the otoliths. *Journal of Biomedical Engineering*, 13(6), 451–458.

Zwart, SR, CR Gibson, TH Mader, K Ericson, R Ploutz-Snyder, M Heer and SM Smith (2012). Vision changes after spaceflight are related to alterations in folate- and vitamin B-12-dependent one-carbon metabolism. *Journal of Nutrition*, 142(3), 427–431.

Lower Body Negative Pressure as a VIIP Countermeasure

11

Jessica M. Scott, PhD and John B. Charles, PhD†*

**Universities Space Research Association, University of Houston-Clear Lake, 3600 Bay Area Blvd, Houston, Texas 77058, USA*
†NASA Johnson Space Center, 2101 E NASA Pkwy, Houston, Texas 77058, USA

1. Introduction

Significant cardiovascular and cerebrovascular challenges occur as a result of both microgravity and returning to Earth-gravity (Fu *et al.*, 2002; Dorfman *et al.*, 2007; Norsk, 2014). Indeed, the cephalad fluid redistribution induced by weightlessness causes an overall decrease in heart size (Perhonen *et al.*, 2001) and perhaps also an increase in cranial fluid volume (Taylor *et al.*, 2013) leading to an elevation of intracranial pressure (ICP).

As illustrated in previous chapters, the cranium acts as a rigid container of virtually incompressible substances including brain (80%), blood (12%), and cerebrospinal fluid (8%) (Haykowsky *et al.*, 2000). These three volumes completely fill the intracranial cavity and remain in a state of dynamic equilibrium with each other. Based on this premise, a significant increase in volume added to the intracranial cavity will increase ICP. Correspondingly, elevations in ICP during spaceflight are likely the consequence of up to 2.0 L of fluid being shifted from the lower body to the upper body accompanied by a lack of gravity to facilitate blood return from the head to the heart. Overall, data from ground-based analogs of spaceflight suggest that there is a significant increase in ICP during a cephalad fluid shift (Murthy *et al.*, 1992; Kawai *et al.*, 1993; Haykowsky *et al.*, 2002).

A gravity-independent means of restoring the gravity-driven fluid distribution in an astronaut's body, application of negative pressure to the lower body has been an important tool for assessing and mitigating these cardiovascular and cerebrovascular changes in spaceflight. Since the first description of this research tool (Stevens and Lamb, 1965), lower body negative pressure (LBNP) has been used in many ways in space and on Earth to assess orthostatic intolerance and responses to vertical acceleration in high-performance aircraft (Scott *et al.*, 2007), to simulate hemorrhage (Hinojosa-Laborde *et al.*, 2014), to alter preload (Esch *et al.*, 2010), to manipulate baroreceptors (Fu *et al.*, 2002), and to serve as a countermeasure against adverse orthostatic changes with short and long-term spaceflight missions (Charles and Lathers, 1994). In this chapter, we discuss the historical use of LBNP and potential visual impairment due to intracranial pressure (VIIP) countermeasures.

2. LBNP Devices

During LBNP, participants usually lie in a supine position with their legs and lower abdomen sealed in the LBNP chamber at the level of the iliac crest (Fig. 1). Various LBNP devices have been constructed including metal cylinders and semi-cylinders, wooden chambers and boxes, and foldable and collapsible devices. Air pressure inside the chamber is reduced by a vacuum pump such as a shop vacuum cleaner, making the pressure inside the chamber less than atmospheric pressure. As a result, blood shifts from an area of relatively high pressure (i.e., the upper body, which is outside the chamber) toward an area of relatively low pressure (i.e., the legs inside the chamber) (Esch *et al.*, 2007a).

3. Physiological Responses to LBNP

LBNP allows for the study of hemodynamic responses to central hypovolemia (Esch *et al.*, 2007b; 2010). Consequently, LBNP has typically been used to examine the physiological responses to orthostasis by quantifying a range of parameters such as heart rate, blood pressure, ventilation, muscle sympathetic nervous activity, hormonal responses, and cerebral hemodynamics (Norsk *et al.*, 1986; Giller *et al.*, 1992; Kuriyama *et al.*, 2000). The physiological responses to LBNP depend on the magnitude of pressure, where LBNP between 40 and 50 mmHg causes similar shifts in blood volume to those of standing posture (Lathers and Charles, 1994). Nonhypotensive pressures are typically less than 40 mmHg, and hypotensive pressures are greater than 40 mmHg (Hinojosa-Laborde *et al.*, 2014). To assess orthostatic tolerance, LBNP is usually applied in a graded fashion starting with 20 mmHg, and increasing by 10 mmHg until the point of presyncope (i.e., a

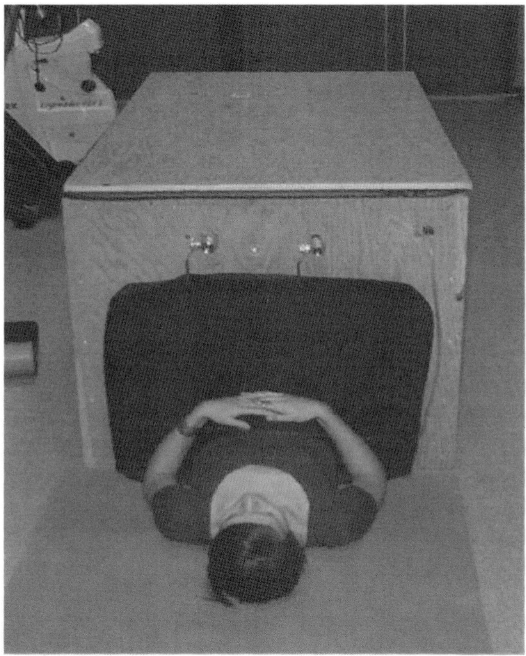

Figure 1. Lower body negative pressure box with a participant inside the chamber. The participant is sealed in the chamber at the iliac crest with a kayak skirt. During LBNP, participants lie in a supine position with their legs sealed in the LBNP chamber at the level of the iliac crest. Air pressure inside the chamber is reduced by a vacuum pump, making the pressure inside the chamber less than atmospheric pressure. By the laws of fluid dynamics, blood shifts from an area of relatively high pressure (i.e., the upper body, which is outside the chamber) toward an area of relatively low pressure (i.e., lower body inside the chamber). Without physiological compensation, blood is shunted away from the thoracic cavity and ultimately pools in the capacitance vessels of the lower limbs and the lower abdomen. From (Esch *et al.*, 2007b)

reduction in mean arterial pressure or heart rate) is reached (Hinojosa-Laborde *et al.*, 2014). As the magnitude of LBNP is increased, more blood accumulates in the lower extremities, with a subsequent reduction in venous return, end diastolic volume and stroke volume (Thomas *et al.*, 2009). A transient reduction in arterial blood pressure elicits reflex responses through stimulation of various baroreceptor populations that result in compensatory elevation in heart and peripheral vascular resistance (Zhang and Levine, 2007).

In one of the first investigations into changes in cerebral hemodynamics during LBNP, Wolthuis *et al.* (1970a, 1970b) reported that plasma bound ^{181}I activity was decreased 7% over the skull in male subjects during LBNP of 50 mmHg. Since this early investigation, subsequent research has demonstrated that the cerebral blood flow (CBF) velocity does indeed decrease during LBNP (Kuriyama *et al.*, 2000; Guo *et al.*, 2006). Notably, CBF velocity is reduced during orthostatic stress even when mean arterial pressure is well maintained. For example, reductions in CBF velocity during LBNP may range from 10% to 30% under steady-state LBNP conditions of about 50 mmHg (Levine *et al.*, 1994; Tobal *et al.*, 2001; Ogawa *et al.*, 2007). Taken together, these studies suggest that LBNP of 40–50 mmHg could be used to draw blood away from the cranium, and thus decrease ICP during microgravity.

3.1. *Nonhypotensive pressures*

Application of LBNP between 5 and 20 mmHg can cause reductions in central venous pressure (CVP) without altering mean arterial pressure. These low pressures can therefore be used to examine the reflex control of peripheral vascular resistance primarily by cardiopulmonary baroreceptors with minimal involvement of arterial baroreceptors. For example, Norsk *et al.* (1986) and Hirsch *et al.* (1989) demonstrated that CVP decreases by ~2 mmHg for every 10 mmHg chamber pressure, up to 30 mmHg, resulted in decreased stroke volume and cardiac output. Higher levels of LBNP (20–40 mmHg) further reduce CVP and splanchnic blood flow while forearm blood flow returns to baseline levels (Hirsch *et al.*, 1989; Wolthuis *et al.*, 1970a, 1970b; Wolthuis and Hoffler, 1970). Injected radioactive iodinated serum albumin was used to determine the rate and severity of regional vascular pooling during LBNP. Pooling occurred in all dependent regions of the lower body, but rates and magnitudes were variable. These data demonstrate regional autoregulation, presumably for the purpose of protecting central blood volumes. There are also several hormonal changes resulting from LBNP. Up to 20 mmHg of LBNP has little effect on arginine vasopressin, aldosterone, or atrial natriuretic factor; however, plasma renin activity increases moderately after prolonged (~20 min) LBNP exposure at 40 mmHg. (Roessler *et al.*, 2011)

3.2. *Hypotensive pressures*

Normally, in response to LBNP of greater than 50 mmHg decompression, the body compensates by peripheral vasoconstriction and an increase in heart rate, which serve to maintain normal circulation (Hirsch *et al.*, 1989). An early study by Beiser *et al.* (1970) outlined the progression to cardiovascular collapse with LBNP by classifying responses into two phases. With this construct, arterial pressures are sustained by appropriate sympathoexcitation to maintain vascular resistance up to the point at which this compensation apparently fails. Without physiological compensations, blood is shunted away from the thoracic cavity and ultimately pools in the capacitance vessels of the lower limbs and the lower abdomen (Wolthuis *et al.*, 1975; Hirsch *et al.*, 1989; Giller *et al.*, 1992). Inadequate physiological compensations in response to increasing negative pressure result in falling arterial blood pressure and, ultimately, syncope (Fu *et al.*, 2009). Therefore, symptoms of impending cardiovascular collapse occur in conjunction with sympathetic withdrawal, loss of peripheral vessel tone, and relative bradycardia (Fu *et al.*, 2009; Ainslie *et al.*, 2009; Thomas *et al.*, 2009). Higher levels of LBNP also result in hormonal changes. Plasma renin activity does not increase significantly until ~50 mmHg during progressive LBNP (Roessler *et al.*, 2011). Arginine vasopressin does not seem to be affected by LBNP in subjects who tolerate negative pressure without showing signs of impending hemodynamic collapse, although it does increase significantly in susceptible subjects (Convertino, 2001). Imam *et al.* (1989) showed that arginine vasopressin only increases in the presence of hypotension, while Norsk (1989) confirmed that although arterial baroreceptor unloading stimulates vasopressin release, the inhibition of arginine vasopressin does not further the development of hypotension during LBNP. Plasma catecholamines increase as a direct linear function of LBNP (Gabrielsen *et al.*, 1996).

4. LBNP During Spaceflight

The application of LBNP has been used for decades as a useful tool in the assessment of the effects of short- and long-duration exposure to microgravity, and as a countermeasure. Russian investigators were the first to adopt LBNP for use in flight by developing, first, a collapsible cylindrical device named "Veter" used only on Salyut-1, and then the "Chibis" system described as "pneumatic trousers" (Fig. 2) starting with Salyut 3 and continuing today on ISS. Cosmonauts slipped into the Chibis and decompressed it by use of a micropump located in the front. The Russian crews were outfitted for blood pressure and ECG monitoring and with rheoencephalography hardware, which uses electrical impedance to measure blood flow and blood distribution to the head (Charles and Lathers, 1994). Typically, cardiovascular responses to increasing levels of LBNP were assessed monthly throughout missions, while during the 2–4 week period before return to Earth, 20 min of low levels of LBNP sessions were scheduled daily. During the final 2 days before return to Earth, LNBP exposure increased to 50 min to a maximum pressure of 40 mmHg (Charles and Lathers, 1994).

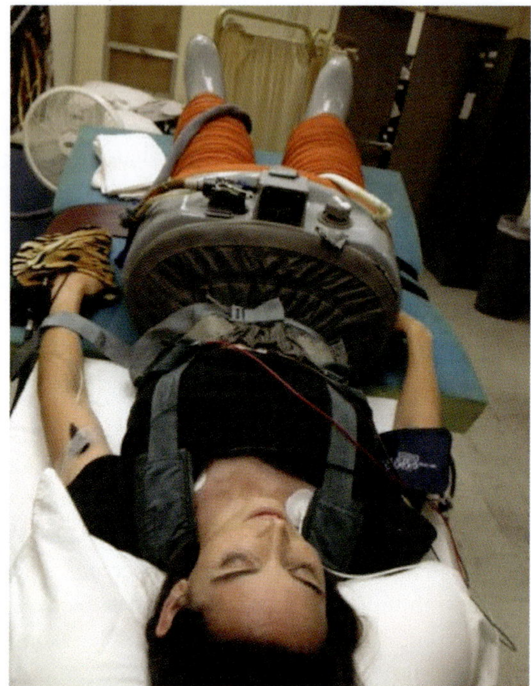

Figure 2. Participant in a Russian chibis (LBNP) suit. The chibis suit provides negative pressure around the lower body to shunt blood away from the thoracic cavity to the lower limbs.

NASA developed a second, collapsible LBNP device, for testing in Space Shuttle flights as a countermeasure for protection against post-flight orthostatic intolerance (Figs. 3 and 4). This LBNP device also provided a standardized stress, allowing researchers to understand the effect of a simulated orthostatic stress on the cardiovascular system at progressive times during short-duration spaceflight. Changes in blood pressure and heart rate were telemetered to the ground, where physicians assessed the condition of the subject's heart and blood vessels. Exaggerated heart rate and blood pressure responses to LBNP were evident within the first few days of spaceflight, corroborating the previous results from Skylab. An experimental countermeasure combining LBNP and fluid ingestion restored in-flight LBNP heart rate and blood pressure responses to pre-flight levels for 1 day after treatment but not for 2 days, and provided protection of post-landing orthostatic function. Unfortunately, any benefits of the combined countermeasure were offset by the complexity of its implementation (e.g., prolonged time for set

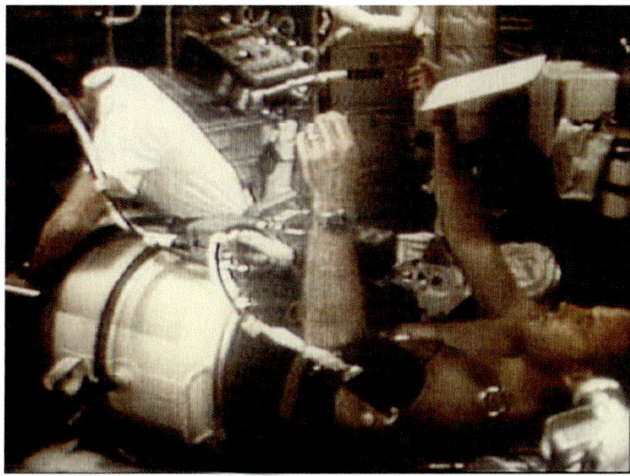

Figure 3. Astronaut Jack R. Lousma, Skylab 3 pilot, in the Lower Body Negative Pressure Device LBNPD, as Astronaut Alan L. Bean, commander, works around the leg band area. NASA Identifier: S73–34180.

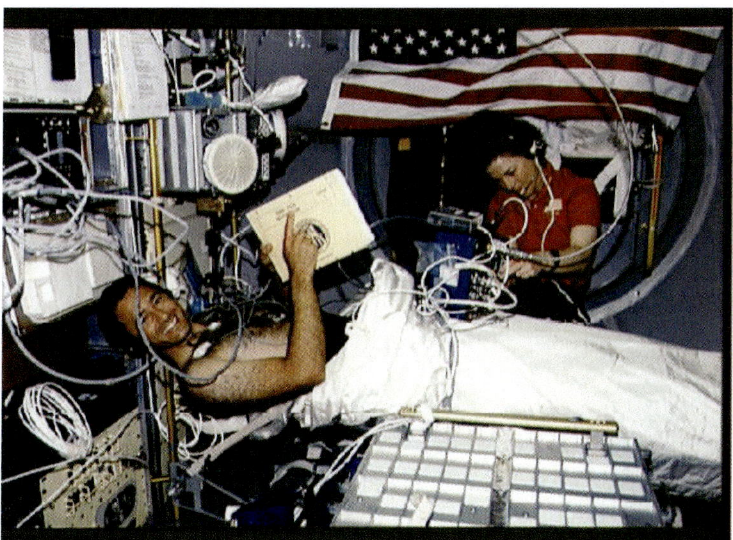

Figure 4. Mission Specialist Bonnie Dunbar and Payload Specialist Lawrence DeLucas in the Spacelab performing a Lower Body Negative Pressure study. DeLucas is encased in the suit and Dunbar is administering and overseeing the procedure. NASA Identifier: sts050–291–017.

up, implementation, and stowing), making it inappropriate for routine application during Shuttle flights (Charles and Lathers, 1994). Nonetheless, these studies demonstrated that LBNP can be used both as a test of the cardiovascular system during spaceflight and as a countermeasure to spaceflight induced orthostatic intolerance.

5. LBNP, Exercise, and Simulated Spaceflight

Bed rest, the most convenient ground-based analog of extended duration weightlessness, has been used to simulate the physiological consequences of spaceflight since the 1960s (Carlson, 1967). The addition of a head down tilt (HDT) component results in a cardiovascular challenge that other models cannot replicate. Prolonged bed rest leads to significant decrements in cardiovascular function, and in the absence of intensive aerobic training, maximal exercise capacity will be impaired even following relatively short exposures to disuse (Trappe *et al.*, 2006). Consequently, NASA has identified a critical need for both equipment and training protocols that will support countermeasures to hypogravity-induced deconditioning while meeting critical parameters related to vehicle space constraints and crew time commitment.

Given that the effects of LBNP are similar to standing, LBNP has been used as an intervention during disuse (Table 1). For example, Stevens and Lamb (Stevens *et al.*, 1966a) used LBNP of 25 and 50 mmHg for 8 h each day during 4 weeks of bed rest and found that this regimen preserved orthostatic tolerance following bed rest. Subsequent studies from this group demonstrated that 30 mmHg LBNP for 12 h per day near the end of bed rest was sufficient to reverse bed rest-induced changes in plasma volume and hematocrit (Stevens *et al.*, 1966b). Fortney (1991) described the benefits of LBNP as a potential countermeasure for orthostatic hypotension by using LBNP 4–6 h per day during bed rest studies, whereas (Guell, 1995, Guell *et al.*, 1990, 1991, 1992) reported the beneficial effects of LBNP by using three sessions of 20 min per day for the first 3 weeks of bed rest.

Another aspect of disuse in weightlessness is loss of exercise capacity. LBNP has been evaluated as a countermeasure for that as well. Riviere and coworkers (Riviere *et al.*, 1990) evaluated effects of resting LBNP during 30 days of bed rest on submaximal exercise responses in five subjects. They employed three 20-min, 35-mmHg LBNP sessions per day for the first 3 weeks of bed rest, and increased the number of LBNP sessions to six per day (2 h total per day) by the end of the 30-day bed-rest period. Despite this substantial time commitment to resting LBNP exposure during bed rest, subjects experienced similar post-bed rest

Table 1. Studies using LBNP as a countermeasure during bed rest.

Authors	Type	Sample	Intervention	Duration (Days)	Results
Lee *et al.* (2014)	Bed rest	8 EX, 8 CON, 8 no EX + PROT	LBNP + exercise; PRO	60	↑leg strength and endurance in EX group; no effect of PRO
Schneider *et al.* (2009)	Bed rest	8 EX, 8 CON	LBNP + exercise	60	VO_{2peak}↓ 21% in CON; no change in EX.
Guinet *et al.* (2009)	Bed rest	8 EX, 8 CON	LBNP + exercise	60	↑blood volume and cardiovascular responses to tilt in EX vs. CONT
Smith *et al.* (2008)	Bed rest	8 EX, 8 CON	LBNP + exercise	60	EX mitigated net bone loss vs. CON
Dorfman *et al.* (2007)	Bed rest	8 EX, 8 CON, 8 no EX + PROT	LBNP + exercise; PRO	60	LV and RV volumes and mass ↓ in CON; no change in EX.
Arbeille *et al.* (2012)	Bed rest	8 EX, 8 CON, 8 no EX + PROT	LBNP + exercise; PRO	60	No difference in CBF between groups during tilt test
Stevens *et al.* (1966a)	Bed rest	CON	8 h Daily LBNP	30	LBNP prevented ↓ in plasma volume
Stevens *et al.* (1966b)	Bed rest	CON	12 h LBNP 2 d before end of bed rest	30	LBNP prevented ↓ in plasma volume, hematocrit
Watenpaugh *et al.* (2007)	Bed rest	Twins: 15 EX, 15 CONT	LBNP + exercise	30	OT ↓ 34% in CON; ↓ 13% in EX.
Lee *et al.* (2009)	Bed rest	Female twins: 7 EX, 7 CONT	LBNP + exercise	30	VO_{2peak}↓ 16% in CON; no change in EX.
Lee *et al.* (2007)	Bed rest	Male twins: 8 EX, 8 CONT	LBNP + exercise	30	VO_{2peak}↓ 23% in CON; no change in EX.

(Continued)

Table 1. (*Continued*)

Authors	Type	Sample	Intervention	Duration (Days)	Results
Arbeille *et al.* (1991)	Bed rest	3 CONT, 3 LBNP	Daily LBNP	30	LBNP maintained OT
Louisy *et al.* (1990)	Bed rest	3 CONT, 3 LBNP	Daily LBNP	30	No difference in leg capacitance between groups
Macias *et al.* (2007)	Bed rest	Twins: 15 EX, 15 CONT	LBNP + exercise	30	↑lumbar spine compressibility in CON; no change in EX.
Zwart *et al.* (2007)	Bed rest	Female twins: 7 EX, 7 CONT	LBNP + exercise	30	EX mitigated net bone loss vs. CON
Monga *et al.* (2006)	Bed rest	Twins: 5 EX, 15 CONT	LBNP + exercise	30	EX mitigated increase in renal stone risk vs. CON
Cao *et al.* (2005)	Bed rest	Twins: 12 EX, 2 CONT	LBNP + exercise	30	EX mitigated increase in lumbar spine deconditioning vs. CON
Maillet *et al.* (1996)	Bed rest	6 EX, 6 CONT	Intermittent LBNP	28	EX maintained OT vs. CON
Sun *et al.* (2005)	Bed rest	6 LBNP 6 CON	LBNP	21	No difference in CBF between groups
Schneider *et al.* (2002)	Bed rest	7 EX, 7 CON	LBNP + exercise	15	↓ OT in EX and CON
Watenpaugh *et al.* (2000)	Bed rest	7 EX, 7 CON	LBNP + exercise	15	VO_{2peak}↓ 10% in CON; no change in EX.
Lee *et al.* (1997)	Bed rest	8 upright EX; 8 supine EX 7 CON	LBNP + exercise; upright EX	5	↓ exercise responses in CON; maintained responses in EX.

EX, exercise; CON, control; LBNP, lower body negative pressure; PRO, protein; OT, orthostatic tolerance; VO_{2peak}, aerobic capacity; CBF, cerebral blood flow; LV, left ventricle; RV, right ventricle.

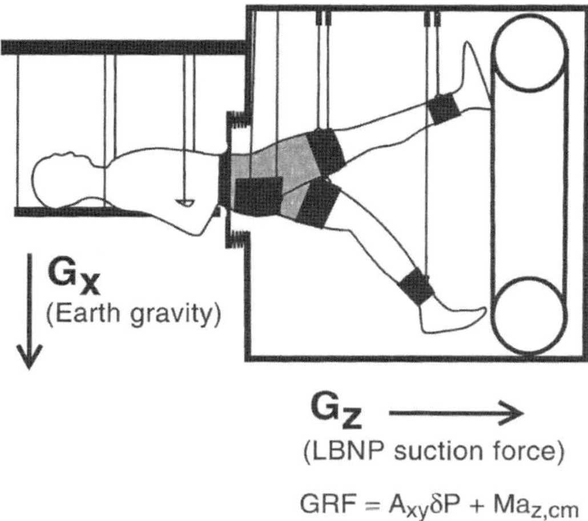

Figure 5. LBNP + Exercise Device. Footward force (Gz) is produced by the suction force of LBNP. Ground reaction force (GRF) during treadmill exercise in LBNP while supine and in microgravity equals the product of the body cross-sectional area (Axy) and the pressure differential (δP) across the LBNP chamber, with additional inertial forces equaling body mass (M) multiplied by footward acceleration (az) at the body center of mass (cm). The subject is suspended at the ankles and thighs by a pulley system, and the hands are holding the suspension cables at waist level. Gx, Earth gravity. From Boda *et al.*, 2000.

hemoconcentration and relative heart rate elevation during submaximal exercise compared with those who underwent bed rest with no daily resting LBNP.

Although LBNP alone does not have a beneficial effect on exercise capacity, numerous experiments have been conducted to determine the efficacy of using exercise with LBNP as a potential combined countermeasure (Table 1). These studies have shown that LBNP and exercise produce Earth-like loading of the musculoskeletal system, approximate gravitational vascular transmural pressures and fluid redistribution, and simulate metabolism, loading, and gait patterns of upright exercise on a treadmill. For example, the treadmill within LBNP protocol (Fig. 5) has been shown to maintain plasma volume and sprint speed, upright exercise capacity, muscle strength, and endurance during 30-day and 60-day (Women's International Space Simulation for Exploration; WISE-2005) bed rest simulations of microgravity (Lee *et al.*, 2007, 2009; Macias *et al.*, 2012). During WISE 60-day HDT studies, the treadmill exercise within LBNP was performed 3–4 days each week along with resistive exercise that was performed 2–3 days each week. Results showed that when treadmill exercise within LBNP was combined with resistive exercises during HDT, cardiac mass actually increased in the exercise group, while it decreased significantly in the nonexercise, control group, as expected (Dorfman *et al.*, 2007). Furthermore, upright peak exercise capacity, (Schneider *et al.*, 2009) muscle strength of the knee, and knee extensor endurance, decreased significantly in the control group but were preserved in the exercise group (Trappe *et al.*, 2008). Together, these investigations elegantly demonstrate that combining LBNP with exercise is an excellent countermeasure against cardiovascular, muscular, and bone deconditioning.

6. LBNP and Exercise as Countermeasures for VIIP

In order to determine if LBNP alone could be used as a possible countermeasure to cerebral fluid shifts, Sun *et al.* (2005) had 12 subjects complete 21 days of HDT bed rest. Six subjects received LBNP at 30 mmHg for 1 h per day, whereas six subjects were controls. They found that there were no differences between groups, with both groups having a significant decrease in CBF velocity throughout bed rest. They hypothesized that with HDT — and, presumably, weightlessness — ICP and therefore, cerebral venous pressure may increase more than arterial pressure. Thus, any role of LBNP in reversing cerebral filling is apparently transient, perhaps lasting only as long as LBNP is being applied.

Moderate and high-intensity aerobic and resistance exercise clearly benefit cardiac, muscle, and bone health (Wisloff *et al.*, 2002; Trappe *et al.*, 2009; Hagen *et al.*, 2012). However, the impact of such exercise — either as a mitigating or an exacerbating factor — on the development of VIIP is unknown. Haykowsky *et al.* (2003) demonstrated that upright resistive exercise without a Valsalva Maneuver (VM) increased ICP by 3 mmHg compared to 18 mmHg with a VM performed alone. Similar increases in intraocular pressure (IOP) have been observed during weight lifting (Bhambhani *et al.*, 2010), indicating that resistance exercise could transiently increase ICP and IOP in microgravity. During moderate intensity aerobic exercise, increases in CBF velocity occur (Querido and Sheel, 2007; Ogoh and Ainslie, 2009), suggesting that such exercise during a cephalad fluid shift could further increase intracranial blood volume and therefore ICP. In contrast, high-intensity aerobic exercise (>70% of peak oxygen uptake) lowers CBF velocity, a consequence which could ultimately decrease ICP (Secher *et al.*, 2008). In addition, it is well established that IOP decreases transiently with aerobic exercise in proportion to intensity and duration (Warburton *et al.*, 1999; Chromiak *et al.*, 2003).

Given the apparent benefit of resistance exercise on the skeletal system in particular (Brooks *et al.*, 2008; 2010), it will likely be a required component of future long-duration missions' countermeasure suite. Nevertheless, if even transient increases in ICP and IOP are determined to be deleterious, perhaps combining LBNP with such exercise might counteract this negative effect. To date, very few studies have examined that pairing of countermeasures. However, Watenpaugh *et al.* (1999) have demonstrated a device in which the intra–LBNP decompression is actually generated by leg extensions, possibly providing the type of combined countermeasure that would protect bone health without excessive increase in IOP and ICP.

7. Conclusions

LBNP has been used extensively in ground and flight research for the assessment of orthostatic tolerance and as a countermeasure for preservation of orthostatic tolerance. Building on this foundation, LBNP could be used as a countermeasure against the elevated intracranial and ocular pressures potentially observed in spaceflight. However, future research is needed to determine the optimal countermeasure pressure and exercise modality required to preserve optimal cranio–ocular pressures.

References

Ainslie, PN, CK Willie and YC Tzeng (2009). Role of SNA in the pathophysiology of cardiovascular collapse during syncope: Muscle vs. brain. *Journal of Physiology*, 587, 5795–5796.

Arbeille, P, D Lebouard, M Massabuau, J Pottier, F Patat, L Pourcelot and A Guell (1991). Effect on the cardiac function of repeated LBNP during a 1-month head down tilt. *Acta Astronautica*, 25, 415–418.

Arbeille, P, K Shoemaker, P Kerbeci, S Schneider, A Hargens and R Hughson (2012). Aortic, cerebral and lower limb arterial and venous response to orthostatic stress after a 60-day bedrest. *European Journal of Applied Physiology*, 112, 277–284.

Beiser, GD, R Zelis, SE Epstein, DT Mason and E Braunwald (1970). The role of skin and muscle resistance vessels in reflexes mediated by the baroreceptor system. *Journal of Clinical Investigation*, 49, 225–231.

Bhambhani, Y, DP Gross, M Haykowsky and S Rashiq (2010). Effect of opioid administration on cardiorespiratory and muscle oxygenation during lifting in chronic back pain patients. *European Journal of Applied Physiology*, 109, 241–250.

Boda, WL, DE Watenpaugh, RE Ballard and AR Hargens (2000). Supine lower body negative pressure exercise simulates metabolic and kinetic features of upright exercise. *Journal of Applied Physiology*, 89(2), 649–654.

Brooks, N, GJ Cloutier, SM Cadena, JE Layne, CA Nelsen, AM Freed, R Roubenoff and C Castaneda-Sceppa (2008). Resistance training and timed essential amino acids protect against the loss of muscle mass and strength during 28 days of bed rest and energy deficit. *Journal of Applied Physiology*, 105, 241–248.

Brooks, NE, SM Cadena, E Vannier, G Cloutier, S Carambula, KH Myburgh, R Roubenoff and C Castaneda-Sceppa (2010). Effects of resistance exercise combined with essential amino acid supplementation and energy deficit on markers of skeletal muscle atrophy and regeneration during bed rest and active recovery. *Muscle Nerve*, 42, 927–935.

Cao, P, S Kimura, BR Macias, T Ueno, DE Watenpaugh and AR Hargens (2005). Exercise within lower body negative pressure partially counteracts lumbar spine deconditioning associated with 28-day bed rest. *Journal of Applied Physiology*, 99, 39–44.

Carlson, LD (1967). Cardiovascular studies during and following simulation and weightlessness. *Life Science of Space Research*, 5, 51–54.

Charles, JB and CM Lathers (1994). Summary of lower body negative pressure experiments during space flight. *Journal of Clinical Pharmacology*, 34, 571–583.

Chromiak, JA, BR Abadie, RA Braswell, YS Koh and DR Chilek (2003). Resistance training exercises acutely reduce intraocular pressure in physically active men and women. *Journal of Strength and Conditioning Research*, 17, 715–720.

Convertino, VA (2001). Lower body negative pressure as a tool for research in aerospace physiology and military medicine. *Journal of Gravitational Physiology*, 8, 1–14.

Dorfman, TA, BD Levine, T Tillery, RM Peshock, JL Hastings, SM Schneider, BR Macias, G Biolo and AR Hargens (2007). Cardiac atrophy in women following bed rest. *Journal of Applied Physiology*, 103, 8–16.

Esch, BT, JM Scott and DE Warburton (2007a). Construction of a lower body negative pressure chamber. *Advances in Physiology Education*, 31, 76–81.

Esch, BT, JM Scott, MJ Haykowsky, DC Mckenzie and DE Warburton (2007b). Diastolic ventricular interactions in endurance-trained athletes during orthostatic stress. *American Journal of Physiology Heart and Circulatory Physiology*, 293, H409–H415.

Esch, BT, JM Scott, MJ Haykowsky, I Paterson, DE Warburton, J Cheng-Baron, K Chow and RB Thompson (2010). Changes in ventricular twist and untwisting with orthostatic stress: Endurance athletes versus normally active individuals. *Journal of Applied Physiology*, 108, 1259–1266.

Fortney, SM (1991). Development of lower body negative pressure as a countermeasure for orthostatic intolerance. *Journal of Clinical Pharmacology*, 31, 888–892.

Fu, Q, BD Levine, JA Pawelczyk, AC Ertl, A Diedrich, JF Cox, JH Zuckerman, CA Ray, ML Smith, S Iwase, M Saito, Y Sugiyama, T Mano, R Zhang, K Iwasaki, LD Lane, JC Buckey, Jr, WH Cooke, RM Robertson, FJ Baisch, CG Blomqvist, DL Eckberg, D Robertson and I Biaggioni (2002). Cardiovascular and sympathetic neural responses to handgrip and cold pressor stimuli in humans before, during and after spaceflight. *Journal of Physiology*, 544, 653–664.

Fu, Q, S Shibata, JL Hastings, A Prasad, MD Palmer and BD Levine (2009). Evidence for unloading arterial baroreceptors during low levels of lower body negative pressure in humans. *American Journal of Physiology. Heart Circulatory Physiology*, 296, H480–488.

Gabrielsen, A, HH Petersen, LB Johansen, N Foldager, NJ Christensen and P Norsk (1996). Relative role of low- and high pressure reflexes on sympathetic activity in humans during simulated gravitational stress. *Journal of Gravitational Physiology*, 3, 29–36.

Giller, CA, BD Levine, Y Meyer, JC Buckey, LD Lane and DJ Borchers (1992). The cerebral hemodynamics of normotensive hypovolemia during lower-body negative pressure. *Journal of Neurosurgery*, 76, 961–966.

Guell, A (1995). Lower body negative pressure (LBNP) as a countermeasure for long term spaceflight. *Acta Astronautica*, 35, 271–280.

Guell, A, A Cornac, MM Faurat, G Gauquelin, A Pavy-Le Traon and C Gharib (1992). Lower body negative pressure as a countermeasure against orthostatic intolerance for long term space flight. *Acta Astronautica*, 27, 103–107.

Guell, A, L Braak and C Gharib (1990). Cardiovascular deconditioning during weightlessness simulation and the use of lower body negative pressure as a countermeasure to orthostatic intolerance. *Physiologist*, 33, S31–33.

Guell, A, L Braak, AP Le Traon and C Gharib (1991). Cardiovascular adaptation during simulated microgravity: lower body negative pressure to counter orthostatic hypotension. *Aviation Space and Environmental Medicine*, 62, 331–335.

Guinet, P, SM Schneider, BR Macias, DE Watenpaugh, RL Hughson, AP Le Traon JY Bansard and AR Hargens (2009). WISE-2005: Effect of aerobic and resistive exercises on orthostatic tolerance during 60 days bed rest in women. *European Journal of Applied Physiology*, 106, 217–227.

Guo, H, N Tierney, F Schaller, PB Raven, SA Smith and X Shi (2006). Cerebral autoregulation is preserved during orthostatic stress superimposed with systemic hypotension. *Journal Applied Physiology*, 100, 1785–1792.

Hagen, KB, H Dagfinrud, RH Moe, N Osteras, I Kjeken, M Grotle and G Smedslund (2012). Exercise therapy for bone and muscle health: An overview of systematic reviews. *BMC Medical*, 10, 167.

Haykowsky, MJ, KK Teo, AH Quinney, DP Humen and DA Taylor (2000). Effects of long term resistance training on left ventricular morphology. *The Canadian Journal of Cardiology*, 16, 35–38.

Haykowsky, MJ, ND Eves, RW De and MJ Findlay (2003). Resistance exercise, the Valsalva maneuver, and cerebrovascular transmural pressure. *Medicine and Science in Sports and Exercise*, 35, 65–68.

Haykowsky, MJ, R Dressendorfer, D Taylor, S Mandic and D Humen (2002). Resistance training and cardiac hypertrophy: Unravelling the training effect. *Sports Medicine*, 32, 837–849.

Hinojosa-Laborde, C, RE Shade, GW Muniz, C Bauer, KA Goei, HF Pidcoke, KK Chung, AP Cap and VA Convertino (2014). Validation of lower body negative pressure as an experimental model of hemorrhage. *Journal of Applied Physiology*, 116, 406–415.

Hirsch, AT, DJ Levenson, SS Cutler, VJ Dzau and MA Creager (1989). Regional vascular responses to prolonged lower body negative pressure in normal subjects. *American Journal of Physiology*, 257, H219–225.

Imam, K, M Maddens, PK Mohanty, JV Felicetta and JR Sowers (1989). Atrial natriuretic peptide attenuates the reflex sympathetic responses to lower body negative pressure. *The American Journal of the Medical Sciences*, 298, 1–7.

Kawai, Y, G Murthy, DE Watenpaugh, GA Breit, CW Deroshia and AR Hargens (1993). Cerebral blood flow velocity in humans exposed to 24 h of head-down tilt. *Journal of Applied Physiology*, 74, 3046–3051.

Kuriyama, K, T Ueno, RE Ballard, PS Cowings, WB Toscano, DE Watenpaugh and AR Hargens (2000). Cerebrovascular responses during lower body negative pressure-induced presyncope. *Aviation, Space, and Environmental Medicine*, 71, 1033–1038.

Lathers, CM and JB Charles (1994). Orthostatic hypotension in patients, bed rest subjects, and astronauts. *Journal of Clinical Pharmacology*, 34, 403–417.

Lee, SM, BS Bennett, AR Hargens, DE Watenpaugh, RE Ballard, G Murthy, SR Ford and SM Fortney (1997). Upright exercise or supine lower body negative pressure exercise maintains exercise responses after bed rest. *Medicine Science Sports Exercise*, 29, 892–900.

Lee, SM, SM Schneider, WL Boda, DE Watenpaugh, BR Macias, RS Meyer and AR Hargens (2007). Supine LBNP exercise maintains exercise capacity in male twins during 30-d bed rest. *Medicine and Science in Sports and Exercise*, 39, 1315–1326.

Lee, SM, SM Schneider, WL Boda, DE Watenpaugh, BR Macias, RS Meyer and AR Hargens (2009). LBNP exercise protects aerobic capacity and sprint speed of female twins during 30 days of bed rest. *Journal of Applied Physiology*, 106, 919–928.

Lee, SM., SM Schneider, AH Feiveson, BR Macias, SM Smith, DE Watenpaugh and AR Hargens (2014). WISE-2005: Countermeasures to prevent muscle deconditioning during bed rest in women. *Journal of Applied Physiology*, 116, 654–667.

Levine, BD, CA Giller, LD Lane, JC Buckey and CG Blomqvist (1994). Cerebral versus systemic hemodynamics during graded orthostatic stress in humans. *Circulation*, 90, 298–306.

Louisy, F., C Gaudin, JM Oppert, A Guell and CY Guezennec (1990). Haemodynamics of leg veins during a 30-days-6 degrees head-down bedrest with and without lower body negative pressure. *European Journal of Applied Physiology Occupational Physiology*, 61, 349–355.

Macias, BR, DD D'lima, A Cutuk, S Patil, N Steklov, TB Neuschwander, S Meuche, CW Colwell and AR Hargens (2012). Leg intramuscular pressures and in vivo knee forces during lower body positive and negative pressure treadmill exercise. *Journal of Applied Physiology*, 113, 31–38.

Macias, BR., P Cao, DE Watenpaugh and AR Hargens (2007). LBNP treadmill exercise maintains spine function and muscle strength in identical twins during 28-day simulated microgravity. *Journal of Applied Physiology*, 102, 2274–2278.

Maillet, A, S Fagette, AM Allevard, A Pavy-Le Traon, A Guell, C Gharib and G Gauquelin (1996). Cardiovascular and hormonal response during a 4-week head-down tilt with and without exercise and LBNP countermeasures. *Journal of Gravity Physiology*, 3, 37–48.

Monga, M, B Macias, E Groppo, M Kostelec and A Hargens (2006). Renal stone risk in a simulated microgravity environment: Impact of treadmill exercise with lower body negative pressure. *Journal of Urology*, 176, 127–131.

Murthy, G, RJ Marchbanks, DE Watenpaugh, JU Meyer, N Eliashberg and AR Hargens (1992). Increased intracranial pressure in humans during simulated microgravity. *Physiologist*, 35, S184–S185.

Norsk, P (1989). Influence of low- and high-pressure baroreflexes on vasopressin release in humans. *Acta Endocrinological (Copenh)*, 121(Suppl 1), 3–27.

Norsk, P (2014). Blood pressure regulation IV: Adaptive responses to weightlessness. *European Journal of Applied Physiology*, 114, 481–497.

Norsk, P, F Bonde-Petersen and J Warberg (1986). Influence of central venous pressure change on plasma vasopressin in humans. *Journal of Applied Physiology*, 61, 1352–1357.

Ogawa, Y, K Iwasaki, K Aoki, S Shibata, J Kato and S Ogawa (2007). Central hypervolemia with hemodilution impairs dynamic cerebral autoregulation. *Anesthesia and Analgesia*, 105, 1389–1396, table of contents.

Ogoh, S and PN Ainslie (2009). Cerebral blood flow during exercise: mechanisms of regulation. *Journal of Applied Physiology*, 107, 1370–1380.

Perhonen, MA, F Franco, LD Lane, JC Buckey, CG Blomqvist, JE Zerwekh, RM Peshock, PT Weatherall and BD Levine (2001). Cardiac atrophy after bed rest and spaceflight. *Journal of Applied Physiology*, 91, 645–653.

Querido, JS and AW Sheel (2007). Regulation of cerebral blood flow during exercise. *Sports Medicine*, 37, 765–782.

Riviere, D, F Crampes, A Pere, M Beauville, A Guell and M Garrigues (1990). Effects of lower body negative pressure on cardiovascular adaptation to one month head-down bedrest. *Physiologist*, 33, S36–S37.

Roessler, A, N Goswami, B Haditsch, JA Loeppky, FC Luft and H Hinghofer-Szalkay (2011). Volume regulating hormone responses to repeated head-up tilt and lower body negative pressure. *European Journal of Clinical Investigation*, 41, 863–869.

Schneider, SM, DE Watenpaugh, SM Lee, AC Ertl, WJ Williams, RE Ballard and AR Hargens (2002). Lower-body negative-pressure exercise and bed-rest-mediated orthostatic intolerance. *Medicine* and *Science* in *Sports* and *Exercise*, 34, 1446–1453.

Schneider, SM, SM Lee, BR Macias, DE Watenpaugh and AR Hargens (2009). WISE-2005: Exercise and nutrition countermeasures for upright VO2pk during bed rest. *Medicine and Science Sports and Exercise*, 41, 2165–2176.

Scott, JM, BT Esch, LS Goodman, SS Bredin, MJ Haykowsky and DE Warburton (2007). Cardiovascular consequences of high-performance aircraft maneuvers: Implications for effective countermeasures and laboratory-based simulations. *Applied Physiology Nutrition and Metabolism*, 32, 332–339.

Secher, NH, T Seifert and JJ Van Lieshout (2008). Cerebral blood flow and metabolism during exercise: Implications for fatigue. *Journal of Applied Physiology*, 104, 306–314.

Smith, SM, SR Zwart, M Heer, SM Lee, N Baecker, S Meuche, BR macias, LC Shackelford, S Schneider and AR Hargens (2008). WISE-2005: Supine treadmill exercise within lower body negative pressure and flywheel resistive exercise as a countermeasure to bed rest-induced bone loss in women during 60-day simulated microgravity. *Bone*, 42, 572–581.

Stevens, PM and LE Lamb (1965). Effects of lower body negative pressure on the cardiovascular system. *American Journal of Cardiology*, 16, 506–515.

Stevens, PM, PB Miller, CA Gilbert, TN Lynch, RL Johnson and LE Lamb (1966a). Influence of long-term lower body negative pressure on the circulatory function of man during prolonged bed rest. *Aerospace Medicine,* 37, 357–367.

Stevens, PM, PB Miller, TN Lynch, CA Gilbert, RL Johnson and LE Lamb (1966b). Effects of lower body negative pressure on physiologic changes due to four weeks of hypoxic bed rest. *Aerospace Medicine,* 37, 466–474.

Sun, XQ, YJ Yao, CB Yang, SZ Jiang, CL Jiang and WB Liang (2005). Effect of lower-body negative pressure on cerebral blood flow velocity during 21 days head-down tilt bed rest. *Medical Science Monitor,* 11, CR1–CR5.

Taylor, CR, M Hanna, BJ Behnke, JN Stabley, DJ Mccullough, RT Davis, 3rd, P Ghosh, A Papadopoulos, JM Muller-Delp and MD Delp (2013). Spaceflight-induced alterations in cerebral artery vasoconstrictor, mechanical, and structural properties: Implications for elevated cerebral perfusion and intracranial pressure. *FASEB Journal,* 27, 2282–2292.

Thomas, KN, JD Cotter, SD Galvin, MJ Williams, CK Willie and PN Ainslie (2009). Initial orthostatic hypotension is unrelated to orthostatic tolerance in healthy young subjects. *Journal of Applied Physiology,* 107, 506–517.

Tobal, N, J Roumy, S Herault, G Fomina and P Arbeille (2001). Doppler measurement of cerebral and lower limb flow during a lower body negative pressure test for predicting orthostatic intolerance. *Journal of Ultrasound in Medicine,* 20, 1207–1217.

Trappe, S, A Creer, K Minchev, D Slivka, E Louis, N Luden and T Trappe (2008). Human soleus single muscle fiber function with exercise or nutrition countermeasures during 60 days of bed rest. *American Journal of Physiology Regulatory Integrative and Comparative Physiology,* 294, R939–947.

Trappe, S, D Costill, P Gallagher, A Creer, JR Peters, H Evans, DA Riley and RH Fitts (2009). Exercise in space: human skeletal muscle after 6 months aboard the International Space Station. (PMID: 19150852). *Journal of Applied Physiology,* 106, 1159–1168.

Trappe, T, S Trappe, G Lee, J Widrick, R Fitts and D Costill (2006). Cardiorespiratory responses to physical work during and following 17 days of bed rest and spaceflight. *Journal of Applied Physiology,* 100, 951–957.

Warburton, DE, MJ Haykowsky, HA Quinney, DP Humen and KK Teo (1999). Reliability and validity of measures of cardiac output during incremental to maximal aerobic exercise. Part I: Conventional techniques. *Sports Medicine,* 27, 23–41.

Watenpaugh, DE, DD O'leary, SM Schneider, SM Lee, BR Macias, K Tanaka, RL Hughson and AR Hargens (2007). Lower body negative pressure exercise plus brief postexercise lower body negative pressure improve post-bed rest orthostatic tolerance. *Journal of Applied Physiology,* 103, 1964–1972.

Watenpaugh, DE, RE Ballard, GA Breit and AR Hargens (1999). Self-generated lower body negative pressure exercise. *Aviation Space and Environmental Medicine,* 70, 522–526.

Watenpaugh, DE, RE Ballard, SM Schneider, SM Lee, AC Ertl, JM William, WL Boda, KJ Hutchinson and AR Hargens (2000). Supine lower body negative pressure exercise during bed rest maintains upright exercise capacity. *Journal of Applied Physiology,* 89, 218–227.

Wisloff, U, JP Loennechen, S Currie, GL Smith and O Ellingsen (2002). Aerobic exercise reduces cardiomyocyte hypertrophy and increases contractility, Ca2+ sensitivity and SERCA-2 in rat after myocardial infarction. *Cardiovascular Research*, 54, 162–174.

Wolthuis, RA and GR Hoffler (1970). Lower body negative pressure as an assay technique for orthostatic tolerance. II. A comparison of the individual response to incremental vs. constant levels of LBNP. *Aerospace Medicine*, 41, 419–424.

Wolthuis, RA, A Leblanc, WA Carpentier and SA Bergman Jr (1975). Response of local vascular volumes to lower body negative pressure stress. *Aviation, Space and Environmental Medicine*, 46, 697–702.

Wolthuis, RA, GW Hoffler and RL Johnson (1970a). Lower body egative pressure as an assay technique for orthostatic tolerance. 3. A comparison of the individual response to incremental leg negative pressure vs. incremental lower body negative pressure. *Aerospace Medicine*, 41, 1354–1357.

Wolthuis, RA, GW Hofflcr and RL Johnson (1970b). Lower body negative pressure as an assay technique for orthostatic tolerance: I. The individual response to a constant level (–40 mm. Hg) of LBNP. *Aerospace Medicine*, 41, 29–35.

Zhang, R and BD Levine (2007). Autonomic ganglionic blockade does not prevent reduction in cerebral blood flow velocity during orthostasis in humans. *Stroke*, 38, 1238–1244.

Zwart, SR, AR Hargens, SM Lee, BR Macias, DE Watenpaugh, K Tse and SM Smith (2007). Lower body negative pressure treadmill exercise as a countermeasure for bed rest-induced bone loss in female identical twins. *Bone*, 40, 529–537.

A Pressure Theory Links the VIIP Syndrome and Eye Diseases

12

John H. K. Liu, PhD

Department of Ophthalmology, University of California San Diego, 9415 Campus Point Drive, La Jolla, California, USA

1. Introduction

This chapter reviews major changes in ocular structures and visual function associated with the visual impairment intracranial pressure (VIIP) syndrome and four well-known diseases affecting the eye: idiopathic intracranial hypertension, glaucoma, ocular hypertension, and hypotony maculopathy. Considering their associated characteristics of change and/or mechanisms of action, one can draw up a unified pressure theory that links the VIIP syndrome and these diseases. Since sufficient knowledge is available to manage pressure conditions related to these diseases, one may explore ways to counter the VIIP syndrome by an approach from the eye if the unified pressure theory is validated.

- VIIP syndrome
- Idiopathic intracranial hypertension
- Glaucoma
- Ocular hypertension
- Hypotony maculopathy
- A unified pressure theory
- Countermeasures of the VIIP syndrome

2. VIIP Syndrome

Recent ophthalmic evaluations of American astronauts after their missions to the International Space Station revealed unexpected ocular and visual abnormalities (Fogarty *et al.*, 2011; Mader *et al.*, 2011, 2013; Marshall-Bowman *et al.*, 2013). Seven astronauts (aged 50.2 ± 4.2; mean ± standard deviation) had an eye examination including visual acuity, refraction, and fundus photography before and after the 6-month spaceflights. Six of them underwent postflight procedures of optical coherence tomography (OCT) and orbital magnetic resonance imaging (MRI) and four of them had lumbar punctures to measure the opening cerebrospinal fluid (CSF) pressure in the lateral decubitus position. Results of these examinations presented ocular abnormalities including decreased near vision in six, globe flattening in five, optic nerve disc edema in five, peripapillary nerve fiber layer thickening by OCT measurement in six, choroidal folds in five, and retinal cotton wool spots in three. Five astronauts with postflight near vision changes had a hyperopic shift of 0.5 diopter or more during the flight in one or both eyes. They also showed globe flattening on orbital MRI. Lumbar punctures performed in the four astronauts with optic disc edema showed moderate elevations of CSF pressure to 15.5–21 mmHg (21–28.5 cm water column) after returning to Earth for 12–66 days. For a comparison, the average lumbar CSF pressure in healthy individuals is around 11 mmHg.

In addition, approximately 300 astronauts were queried for vision changes in near and distant visual acuity after their missions (Mader *et al.*, 2011). Degradations were reported for 29% and 60% of astronauts during short-duration and long-duration spaceflights, respectively. Some vision changes persisted for more than 1 year after the spaceflight. This survey affirmed the tendency for a hyperopic shift in flying astronauts. Among many possible explanations, elevated intracranial pressure (ICP) due to head-ward body fluid shift under microgravity (Watenpaugh and Hargens, 1996) is the leading mechanism for the observed optic disc edema/nerve fiber layer thickening, globe flattening, choroidal folds, and hyperopic shift (Mader *et al.*, 2011). Thus, this spaceflight-related problem has been named VIIP syndrome (Fogarty *et al.*, 2011).

It is also known that, when the vertical distance between the eye and heart shortens, an elevation of intraocular pressure (IOP) occurs due to the redistribution of blood to the choroid and the increase of episcleral venous pressure (Liu and Weinreb, 2014). While an elevation of ICP due to head-ward body fluid shift is generally accepted during spaceflight, little is documented about the changes of IOP in astronauts under the same microgravity environment in the International Space Station. Available data in the literature indicate that an IOP elevation may or may not happen in long-duration spaceflight. Ground-based, head-down bed rest experiments for simulating body fluid shift under microgravity showed that an initial posture-dependent IOP elevation remained for hours (Linder and Trick, 1987), but may or may not return to the baseline after a few days (Mader, 1991; Chiquet *et al.*, 2003). During the German-Russian MIR mission and later the German Spacelab D2 mission, measurements of IOP using the self-tonometer in one astronaut and later in three astronauts showed that IOP gradually returned to the preflight levels in 5 days (Schwartz *et al.*, 1993; Draeger *et al.*, 1994, 1995; Draeger, 2010). However, later data from one Korean astronaut using the pressure phosphene tonometer showed that the elevated IOP on the fourth day spaceflight persisted on the eighth day (Chung *et al.*, 2011). The total number of astronauts who have had their IOP measurements performed during the spaceflights is very small, and no general conclusion can be made regarding the time-dependent IOP change. However, it is noted that the preflight and postflight IOP levels for those seven American astronauts showing the VIIP syndrome were all relatively low in the range of 10–16 mmHg, considering their older ages (Mader *et al.*, 2011). The average IOP in general population is approximately 16 mmHg.

3. Idiopathic Intracranial Hypertension

In clinical ophthalmology, such structural changes around the optic disc observed in astronauts having the VIIP syndrome are frequently presented in patients with idiopathic intracranial hypertension, also called benign intracranial hypertension or pseudotumor cerebri (Dhungana *et al.*, 2010). This disease affects predominantly overweighted young to middle-aged women characterized by elevated ICP without an abnormal CSF composition or identifiable brain pathology based on MRI neuroimaging. Headache is the most common symptom preceding the ophthalmological changes. A long-term ICP elevation seems to be needed for the patients showing characteristic changes around the optic nerve head as papillary edema. Although the detail mechanism is not clear, the ICP elevation is believed to be due to an abnormal CSF dynamics or an impaired CSF absorption. The diagnosis of idiopathic intracranial hypertension relies on an elevated opening CSF pressure using lumbar puncture in the lateral decubitus position. The pressure is commonly set to be more than 18.5 mmHg (25 cm water column). There is no report of an abnormal IOP level in patients with idiopathic intracranial hypertension.

Although not life-threatening, idiopathic intracranial hypertension may lead to visual impairment. Visual acuity remains normal in the early stage but can deteriorate rapidly in severe and advanced cases. The disease can be a self-limiting condition that resolved spontaneously or after initial lumbar puncture in some patients because of lowering of the ICP/CSF pressure. Weight loss is helpful to reduce clinical symptoms. Weight loss is also likely accompanied with a lowering of ICP (Berdahl *et al.*, 2012a). Evidence of structural changes in the optic nerve head is an indication to initiate a treatment with medication. The standard treatment includes the use of systemic carbonic anhydrase inhibitor, most notably acetazolamide, which reduces CSF production and ICP. Surgical procedures for optic nerve sheath decompression or CSF diversion may also be used in more advanced cases to lower ICP. When idiopathic intracranial hypertension is treated with medication or surgery to lower ICP, the local appearance of papillary edema has less of a tendency to advance to other ocular damages. Thus, characteristic changes associated with the VIIP syndrome such as globe flattening, choroidal folds, and hyperopic shift are not evident in patients with early stage of idiopathic intracranial hypertension.

4. Glaucoma

Glaucoma, an age-related eye disease, is a leading cause of blindness. Elevation of IOP is a major risk factor for glaucoma and lowering IOP is the only proven method to reduce the incidence of glaucoma onset and slow down the disease progression (Weinreb *et al.*, 2014). A hallmark of glaucomatous damage is optic disc cupping, a backward displacement of optic nerve disc. Although a hypothetical role of ICP in glaucoma pathogenesis has existed for many years, not enough data were available to evaluate the hypothesis until recently. Recent reports have indicated a role of low ICP in the pathogenesis of primary open-angle glaucoma. Investigators reviewed Mayo Clinic charts of the opening CSF pressure in 62,468 neurological patients receiving lumbar puncture from 1985 to 2007 and found a significant correlation between a low lumbar CSF pressure and primary open-angle glaucoma (Berdahl *et al.*, 2008a, 2008b). The correlation appeared in patients with elevated IOP as well as with normal IOP, but all related glaucoma patients had a mean low lumbar CSF pressure. Confirmative evidence came from a prospective study that measured CSF pressures in glaucoma patients receiving lumbar punctures in Beijing, China (Ren *et al.*, 2010). These investigators proposed that a high translaminar pressure difference (see Fig. 1 for the definition) at the optic nerve head, the junction where the cephalic and the intraocular fluids interact, is a more precise risk factor than a high IOP for developing optic disc cupping in glaucoma patients.

There are limitations upon the use of opening CSF pressure obtained from lumbar puncture for the calculation of translaminar pressure difference. Standard lumbar puncture is performed with patients in the lateral decubitus position, but

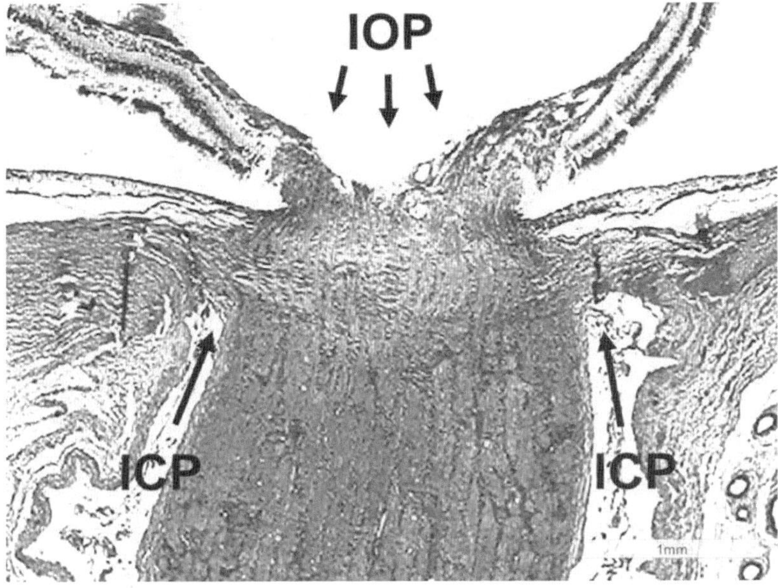

Figure 1. Translaminar pressure difference = intraocular pressure (IOP) minus intracranial pressure (ICP). (Specimen provided by Dr. Yeni Yucel, Director, Ophthalmic Pathology, University of Toronto)

humans spend approximately two thirds of daily life in a vertical body position during the diurnal/wake period. Normal ICP is probably near 0 mmHg at eye level in a vertical body position and about 11 mmHg in the lying position (Magnaes, 1976a, 1976b). The lumbar CSF pressure reading is close to the habitual ICP in a recumbent person who is asleep, but the level should be much higher than the resting ICP at eye level for the same person during the diurnal/wake period in a vertical body position. For IOP, the increase from a vertical body position during the diurnal/wake period to a recumbent body position during the nocturnal/sleep period is in the range of 3–5 mmHg (Liu *et al.*, 2003; Liu and Weinreb, 2014). Therefore, there is a net shift of translaminar pressure difference approximately 6–8 mmHg downward from the diurnal/wake period to the nocturnal/sleep period. This daily cycle of translaminar pressure difference is a part of biological nature for healthy individuals without ocular abnormalities. Reports have also showed that a short-term (hours) high degree of head–down tilt leads to no ocular pathological consequences (Liu and Weinreb, 2014). Thus, a critical limitation is that a single lumbar puncture provides pressure reading at one moment of time. Like many biological parameters, ICP is dynamic in real life. Repeated lumbar punctures in the same person over a short time period are technically impossible. In addition, a broad use of lumbar punctures to prospectively collect CSF pressure data in glaucoma patients is hard to justify since the invasive procedure does carry some risks with little proved medical benefits to the patients. Despite these limitations, new reports have supported a broader pressure theory that includes an ICP role in glaucoma pathogenesis.

Some glaucoma patients always present their office-hour sitting IOP readings in a normal level (e.g., <21 mmHg), but develop glaucomatous damages anyway. These patients were regarded as having normal-tension glaucoma or low-tension glaucoma to indicate their office-hour sitting IOP is lower than those patients who have glaucomatous damages and a high IOP. In Japan, the prevalence of normal-tension glaucoma is very high. Since the office-hour IOP in these patients are normal, the diagnosis of normal-tension glaucoma requires visual function test and sophisticated tools for evaluating ocular structures. Therefore, the prevalence of normal-tension glaucoma is probably underestimated in some other countries. Interestingly, if one considers the recumbent IOP during sleep in a Japanese group, a significant portion of the normal-tension glaucoma patients actually have IOP elevation more than the average during sleep (Hara *et al.*, 2006). We may recall that the recumbent ICP in the normal-tension glaucoma patients is also low upon the retrospective review of Mayo Clinic records (Berdahl *et al.*, 2008a, 2008b). Therefore, the translaminar pressure difference, IOP minus ICP, is probably a better risk factor than IOP alone for causing the characteristic cupping of the optic disc.

Based on observations of the opposite characteristic changes in the optic nerve head, Berdahl, Yu, and Morgan have put forth a hypothesis that describes the role of translaminar pressure difference for the pathogenesis of glaucoma as well as the VIIP syndrome (Berdahl *et al.*, 2012b). The characteristics around the optic nerve head in glaucoma patients are on the opposite direction of the VIIP syndrome and idiopathic intracranial hypertension. There is optic disc cupping associated with glaucoma and papillary edema associated with the VIIP syndrome and idiopathic intracranial hypertension. In adult-onset glaucoma cases, there is no correlation between IOP and eyeball size. However, a significant increase of eyeball size is associated with an elevated IOP in childhood glaucoma due to a relatively weak sclera in young children. On the contrary, globe flattening is observed in astronauts with the VIIP syndrome.

5. Ocular Hypertension

Individuals with a high IOP, but no ocular pathologies related to glaucoma are referred as having "ocular hypertension". The prevalence of ocular hypertension is a few times greater than the prevalence of glaucoma with a high IOP. It is generally believed that some individuals with ocular hypertension, for example, certain individuals without a family history of glaucoma, may never develop glaucoma during their lifetime. A higher mean lumbar CSF pressure was found in patients having an elevated IOP but no glaucomatous damage in the Mayo Clinic records indicating that a higher ICP/CSF pressure may counter the conversion from ocular hypertension to glaucoma (Berdahl *et al.*, 2008b). In a small prospective study that included individuals with "ocular hypertension" in Beijing, China, their mean lumbar CSF pressure is higher than the healthy individuals (Ren *et al.*, 2011). Therefore, realistically more than the usual magnitude of ICP increase during the sleep period may counter the impact of high IOP on ocular structures daily and prevent the development of glaucomatous optic nerve disc cupping.

The 24-h IOP pattern in patients with ocular hypertension is somewhat similar to those patients with primary open-angle glaucoma (Grippo *et al.*, 2013). Therefore, IOP alone may not determine whether or not a patient with an elevated IOP will lead to glaucomatous damages eventually. The level of ICP should also be considered, which supports the role of translaminar pressure difference in maintaining the normal ocular structures and visual function. During the night, at least, a higher CSF pressure provides a protective role against the development of glaucoma when the IOP is high, as opposed to a lower CSF pressure being associated with glaucoma regardless of what the IOP level is. The overall new evidence of ICP/CSF pressure information from recent studies in patients with primary open-angle glaucoma and ocular hypertension supports the concept that a high pressure difference across the lamina cribrosa represents a major risk factor for causing the backward movement of optic nerve disc more accurately than the traditional thinking of an elevated IOP.

6. Hypotony Maculopathy

Hypotony maculopathy, also called hypotony chorioretinopathy, is an eye disease due to a very low IOP (e.g., 6.5 mmHg) associated with ocular trauma or invasive anterior segment surgeries (Costa and Arcieri, 2007). Historically, the incidence of hypotony maculopathy increased after the introduction of antimetabolites during invasive glaucoma surgery to lower IOP. A slow healing of the surgical wound due to the antimetabolite may unintentionally keep the postsurgical IOP very low and cause hypotony maculopathy. Many ocular characteristics observed in the VIIP syndrome are observed in hypotony maculopathy including papillary edema, globe flattening, choroidal folds, and hyperopic shift. Early detection based on these characteristics and determination of the cause is essential to prevent visual impairment through appropriate measures to restore IOP. If hypotony maculopathy is not treated promptly, prolonged hypotony may lead to irreversible fibrosis in the retina, choroid, and sclera.

Translaminar pressure difference is low with hypotony maculopathy. Papillary edema is probably the result of anterior bowing of the lamina cribrosa, constricting axonal bundles in the lamina scleralis, and reducing axoplasmic transport due to the increase of pressure gradient from the retrolaminar subarachnoid space to the eye. Ultrasonography usually demonstrates flattening and thickening of the posterior sclera and choroid. As the anterior-posterior diameter of the vitreous cavity decreases, hyperopic shift occurs. The thick perifoveal retina surrounding the thin fovea is thrown into radial folds. The pressure theory indicates that a low IOP causes the scleral wall to collapse inward. Therefore, a low scleral rigidity can facilitate the collapse of the scleral wall during hypotony maculopathy. The sclera of younger patients is more elastic than that of older patients and may shrink more upon a low IOP condition. Similarly, the sclera in a myopic eye is thinner and likely to shrink more in hypotony maculopathy.

Hypotony maculopathy is treated with procedures designed to elevate IOP. An increase in IOP can counter the shift of translaminar pressure difference and reverse papillary edema, globe flattening, choroidal folds, and the hyperopic shift associated with hypotony maculopathy. The procedure of elevating IOP should be employed once the cause is determined since a delay may result in permanent structural changes and vision impairment. As IOP is elevated in patients with hypotony maculopathy, for example, the choroidal folds straighten out and may completely disappear. The choroid and sclera recover their original thickness, and the tortuosity and engorgement of the retinal vessels disappear. It supports the pressure theory that return of the normal translaminar pressure difference can restore normal ocular structures and visual function. A similar strategy but in the opposite direction seems to work by nature in patients with ocular hypertension using a high ICP to counter the impact of an elevated IOP and to avoid the optic nerve disc cupping.

7. A Unified Pressure Theory

Table 1 summarizes major changes in ocular structures and visual function by the VIIP syndrome, idiopathic intracranial hypertension, glaucoma, ocular hypertension, and hypotony maculopathy. The VIIP syndrome and idiopathic intracranial hypertension share the structural characteristics around the optic nerve head, mainly the papillary edema. The change is due to the ICP increase in the retrolaminar subarach-

Table 1. Major ocular characteristics related to the VIIP syndrome and eye diseases.

	VIIP	Idiopathic intracranial hypertension	Glaucoma	Ocular hypertension	Hypotony maculopathy
Optic nerve head	Edema	Edema	Cupping	Normal	Edema
ICP	Increase	Increase	Decrease	Increase	Normal
IOP	May increase	Normal	Usually increase	Increase	Decrease
Translaminar pressure change	Decrease	Decrease	Increase	Normal	Decrease
Globe flattening	Flattening	Some	Enlargement (young children)	Normal	Flattening
Choroidal folds	Yes	Some	No	No	Yes
Refractive shift	Hyperopic shift	Rarely reported	Not significant	No	Hyperopic shift
Time course	Long duration	Various	Long duration	Long duration	Short duration

noid space for the idiopathic intracranial hypertension and presumably for the VIIP syndrome. However, the damage does not seem to advance beyond this area and affect visual function in effectively treated patients with early idiopathic intracranial hypertension. Structural characteristics of optic nerve head in patients with glaucoma are on the opposite side (cupping) as the VIIP syndrome (papillary edema) due to the opposite changes in the translaminar pressure difference. When both the ICP and IOP are high in patients with ocular hypertension, ocular structures can remain normal for a long time due to the absence of net change in the translaminar pressure difference. There are many similarities for the changes in ocular structures and visual function between the VIIP syndrome and hypotony maculopathy (optic nerve head edema, globe flattening, choroidal folds, and hyperopic shift) despite each condition involves only a different component of the translaminar pressure difference. Clinical course of hypotony maculopathy usually develops within a short period of time, but similar changes in ocular structures and visual function in the VIIP syndrome may take a longer time to develop.

Taken together, clinical observations indicate that a balanced translaminar pressure difference at the optic nerve head is critical to maintain the structures of the optic nerve head initially and then other ocular structures for these seemly separated conditions and diseases. Visual impairment observed in those astronauts with the VIIP syndrome after long-duration spaceflight is probably associated with a persistent, abnormal pressure from the brain against the optic nerve head and other ocular structures due to a higher ICP. While other mechanisms may also be involved, such as an elevation of central venous pressure for altering ocular circulation as well as ocular lymphatic system, an abnormal translaminar pressure difference is likely the major cause at least in the early stage.

This unified pressure theory is straightforward and comprehensive, but remains as a theory and requires validity. Careful examinations of ICP, IOP, optic nerve head, macula, and associated structures and visual function during the spaceflight should provide data to validate this theory for the VIIP syndrome. A critical step is to confirm an elevated ICP in astronauts during spaceflight. To achieve this goal, a leap forward is to develop a reliable noninvasive device for monitoring ICP under microgravity. Stronger evidences for the ICP levels in patients having glaucoma with high IOP, normal-tension glaucoma, and ocular hypertension in different body positions using a reliable noninvasive measuring device are also helpful to validate the unified pressure theory.

As discussed, the current IOP data during spaceflight is insufficient. Unless new data indicate differently, a reduction of translaminar pressure difference is assumed to occur during the spaceflight in the International Space Station. As an elevated ICP is likely consistent during the spaceflight, an elevated IOP may gradually return to normal. It would also be interesting to examine whether or not the baseline IOP is correlated negatively with the occurrence of VIIP syndrome in astronauts. A lower than usual baseline IOP would reduce the baseline translaminar pressure difference. In other words, a lower than usual baseline IOP would increase the impact of ICP against the optic nerve head and other ocular structures at all time. Baseline IOP and the degree of IOP change under microgravity can impact the translaminar pressure difference at a fixed time interval and the impact may be time dependent. These IOP-related factors should be examined along with ICP changes. Tonopen, a portable tonometer, and a spectral-domain OCT are currently onboard the International Space Station to monitor the change of IOP and ocular structures. Anticipated new data from these devices will be very valuable for evaluating the unified pressure theory.

Since the translaminar pressure difference is dynamic due to routine daily change of body positions, the VIIP syndrome, idiopathic intracranial hypertension, glaucoma, and probably other eye conditions discussed must involve abnormally low or high translaminar pressure difference for a significant portion of the daily life. Considering the endogenous daily fluctuations in translaminar pressure difference, it is unclear how long a low translaminar pressure difference is needed for the development of the VIIP syndrome. It should also be noted that this unified pressure theory covers a majority of ocular characteristics related to the VIIP syndrome and eye diseases, but not all of them. For example, the cotton wool spots for the VIIP syndrome may require the involvements of not only the translaminar pressure difference, but also the retinal and choroidal blood circulations.

8. Countermeasures of the VIIP Syndrome

The VIIP syndrome does not present as a serious medical issue for the astronauts so far. The hyperopic shift, even long lasting, can be corrected with appropriate reading glasses during the spaceflight and afterward. Changes in ocular structures do not seem to worsen after the spaceflight. The cotton wool spot, though may be a permanent damage, is localized and does not affect essential daily activities. However, there is an increasing concern that the VIIP syndrome can accelerate when taking repeated spaceflights to the International Space Station or taking a spaceflight of much longer than 6 months (Mader *et al.*, 2013). While a high percentage of astronauts onboard the International Space Station is developing visual abnormalities, there is no clinical strategy to prevent the damage. Without a strategy to treat the VIIP syndrome, our future space exploration including a manned mission to Mars that requires spaceflight of a few years will be in jeopardy.

Therefore, a timely evaluation of strategies and countermeasures is essential. Since the leading cause for the VIIP syndrome is the body fluid shift, one approach to counter the VIIP syndrome is to shift the body fluid away from the head during the spaceflight using the lower body negative pressure. This systemic approach has been discussed in another chapter of this book. With a systemic approach, it is expected that less accumulation of tissue fluid occurs in the brain as well as in the eye. Thus, both ICP and IOP would be affected as observed during a ground-based simulated experiment using the head–down tilt model (Macias *et al.*, 2015). No experimental data or theoretical model has yet showed how ICP, IOP, and the translaminar pressure difference may change during the spaceflight. The unified pressure theory predicts that the mechanism causing the VIIP syndrome would be modified only when there is a net change of translaminar pressure difference. Practically, the lower body negative pressure may need to be applied for hours daily in order to be effective since the VIIP syndrome takes a long time to develop. The latter consideration is also valid for the use of other systemic countermeasures.

An alternative countermeasure for the VIIP syndrome is by an ocular approach. If the unified pressure theory presented in this chapter is correct, an ocular approach to increase the translaminar pressure difference should be considered. As discussed earlier, structural and functional characteristics of hypotony maculopathy can be reversed by surgical intervention of the very low IOP. It is a real possibility that the VIIP syndrome-related ocular changes can be reversed by an increase of IOP for the purpose of maintaining a normal translaminar pressure difference when the VIIP syndrome is developing. Although there is a concern that an elevated IOP can cause damage to the optic nerve head as seen in glaucoma, it is possible that an elevated IOP may not cause any damage since the ICP of astronauts is high under microgravity to provide the needed pressure balance. Raising IOP is possible by pharmacological or physiological ways using a local approach. It is well known that IOP can be increased using topical medications such as glucocorticoids (Kass and Sears, 1977). There are probably other topical pharmaceuticals that can increase IOP under an appropriate dose and regimen for each individual astronaut. Also, physiologically acceptable IOP elevation is probably achievable using an adjustable pressure goggles that raises orbital pressure (Ragauskas, 2012). When an elevation of IOP is used to counter an elevated ICP in flying astronauts, IOP in a safe range will need to be monitored. An elevated IOP will only affect local tissues with less safety concern for systemic consequences. In contrast, a systemic approach to counteract the VIIP syndrome may affect many organs and tissues.

The strategy of treating VIIP syndrome based on the unified pressure theory is testable under the current 6 month deployment to the International Space Station and when a longer mission to Mars is taken place. The ocular approach has advantages and limitations. The unified pressure theory can be tested using a relatively simple experimental design with one eye to perform the experiment and the contralateral eye as the control. Such an experimental design may significantly reduce the number of subjects needed for a valid statistical analysis. Since the VIIP syndrome develops slowly over a few months, a long-term application of countermeasure for the VIIP syndrome is necessary. For this consideration, an ocular approach is preferable since it impacts the human activities much less than a systemic approach in the International Space Station and for longer future spaceflights. The ocular approach has a limitation that the treatment outcomes are limited to the associated ocular structures and visual function. The ocular approach does not counter all the physiological consequences related to head-ward body fluid shift and the VIIP syndrome such as the pathology in the brain. Lastly, the unified pressure theory may be verified in ground-based laboratory studies such as the use of head-down tilt model to alter the translaminar pressure difference. However, these ground studies can probably include only relatively short-term experiments and the VIIP syndrome-related changes in ocular structures and visual function may not be significant enough to be useful.

References

Berdahl, JP, D Fleischman, J Zaydlarova, S Stinnett, RR Allingham and MP Fautsch (2012a). Body mass index has a linear relationship with cerebrospinal fluid pressure. *Investigative Ophthalmology and Visual Science*, 53(3), 1422–1427. doi:10.1167/iovs.11-8220.

Berdahl, JP, DY Yu and WH Morgan (2012b). The translaminar pressure gradient in sustained zero gravity, idiopathic intracranial hypertension, and glaucoma. *Medical Hypotheses*, 79(6), 719–724. doi:10.1016/j.mehy.2012.08.009.

Berdahl, JP, RR Allingham and DH Johnson (2008a). Cerebrospinal fluid pressure is decreased in primary open-angle glaucoma. *Ophthalmology*, 115(5), 763–768. doi:10.1016/j.ophtha.2008.01.013.

Berdahl, JP, MP Fautsch, SS Stinnett and RR Allingham (2008b). Intracranial pressure in primary open angle glaucoma, normal tension glaucoma, and ocular hypertension: A case-control study. *Investigative Ophthalmology and Visual Science*, 49(12), 5412–5418. doi: 10.1167/iovs.08-2228

Chiquet, C, MA Custaud, AP Le Traon, C Millet, C Gharib and P Denis (2003). Changes in intraocular pressure during prolonged (7 day) head-down tilt bedrest. *Journal of Glaucoma*, 12(3), 204–208.

Chung, KY, SJ Woo, S Yi, GH Choi, CH Ahn, GC Hur, JG Lim and TW Kim (2011). Diurnal pattern of intraocular pressure is affected by microgravity when measured in space with the pressure phosphene tonometer (PPT). *Journal of Glaucoma*, 20(8), 488–491. doi:10.1097/IJG.0b013e3181f464d2.

Costa, VP and ES Arcieri (2007). Hypotony maculopathy. *Acta Ophthalmological Scandinavia*, 85(6), 586–597. doi:10.1111/j.1600-0420.2007.00910.x.

Dhungana, S, B Sharrack and N Woodroofe (2010). Idiopathic intracranial hypertension. *Acta Neurologica Scandinavia*, 121(2), 71–82. doi:10.1111/j.1600-0404.2009.01172.x.

Draeger, J (2010). The diurnal variation of intraocular pressure-the most important symptom for early detection and follow-up of the glaucomas. *Graefes Archive for Clinical Experimental Ophthalmology*, 248(10), 1367–1370. doi:10.1007/s00417-010-1439-1.

Draeger, J, R Schwartz, S Groenhoff and C Stern (1994). Self tonometry during the German 1993 Spacelab D2 mission. *Ophthalmologe*, 91(5), 697–699.

Draeger, J, R Schwartz, S Groenhoff and C Stern (1995). Self-tonometry under microgravity conditions. *Aviation, Space, and Environmental Medicine*, 66(6), 568–570.

Fogarty, JA, C Otto, E Kerstman, C Oubre and J Wu (2011). The visual impairment intracranial pressure summit report. *NASA/TP-2011-216160*. Houston.

Grippo, TM, JH Liu, N Zebardast, TB Arnold, GH Moore and RN Weinreb (2013). Twenty-four-hour pattern of intraocular pressure in untreated patients with ocular hypertension. *Investigative Ophthalmology and Visual Science*, 54(1), 512–517. doi:10.1167/iovs.12-10709.

Hara, T, T Hara and T Tsuru (2006). Increase of peak intraocular pressure during sleep in reproduced diurnal changes by posture. *Archives of Ophthalmology*, 124(2), 165–168. doi:10.1001/archopht.124.2.165.

Kass, MA and ML Sears (1977). Hormonal regulation of intraocular pressure. *Survey of Ophthalmology*, 22(3), 153–176.

Linder, BJ and GL Trick (1987). Simulation of spaceflight with whole-body head-down tilt: influence on intraocular pressure and retinocortical processing. *Aviation Space and Environmental Medicine*, 58(9 Pt 2), A139–A142.

Liu, JH, X Zhang, DF Kripke and RN Weinreb (2003). Twenty-four-hour intraocular pressure pattern associated with early glaucomatous changes. *Investigative Ophthalmology and Visual Science*, 44(4), 1586–1590.

Liu, JHK and RN Weinreb (2014). Posture, intraocular pressure and visual function. *British Journal of Ophthalmology*, 98, 288–289.

Macias, BR, JH Liu, N Grande-Gutierrez and AR Hargens (2015). Intraocular and intracranial pressures during head-down tilt with lower body negative pressure. *Aerospace Medicine and Human Performance*, 86(1), 3–7. doi:10.3357/AMHP.4044.2015.

Mader, TH (1991). Intraocular pressure in microgravity. *Journal of Clinical Pharmacology*, 31(10), 947–950.

Mader, TH, CR Gibson, AF Pass, AG Lee, HE Killer, HC Hansen, JP Dervay, MR Barratt, WJ Tarver, AE Sargsyan, LA Kramer, R Riascos, DG Bedi and DR Pettit (2013). Optic disc edema in an astronaut after repeat long-duration space flight. *Journal of Neuro-ophthalmology*, 33(3), 249–255. doi:10.1097/WNO.0b013e31829b41a6.

Mader, TH, CR Gibson, AF Pass, LA Kramer, AG Lee, J Fogarty, WJ Tarver, JP Dervay, DR Hamilton, A Sargsyan, Phillips JL, D Tran, W Lipsky, J Choi, C Stern, R Kuyumjian and JD Polk (2011). Optic disc edema, globe flattening, choroidal folds, and hyperopic shifts observed in astronauts after long-duration space flight. *Ophthalmology*, 118(10), 2058–2069. doi:10.1016/j.ophtha.2011.06.021.

Magnaes, B (1976a). Body position and cerebrospinal fluid pressure. Part 1: Clinical studies on the effect of rapid postural changes. *Journal of Neurosurgery*, 44(6), 687–697. doi:10.3171/jns.1976.44.6.0687.

Magnaes, B (1976b). Body position and cerebrospinal fluid pressure. Part 2: Clinical studies on orthostatic pressure and the hydrostatic indifferent point. *Journal of Neurosurgery*, 44(6), 698–705. doi:10.3171/jns.1976.44.6.0698.

Marshall-Bowman, K, MR Barratt and CR Gibson (2013). Ophthalmic changes and increased intracranial pressure associated with long duration spaceflight: An emerging understanding. *Acta Astronautica*, (87), 77–87.

Ragauskas, A, V Matijosaitis, R Zakelis, K Petrikonis, D Rastenyte, I Piper and G Daubaris (2012). Clinical assessment of noninvasive intracranial pressure absolute value measurement method. *Neurology*, 78(21), 1684–1691. doi:10.1212/WNL.0b013e3182574f50.

Ren, R, JB Jonas, G Tian, Y Zhen, K Ma, S Li, H Wang, B Li, X Zhang and N Wang (2010). Cerebrospinal fluid pressure in glaucoma: A prospective study. *Ophthalmology*, 117(2), 259–266. doi:10.1016/j.ophtha.2009.06.058.

Ren, R, X Zhang, N Wang, B Li, G Tian and JB Jonas (2011). Cerebrospinal fluid pressure in ocular hypertension. *Acta Ophthalmologica*, 89(2), e142–e148. doi:10.1111/j.1755-3768.2010.02015.x.

Schwartz, R, J Draeger, S Groenhoff and KD Flade (1993). Results of self-tonometry during the 1st German-Russian MIR mission 1992. *Ophthalmologe*, 90(6), 640–642.

Watenpaugh, DE and AR Hargens (1996). The cardiovascular system in microgravity. In *Handbook of Physiology: Environmental Physiology*, MJ Fregly and CM Blatteis (eds.), Vol. 1, pp. 631–674. New York: Oxford University Press.

Weinreb, RN, T Aung and FA Medeiros (2014). The pathophysiology and treatment of glaucoma: a review. *Journal of the American Medical Association*, 311(18), 1901–1911. doi:10.1001/jama.2014.3192.

Index